AGRAMMATISM

AGRAMMATISM

Edited by

Harry A. Whitaker, Ph.D.

Department of Psychology
University of Quebec at Montreal
Montreal, Quebec, Canada

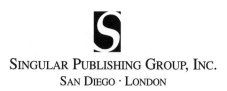

SINGULAR PUBLISHING GROUP, INC.
SAN DIEGO · LONDON

Singular Publishing Group, Inc.
401 West "A" Street, Suite 325
San Diego, California 92101-7904

Singular Publishing Ltd.
19 Compton Terrace
London, NI 2UN UK

e-mail:singpub@mail.cerfnet.com
Website: http://www.singpub.com

Library of Congress Cataloging-in-Publication Data

Agrammatism / [edited by] Harry A. Whitaker.
    p.   cm.
    Includes bibliographical references.
    ISBN 1–56593–744–9
    1. Agrammatism. I. Whitaker, Harry A.
    [DNLM: 1. Aphasia, Broca. WL 340.5 A2771 1977]
  RC425.5.A372 1997
  616.85'52—dc21
  DNLM/DLC
  for Library of Congress   91–1040
                                                  CIP

CONTENTS

Preface

Over the last 23 years that I have been Editor of the journal *Brain and Language,* there have been many opportunities to collect thematically related research papers. Usually done as a special issue of the journal, the first of these collections was on the dichotic listening technique and the role of the thalamus in language, hot topics in the mid-1970s. The response to thematic special issues has been quite positive; they provide colleagues with an up-to-date review of a variety of typical research questions without wasting space on textbook-type surveys and summaries. Space is limited in a journal number, however, and on occasion a book format is appropriate for a topic of sufficient relevance to current neuropsychological work.

When I first approached Sadanand Singh with the idea of reprinting key papers from *Brain and Language* in topical collections, his enthusiasm for the project convinced me that it was worthwhile. The very gracious response and assistance on the part of Academic Press, publisher of *Brain and Language* and of *Brain and Cognition,* removed all administrative and technical barriers. We are all, collectively, pleased to bring you the first of this series, a collection of papers on agrammatism.

I wish also to thank Vicki Fromkin, my Ph.D. thesis advisor, colleague, and friend, for all of her help in choosing the many papers in this volume. Thanks, too, to Yosef Grodzinski and to Gonia Jarema for their helpful and timely consultations. Finally, I wish to thank all of the authors of the papers herein: It is their work that passed the peer review process and brought their insights and analyses to our attention.

Harry Whitaker

An Introduction to Premodern
Agrammatism Research

HARRY A. WHITAKER

Grammatical impairments are the quintessentially linguistic aspects of aphasia, applicable to the structure of the language at the word, phrase, sentence, and discourse levels, rather than its sound or meaning. Historical discussions of neuropsychology, in particular neurolinguistics (e.g., Arbib, Caplan, & Marshall, 1982; Benton, 1988, 1991; Bouton, 1991; Eling, 1994) have always mentioned the principal figures in the history of agrammatism research, but nevertheless have not completely situated that research in the context of classical aphasia studies. In this essay we suggest that the model of sentence structure proposed by John Hughlings Jackson [1834–1911] and employed by both Arnold Pick [1851–1924] and Henry Head [1861–1940] in their ideas on agrammatism and syntactical aphasia, respectively, represents a different line of historical development in neurolinguistics than the so-called classical views of their colleagues. This difference in the premodern work on agrammatism employed abstract (mental) models of sentence structure which were presumed to underlie observed speech, models that seem to be formally equivalent to today's cognitive neuropsychological models of language, albeit vastly less detailed, whereas the classical aphasia studies of their contemporaries, Broca, Wernicke, Lichtheim, Dejerine, Marie, and others, were typically limited to taxonomic analyses of observable word- and subword-level phenomena, which were correlated with specific, and thus observable, brain sites.

Although what we now call agrammatism must have been noticed whenever aphasic impairments were noticed, the first published case description that we have been able to find is from the 17th century. *The Medical-Practical Observations of Effects Inside and Outside the Head* by J. J. Wepfer [1620–1694] is a compendium of well-documented neuropsychological case histories, published posthumously in 1727 by two of Wepfer's descendants, Bernhardinus and Georg Michael Wepfer. The book is notable for its accuracy, colorful clinical descriptions, and systematic organization. In their study of Wepfer, Luzzatti and Whitaker (1996) identified several cases with clear language disorders. "Observation #98, "loss of memory," is the description of a transient language disorder with anomia (a selective impairment of proper names) and a syntactic disorder (agrammatism). No acalculia or other neuropsychological deficits were reported. The following is translated from the Latin original:

1

R.N.N. is a 53-year-old man . . . in July 1683 he complained that he had suddenly forgotten all names, and in fact he could not even express his own name. He could not designate any object with its name, neither in Latin nor in German. He gave the impression he could recognize things and people, but their names could not be produced; he tried and tried with all his will to explain what he was thinking on various topics, but he was destitute of words; those words he could utter were alien and incoherent . . . Sometimes, he could not find proper names for people and places as quickly as customary, and from time to time he could not find some of the little words [verbulum = function words?]. *When he was talking, I could observe him from time to time violate syntactic rules and, contrary to the structure of German sentences, he would pre-pose one word to another and sometimes he could not complete a word* (= loss of morphological suffixes?). (pp. 367–371)

In addition to its interest as an early study of agrammatism, Wepfer's case is also exemplary of most, but not all, classical aphasia research on grammatical or syntactic disorders up to the 1970s: a descriptive summary of the omission or misuse of function words or inflections in spontaneous or elicited speech samples of patients with an expressive aphasia. It is exemplary as well as an analysis that made no attempt to explain the disorder but rather to describe it, a tradition in neuropsychology which still has its advocates, as Grodzinsky (1993) observed.

We remember John Hughlings Jackson [1835–1911] for his analyses of patients who suffered from severe expressive aphasia ("could not speak") but who retained some measure of cognitive functioning:

(1) that the speechless patient has lost the memory of the words serving in speech and (2) that he has not lost the memory of words serving in other ways. (Taylor, 1958, p. 186)

As part of his preoccupation, Jackson considered how these two aspects of speech, voluntary and involuntary expressions, might be localized in the two sides of the brain, and as an example of involuntary or automatic speech, he spent much of his research energy analyzing the recurrent utterances of the patient with severe expressive aphasia. Jackson did not seem to have taken much interest in the varieties of aphasia with which his contemporaries were engrossed; in his collected papers on affectations of speech (Taylor, 1958), aside from Broca, there are no discussions of Wernicke, Dejerine, Lichtheim, and others who contributed to the classical model of the aphasias. And yet, curiously, it was Jackson's notion of proposition as the essential unit of internal mental strucuture as well as expressive language which, in the work of Arnold Pick and Henry Head, laid the foundations for the study of agrammatism. In his "Notes on the Phsyiology and Pathology of the Nervous System" (1868), Jackson first develops his notion of the propositional basis of language, as well as his ideas concerning the role of the right hemisphere in automatic (involuntary) expression and perception. That this is clearly a psycholinguistic construct is clear.

The meaning of a proposition does not depend on the mere words which compose it, but on the relations these words have to one another—such a relation that the sentence is a unit. (Taylor, 1958, pp. 234-235)

Here, as well as in his (1893) paper, "Words and Other Symbols in Mentation," Jackson argues that the proposition is the main unit of thought, reasoning or mentation:

When anyone says that words are essential for thought, he may, I suppose, mean that words or some other symbols (or both words and other symbols) are so. Pantomimic actions, for example, are symbols analogous to words, and untrained deaf-mutes use these, not only for inter-communication, but also in thought. There are in all men, I submit, actions not reaching the rank of what would commonly be called pantomime, which are symbols in mentation. In all cases it is meant that propositions of symbols (verbal or pantomimic) serve in mentation; evidently to speak is to propositionize. (Taylor, 1958, p. 2050)

Arnold Pick wrote the first treatise devoted exclusively to agrammatism, only sections of which have been translated from the German (Spreen, 1973; Friederici, 1994). Linguistic theory was not well developed in 1913 when Pick completed this monograph; nonetheless, some of his theoretical assumptions are notable. He assumed that a sentence schema, which logically implied a syntactic structure, precedes the selection of lexical items; he suggested that content words were selected prior to function words, after which surface grammatical form is specified (Friederichi, p. 257; also see Spreen, 1973, pp. 147–152, for a more detailed analysis of the hierarchical order in Pick's microgenesis of language). From Pick's monograph on agrammatism:

That the schematic formulation of the sentence precedes the choice of words, as well as the syntactic and the portion of the grammatical functions that corresponds to it, is shown by the fact that the meaning of a single word, whatever it may be, is determined only by the position it takes or interacts with; therefore the mental framework should in principle be ready in a grammatical sense as well: before the choice of words ensues, the plan has to be determined before the different pieces are put together. (Friederici, 1994, p. 267)

Pick's discussion of agrammatism in the 1913 monograph was taken up again in a chapter published posthumously in 1931. According to Jason Brown (1973), Pick contributed a chapter on aphasia to a handbook on normal and pathological physiology in 1931, a chapter that had originally been written just before Pick's death in 1924, and was subsequently edited by Otto Sittig and then again by Rudolf Thiele.

The section on agrammatism (Brown, 1973, pp. 76–86) would thus represent his final ideas on this subject—noting, of course, that he would have read Henry Head's ideas on the subject by this time. Pick focused on two forms of expressive agrammatism, motor or quantitative and sensory or qualitative. He attributed both to the loss of, and/or impaired motor control over, grammatical devices (Friederici, pp. 258–259). He associated "motor agrammatism" with motor aphasia, frontal lesions, and a telegraphic style; whereas he linked "sensory agrammatism" with Kleist's "paragrammatism" (thus, with lesions of the temporal lobe), although emphasizing speech output, or what he called "the expressive side" (Brown, 1973, p. 76). From the 1931 chapter:

This temporally determined form is characterized, in pure cases, by disturbances in the use of auxiliary words, incorrect word inflections, and erroneous prefixes and suffixes. In other words, it concerns all those linguistic devices which serve to express relationships between objects, which differ widely and numerically from one language to another. . . . Regarding telegraphic style of primary origin, discussed in relation to motor agrammatism, in which the word order is not appreciably disturbed, alterations of word order have occasionally been reported as due to a discrepancy between the normal order (most important element first) and the grammatically required order (final position of the verb as in the languages of children). However, a thorough investigation of this question, based upon linguistics. . . . is not yet available. . . . absense of or defect in the auxiliary words which are normally produced in automatic fashion. It is probable that the patient with motor agrammatism at times retains the sentence skeleton since he may not comprehend the prepositions nor be able to write them. . . . The patient attempts to produce the best possible results (that which best makes him understood) with the least expenditure of effort, utilizing the optimal but still automatic application of his linguistic resources. . . . Another likely factor is the attention fixed on the effortful production of speech. If the prepositions are either not automatic or only incompletely so, attention will not suffice for their voluntary production. . . . In paragrammatism, the temporal form of expressive agrammatism, it must be remembered that grammar is by no means a unified process, but contains many factors which may be affected separately or in combination. In this form, the disorder lies one stage deeper than telegrammatism. . . . There is a discrepancy between poor agrammatical speech and better appraisal of ungrammatical sentences presented to the patient. This is explained by the contrast between defective or absent feeling for the language [and] the fact that the patient recognizes what he sees as incorrect, but is incapable of putting it into correct grammatical form. (Brown, 1973, pp. 74–84)

And in the next chapter on word deafness and speech deafness, Pick continues the discussion of agrammatism:

Disorders of the second type concern what is called sensory (impressive) agrammatism (in the narrow sense). Disturbance of stages in the comprehension of sentence meaning which correspond to the grammaticazation of the sentence, insofar as both characterize relationships, will disturb to a varying extent the comprehension of those relationships. There may also be a loss of knowledge of sentence form. . . . this latter form is generally not separated from the others, both for clinical considerations (e.g., the coexistence of expressive and sensory agrammatism) as well as psychological considerations (e.g. the same process is at one time centrifugal and at another centripetal). . . . A distinction should be made between lack of comprehension of the grammatical forms of correct speech and inadequate recognition of incorrect forms. (Brown, 1973, pp. 94–95)

Thus, it is apparent that, in his 1931 chapter, Pick, using some of the arguments from Head (below), had placed syntactic organization in a central position between sound and meaning and had given it a clear role in both expression and comprehension. As well, he recognized that there are multiple components to this syntactic organization, not all of which are affected together in the various forms of expressive and impressive grammatical disorders. Finally, borrowing from Jackson, Pick also distinguishes between automatic and voluntary dimensions of syntactic organization, which he employs in part to explain the observed variation between agrammatic output and comprehension.

We often remember Henry Head for his rather spirited, although inaccurate and somewhat misdirected, attack on the "diagram makers," the classical aphasiologists; he is not often cited for his efforts to criticize superficial descriptions of aphasic disturbances, such as "motor" or "sensory," nor for his efforts to avoid inaccurate clinical accounts, such as, "the patient was said to be able to read and write, although he could not speak" (Head, 1925, Vol. I, pp. 197–217), problems that continue to plague aphasia research. Caplan (1987) has a thoughtful discussion of Head's critique of inclusive diagnostic categories of aphasia; he points out that Head had observed that actual aphasic performance usually crosses descriptive boundaries, that specific aphasia syndromes are often transient, and that there is wide variation in aphasic performance in patients with quite similar lesion (Caplan, 1987, pp. 83–88). As Caplan observed, these problems remain unsolved.

Contemporary researchers have, erroneously we think, correlated Head's syntactical aphasia with the syndrome of Wernicke's aphasia (for example, cf. LeCours, Lhermitte, & Bryans, 1983, pp. 254–255; Goodglass and Kaplan, 1983, p. 77; Goodglass, 1993, p. 24; Benson and Ardilla, 1996, pp. 114–115); it is not at all clear that this does justice to Head's clinical observations nor to his theoretical analysis of aphasia. Weisenburg and McBride (1935) observed, "The syntactical form in Head's conception differs from the sensory aphasia which shows pronounced disturbances of speaking and also from the so-called agrammatism or paragrammatism, but partakes of the nature of these" (p. 50); they credit a French researcher, Delacroix, with noting the correspondence between Head's four aspects of aphasia and the hypothetical stages from thought to spoken expression. This is very similar to Pick's (1913) conception, which, according to Spreen (1973), was drawn from contemporary psychological research by Wilhelm Wundt, Karl Buhler, William James, and others. In this model, Head characterized syntactical aphasia as a defect in (internal) grammatical arrangement (1935, pp. 50–51). In comparing Head's ideas about aphasia to others that were more popularly received, Weisenburg and McBride (1935) suggest that it is "superior to them in theory and inferior in practice"; their reasoning: "that it is generally regarded as unsatisfactory may be judged from the fact that it has not been adopted" (1935, pp. 50–51). Weisenburg and McBride wrote of Head's system as though it was a classification of aphasias; we believe, on the other hand, that Head is not actually trying to classify aphasic disorders but rather trying to develop a psycholinguistically based theory with which to describe aphasic disorders. Thus for Head there are not four types of aphasia but four components to symbolic formulation and expression, each or any of which may break down.

What Head attempted was to characterize the nature of language impairments in their psychological context, albeit without the benefit of well-constructed linguistic or psycholinguistic theories. He proposed four types of aphasia: verbal, syntactical, nominal, and sematic, of which syntactical attempted to comprehend the various aspects of agrammatism. It is clear that Head (1925) intended these four categories as exemplars, not absolute types:

> No two examples of aphasia exactly resemble one another; each represents the response of a particular individual to the abnormal conditions. But, in many cases, the morbid manifestations can be roughly classed under such descriptive categories as Verbal, Syntactical, Nominal or Semantic defects of symbolic formulation and expression. (Vol. II, p. x)

For Head, syntactical defects (Vol. I, pp. 230–240) represented impaired grammatical structure of the phrase as well as impaired rhythmic (what we would now call "prosodic") aspects of symbolic formulation. As an example of this disorder, he observed that "the patient talks rapidly, his speech is jargon, and prepositions, conjunctions and articles tend to be omitted (Vol. II, p. xiv). He used the term "syntactical" in lieu of "agrammatic" because he thought that the language problems go deeper than the surface, observable grammatical words; he thought that they affected the basic (and, of course, internal and mental) formation and use of language (Vol. I, p. 240). Three cases of syntactical aphasia (Cases 13, 14, and 15) presented in Vol. II (pp. 198-247) are also of interest for his follow-up studies, one having been re-examined 7 years after initial injury. The patients' agrammatic output, verbal and written, is well described although it is not theoretically linked with their evident comprehension difficulties, a theoretical lapse which Pick did not make. Consider, for example, Head's case of syntactical aphasia #15:

> *Asked what he had done since he came to the London Hospital, he replied, "To here; only washing, cups and plates." Have you played any games? "Played games, yes, played one daytime, garden." . . . He did not usually employ wrong words and, if the subject under discussion was known, it was not difficult to gather the sense of what he wished to say. Thus, when I was testing his taste and placed some quinine upon his tongue, he said, "Rotten to drink it. Something medicine or that. Make you drop of water after it, so to take out of your mouth." . . . . when asked to say after me short sentences, which he had not heard before, his defective syntax became evident . . . In this case the disorder of language mainly affected syntax and rhythm. The production of single words and their use as names were not materially disturbed; but groups of words could not be combined into coherent and effective phrases. (Vol. I, pp. 174–178)*

By the time Weisenburg and McBride (1935) completed their clinical psychological study of aphasia, both the concepts of agrammatism and paragrammatism were incorporated into general models of language disorders due largely to the efforts of German researchers such as Bonhoeffer, Goldstein, Salamon, Isserlin, Kleist (who had coined the term "paragrammatism"), and Pick. In their review of the research on agrammatism, Weisenburg and McBride (1935, pp. 60-61, 71–72) remarked on the omission of grammatical words ("telegram style"), altered word-order, and the omission or confusion of prefixes, suffixes, and inflections, of course. They also took the next step of discussing models of grammatical disturbances, debating in particular the "economy of effort" principle as the cause of agrammatic aphasia. Weisenburg and McBride took sufficient interest in this topic to have included in their case reports an agrammatic aphasic patient (predominantly expressive disorder) (Case No. 20, pp. 483-491); and several of the tests in their aphasia battery explicitly addressed the evaluation of grammatical abilities, as well. Weisenburg and McBride did understand the central nature of grammatical disturbances as the following comments demonstrate:

> *The question of paragrammatism has already been touched on in connection with agrammatism and the cortical form of motor aphasia. It has been said that paragrammatism is characterized by confusions of grammatical forms, of auxiliaries, pronouns, prepositions, and so forth, and by changes in word order. A consideration of the nature and extent of these errors makes it evident that they are not simply the result of word-substitutions, and consequently not like the paraphasic errors. They involve a more extensive change which shows uncertainty, not so much in the choice of words, as in the grammatical and formal aspects of the sentence structure. (1935, p. 72)*

However, the most insightful aspect of Weisenburg and McBride's study is their recognition that Henry Head had attempted a psycholinguistic analysis of the aphasias, that Arnold Pick had proposed an abstract structural model of agrammatism, and that both Head and Pick had based their ideas on those of Jackson. Perhaps one should regard their commentary as the first recognition of the nascent cognitive tradition in neurolinguistics. What remained in the development of theories of agrammatism from the second World War to the 1970s could be described in two major developments (cf. Goodglass & Menn, 1985; Benton, 1991): First, the increased use of linguistic theory in the analysis of aphasia (Roman Jacobson's in the 1950s and 1960s, Noam Chomsky's in the 1970s and after) led to increased awareness of the pervasiveness of syntactic and grammatical impairments in aphasia and, second, to the development of cognitive science modeling to try to explain why aphasic language and, in particular, grammatical impairments are the way they are: an underlying deficit in X causes language impairments a, b, and c. Modern linguistic analyses and cognitive science approaches in general rely on abstract structural models thought to underlie the overt manifestations of language behavior.

The papers collected in this volume represent some of the bet exemplars of this current research, all drawn from papers published in the last few years in the journal *Brain and Language*. The reader who is interested in situating this work within the contemporary debates and controversies on agrammatism is encouraged to read the overviews by Grodzinsky (1993) and Fromkin (1995).

REFERENCES

Arbib, M., Caplan, D., & Marshall, J. 1982. Neurolinguistics in historical perspective. In M.A. Arbib, D. Caplan, & J.C. Marshall (Eds.), *Neural models of language processes*. New York: Academic Press. Pp. 5–24.

Benson, F., & Ardila, A. 1996. *Aphasia*. New York: Oxford University Press.

Benton, A. 1988. Neuropsychology: Past, present and future. In F. Boller & J. Grafman (Eds.), *Handbook of neuropsychology*. Amsterdam: Elsevier. Vol. 1, Pp 3–27.

Benton, A. 1991. Aphasia: Historical perspective. In M.T. Sarno (Ed.), *Acquired aphasia*. San Diego: Academic Press. Second Edition, Pp. 1–26.

Bouton, C. 1991. *Neurolinguistics: Historical and theoretical perspectives*. New York: Plenum.

Brown, J. 1973. *Aphasia by Arnold Pick*. Springfield, IL: Charles C. Thomas.

Caplan, D. 1991. *Neurolinguistics and linguistic aphasiology*. Cambridge: Cambridge Unversity Press.

De Bleser, R. 1994. Kurt Goldstein. In P. Eling (Ed.), *Reader in the history of aphasia*. Amsterdam: Benjamins. Pp. 319–347.

Eling, P. (Ed.). 1994. *Reader in the history of aphasia*. Amsterdam: Benjamins.

Friederici, A. 1994. Arnold Pick. In P. Eling (Ed.), *Reader in the history of aphasia*. Amsterdam: Benjamins. Pp. 252–280.

Fromkin, V. 1995. Introduction (to the Special Issue: Linguistic Representational an Processing Analyses of Agrammatism. Guest Editor: Victoria A. Fromkin). Brain and Language, **50**, 1–9.

Goodglass, H., & Kaplan, E. 1983. *The assessment of aphasia and related disorders*. Philadelphia: Lea & Febiger. Second Ed.

Goodglass, H., & Menn, L. 1985. Is agrammatism a unitary phenomenon? In M.L. Kean (Ed.), *Agrammatism*. Orlando: Academic Press. Pp. 1–26.

Goodglass, H. 1993. *Understanding aphasia*. San Diego: Academic Press.

Grodzinsky, Y. 1993. Introduction (to the Special Issue: Grammatical Investigations of Aphasia. Guest Editor: Yosef Grodzinsky). *Brain and Language,* **45**, 299–305.

Head, H. 1925. *Aphasia and kindred disorders of speech*. Cambridge: Cambridge University Press. Vols. I and II.

Hudson, P. 1994. Henry Head. In P. Eling (Ed.), *Reader in the history of aphasia*. Amsterdam: Benjamins. Pp. 281–318.

Jackson, J. 1868. Notes on the physiology and pathology of the nervous system. *Medical Times and Gazette,* **2**, 208, 358, 526, 696; **1**, 245, 699l **2**, 481. Reprinted in Taylor (1958).

Jackson, J. 1878–80. On affections of speech from disease of the brain. *Brain,* **1**, 304–330. *Brain,* **2**, 203–222, 323–356. Reprinted in Taylor (1958)

Jackson, J. 1893. Words and other symbols in mentation. *Medical Press and Circular,* **2**, 205. Reprinted in Taylor (1958).

Lecours, A.R., Lhermitte, F., & Bryans, B. 1983. *Aphasiology.* London: Bailliere Tindall.

Luzzatti, C., & Whitaker, H. 1996. Johanns Schenk and Johannes Jakob Wepfer: Clinical and anatomical observations in the prehistory of neurolinguistics and neuropsychology. *Journal of Neurolinguistics,* **9**(3), 2–8.

Pick, A. 1913. *Die agrammatischen Sprachstorungen.* Berlin: Springer.

Spreen, O. 1973. Psycholinguistics and aphasia: The contribution of Arnold Pick. In H. Goodglass & S. Blumstein (Eds.), *Psycholinguistics and aphasia.* Baltimore: Johns Hopkins. Pp 141–170.

Taylor, J. 1958. *Selected writings of John Hughlings Jackson.* London: Staples Press.

Wepfer, J. 1727. *Observationes medico-practicae de affectionis capitis internis & externis.* Schaffhausen: Ziegler.

Weisenburg, T., & McBride, K. 1935. *Aphasia.* New York: Hafner. Second reprint, 1973.

BRAIN AND LANGUAGE **45**, 306–317 (1993)

Relevance of Adverb Distribution for the Analysis of Sentence Representation in Agrammatic Patients

LIDIA LONZI AND CLAUDIO LUZZATTI

Department of Neurology and Department of Psychology, Università degli Studi, Milan, Italy

In this study, it is shown that functional categories are present in agrammatic grammar. Specifically, the verb–adverb order is investigated in three agrammatic patients by means of a constituent ordering task. It is shown that when the verb is in a nonfinite form, it either precedes or follows the specifier-like adverb (both positions are correct), but when the verb is finite, the adverb always follows it (which is the only possible order). The conclusions are that (i) a functional category (namely Inflection), which is responsible for the relative order verb-–adverb (of the relevant class), must exist in agrammatic grammar, and (ii) agrammatic aphasia cannot be described as a syntactic impairment involving basic sentence structure. © 1993 Academic Press, Inc.

INTRODUCTION

In the past, some authors have argued for the total loss of syntax in agrammatism (e.g., Caramazza & Zurif, 1976; Caplan & Futter, 1986; see Grodzinsky, 1990, for a detailed discussion), and this view is now being reproposed under the heading of a total loss of functional categories (Ouhalla, 1990). According to the proponents of this analysis, the functional category of Inflection—projecting as I(nfl)P(hrase) in a generalized X-bar format—is necessary to preserve the correct word order in the sentence; in particular, the respective order of the verb and its complements. Ouhalla (1992), for instance, makes the claim that the O–V–S order of sentences documented in Saffran, Schwartz, and Marin (1980) in English

This paper was presented as a poster at the 29th Annual Academy of Aphasia (Rome, 13–15 October, 1991). We are indebted to Josef Bayer, Ria De Bleser, Yoseph Grodzinsky, and an anonymous reviewer, who made detailed comments on previous versions of the paper and strongly contributed toward its improvement. Thanks are also due to Nadia Allamano and Lorena Lorenzi of the Medical Centre of Veruno, for their help in selecting the patients and administering the task. Address reprint requests to Claudio Luzzatti, Department of Psychology, Università degli Studi, Via F. Sforza 23, 20122 Milan, Italy.

9

speaking agrammatics is to be taken as evidence that the functional category Infl lacks in agrammatic patients.

Here, we would like to exploit another aspect of Inflection that might enable us to obtain better and more straightforward evidence of its presence in the structure of the sentence: its effective role in the morphological realization of the finite verb.

THEORETICAL BACKGROUND

In Italian, tensed verbs always precede the adverbs, even if they are adverbs generated in the left periphery of VP (henceforth, specifier-like adverbs); see Figs. 1 and 2.

An explanation of this phenomenon is given by the theory of Verb Movement to Infl in finite sentences (Pollock, 1989). In Pollock's (1989) proposal, I(nfl)P is split in two projections, F1 and F2.[1] For French, he assumes Verb Movement to the highest projection (F1) for the finite verb and an optional Short Movement to the lower projection (F2) for the infinitive. According to this theory, endorsed by many authors, the verb, in Italian and French finite sentences, moves to the head of F1 to get the relevant morphological features (or simply to check them, see Chomsky, 1992). Thus, a tensed verb always precedes the adverb, even though it is the adverb—in the base structure—that precedes, being the specifier. This is the case with the adverbs seen in Figs. 1 and 2. However, non-tensed verbs can either precede or follow the specifier-like adverb, for they can either undergo Short Movement or remain in their base position (see Fig. 3).

The prediction follows that patients can get the relevant pattern correct (i.e., *finite verb–adverb*) only if they have the sentence structure preserved—more specifically the functional category Infl. The sequence *adverb–finite verb* would be possible only if syntax or functional categories were lost.

In Pollock's analysis, evidence of Verb Movement in French is lent also by the negative marker *pas*. In his analysis, NegP is between F1 and F2, and *pas* is in the specifier position of NegP. Whereas *pas* never moves, the negative head itself, *ne*, being a clitic (as, possibly, the Italian negative head *non*), is always adjoined to the left of the (± finite) verb. Italian, on the other hand, lacks an obligatory specifier of NegP like the French *pas*, therefore, compared to French, it lacks further evidence concerning Verb Movement. Whereas *pas*, like all specifier-like adverbs,

---

[1] For the two Infl projections, we adopt the alternative notation F1 and F2, proposed by Pollock (1989), because their respective nature of T(ense)P and AgrP is controversial. Chomsky (1992), for instance, adopts the opposite order (AgrP and TP, respectively). The solution to the question has no bearing on our issue.

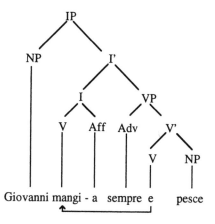

'John eats always fish'

Fɪɢ. 1. Structure underlying an Italian transitive sentence.

always follows the tensed verb, it always precedes the nontensed verb that never moves to a projection higher than F2.

It is precisely an analysis of the relative order between the (± finite) verb and the specifier-like adverb, as well as that of the relative order between the verb and the negative marker *pas,* that should allow us to verify the hypothesis of the lack of the functional category Infl in the language of patients with agrammatic speech output.

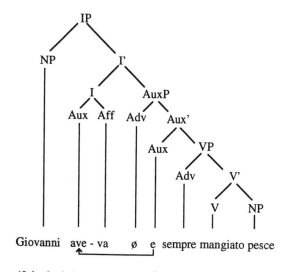

'John had always eaten fish'

Fɪɢ. 2. Structure underlying an Italian sentence with a complex verbal form finite Auxiliary + Past Participle (Aux + PstPrt).

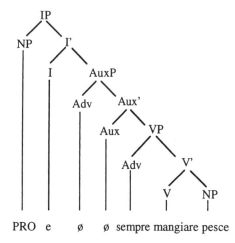

PRO   e   ∅   ∅   sempre mangiare pesce

'to always eat fish ...'

Fig. 3. Structure underlying an Italian infinitival sentence.

THE STUDY

We will start by analyzing the spontaneous speech in the few Italian and French agrammatic subjects described in the literature, and in three subjects studied in our laboratory. We will then present an experiment on word ordering.

Subjects

Four French subjects are described in Tissot, Mounin, and Lhermitte (1973), and two in Nespoulous, Dordain, Perron, Jarema, and Chazal (1990); two Italian subjects are described in Miceli, Mazzucchi, Menn, and Goodglass (1983), and two in Miceli and Mazzucchi (1990).

As for our patients, they were selected from a pool of 216 aphasic subjects, for the presence of typical agrammatic speech output, i.e., short sentences with omission of function words and substitutions (and omissions) of bound morphemes. One agrammatic patient did not use any predicate adverbs in about 40 min of conversation; therefore, he was excluded from the study.

AD is a 19-year-old school girl. Eight months before entering this study, she underwent neurosurgical treatment for the rupture of a cerebral aneurysm. She presented with faciobrachial right hemiparesis and aphasia. A CT scan showed the presence of a left frontoinsular hypodense area. A language examination made with the Italian version of the AAT showed a language disorder with the features of Broca's aphasia. Speech output was agrammatic, and there was anomia and mild dyslexia.

EB is a 15-year-old school boy. Six months before entering our study, he was a victim of a stroke, due to a thrombosis of the left internal carotid artery. A CT scan showed a left frontoinsular hypodense cerebral lesion. He presented with right hemiplegia. The AAT examination showed a medium-degree language disorder with the features of Broca's aphasia. Spontaneous speech output was rich but severely agrammatic.

CM is a left-handed medical student; about 8 months before entering our study, he was the victim of a car accident. When he came out of his coma, he presented a left hemiplegia and aphasia. CT scan showed an intraparenchimal frontoinsular hematoma in the right hemisphere. The language disorder was compatible with Broca's aphasia with agrammatic spontaneous speech.

The features of the spontaneous speech of the cases reported in the literature are described in the respective studies; Table 1 summarizes the relevant features for our three patients.

Although zero-inflection is not an option in Italian, the label "omission of inflectional affixes" is not at odds with Grodzinsky's (1990) well-known prediction that word parts are omitted in agrammatic speech only if zero-inflection is an option of the language. Under this label, in fact, we simply recorded the peculiar occurrences in which patients struggled with their difficulty with the appropriate word-ending, eventually giving up and leaving the word "unfinished."

Preliminary Evidence from Spontaneous Speech

We considered (i) the verb–adverb order for the French and Italian subjects in the literature and our Italian subjects, and (ii) the verb-negative marker order for the French subjects in the literature.

1. Adverbs. We analyzed the relative order of the ($\pm$ finite) verb with respect to the specifier-like adverb. All the relevant strings were correct, both in the transcriptions (and relevant glossae[2]) of French and Italian agrammatic cases and in our patients' spontaneous speech production (see Appendix 1).

The specifier-like adverb occurrences are 22 in the literature and 20 in our patients' speech output.

In all cases but one, the finite verbs precede the adverb, and not the other way around. The only Adv + V(+finite) sequence was produced by CM: *non più, eh, posso parlare* ("Not anymore, uh, can (1stP) speak"). In this case, however, the hesitation marked by *eh* seems to reflect the patient's late decision to provide the auxiliary-like verb "posso" ("can" 1stP). The patient was close to using the agrammatic infinitival sequence *non più parlare* ("Not anymore to speak"), instead of *non posso più parlare* ("I cannot speak anymore"), and, according to his self-correcting attitude, introduced the missing auxiliary too late.

2. Negation. For French, as stated above, we then considered the position of the negative marker *pas* with respect to the verb, whether tensed or not. In this case, also, no wrong sequence was found. One hundred percent of the eight relevant occurrences were correct.

Experiment

Materials. In order to see whether data from spontaneous speech are reliable and can be replicated in an experimental situation, we tested the three agrammatic patients by means of a constituent ordering task, made up of 75 sentences requiring different positions of the adverb with respect to the ($\pm$ finite) verb.

---

[2] We disregarded a sequence registered by Miceli et al. (1990) as "wrong word order" (i.e., Adv + Finite Verb): *lo.guido. . . poco.corro, corro.* "I.drive . . . little.run1stP, run." This sequence is at least ambiguous, since the adverb *poco* ("little") (i) is followed by a short pause, (ii) follows another finite verb, and, crucially, (iii) is an adverb parenthetically used in agrammatic speech, instead of *per un poco,* "for a little."

TABLE 1

Main Features of the Agrammatic Spontaneous Speech of the Three
Patients Described in This Study

Patient	AD	EB	CM
Omissions			
Articles	+	+	+
Prepositions	+	+	+
Auxiliaries	(+)	+	+
Verbs	+ +	+	+
Clitic pronouns	(+)	+	±
Negations	+	−	±
Inflect. affixes	±	±	−
Unstressed initial sounds	−	+	−
Substitutions			
Infinitives	+	+	±
3rd pers.	±	±	−
Prepositions	±	−	+
Agreement (Gen., Num.)	−	+	±
Token Test (AAT % ranks)	66	69	99

Note. +, Presence of the feature; −, absence of the feature; ±, one/two occurrences;
+ +, marked presence of the feature. Features which may not be fully evaluated due to
the wide concomitant omission of lexical verbs are in parentheses

We selected 17 complement-like adverbs and 9 specifier-like adverbs (see Appendix 2).[3,4]
We constructed 75 sentences, in which each adverb appeared as a predicate modifier, and
the lexical verb (30) was given in the finite, infinitival, and Aux + PstPrt forms, respectively.[5]

The sentences were constructed according to the following schemes:

(1) (Det)Noun − Verb(+ fin) − Adverb − ((Det) Noun)

$$(2)\ (Det)Noun\ -\ Aux(+fin)\ -\ \begin{cases} Participle\ -\ Adverb \\ \\ Adverb\ -\ Participle \end{cases}$$

---

[3] The terminology adopted in this paper may seem unorthodox since it is relatively new
(for the specifier-like adverbs see Pollock, 1989; Belletti, 1990; Lonzi, 1990; for complement-
like adverbs, Larson, 1988; Lonzi, 1992). Specifier-like adverbs (essentially quantifiers or
degree adverbs) have their base position to the left of the verb, complement-like adverbs
to the right. It has also been proposed that specifier-like adverbs be left-adjoined to maximal
projections rather than base-generated in the relevant specifier positions (Belletti, 1990).
Both solutions may be safely adopted, with respect to our conclusion.

[4] We included complement-like (virtually, manner) adverbs, for, in Italian, they represent
the large majority of adverbs (Lonzi, 1991), and, furthermore, they can lend evidence to
the effect that the head-complement parameter is respected also in infinitival sentences,
where the expected behavior of the two types of adverbs is different.

[5] For example: Finite V: *Pietro gioca solamente* ("P. only plays"); Infinitival V: *Solamente giocare/giocare solamente non va bene* ("To play only is not good"); Aux + PstPrt:
Pietro ha solamente giocato ("P. has only played"). Since sentences with a simple finite
form do not allow for the presence of certain specifier-like adverbs (Lonzi, 1990), we have
constructed the relevant Aux + PstPrt strings (2 × 4) and infinitival sentences (2 × 4) twice.

(3) V(+ fin) + Prep − Verb(− fin) − Adverb

(4) $\left.\begin{array}{l} \text{Verb}(-\text{fin}) \ - \ \text{Adverb} \\ \text{Adverb} \ - \ \text{Verb}(-\text{fin}) \end{array}\right\}$ − ((Det)Noun) − Copula + Adj

(5) ((Det)Noun − Modal − Verb(− fin) − Adverb − (Prep + Noun or (Det)Noun)

Each sentence, of three to six words including determiners, was divided into three to four constituents. Stimuli were presented on separate cardboard cards and read aloud in a random order by the examiner. The subject was asked to order them in such a way as to form a correct Italian sentence. While the patient was informed that more than one solution might have been allowed, s/he was invited to select the "best" of all (i.e., in our view, the unmarked option). Since the four subjects had a variable reading deficit, the examiner read aloud the solution adopted by the patient, without providing intonational cues, before s/he decided that it was her/his definitive choice. In each sentence, the adverb could precede and/or follow the verb according to the rules described above.

If there were no functional categories, we might predict that any order would be possible for agrammatics, or that specifier-like adverbs will always precede the verb independently from its tense, due to the lack of Verb Movement.

Results

Table 2 summarizes the performance of the three subjects on the constituent ordering task. The patients' responses are classified by the possible sources of errors. Under (i), the number of unacceptable sentences are listed; under (ii), the number of sentences with a specific violation of the reciprocal order verb–adverb are shown; under (iii), the number of sentences involving a marked order verb–adverb (as, for instance, in exclamations) are given; under (iv), the number of errors compatible with a switch from one class (specifier-like) to another (complement-like) are listed. More precisely, errors of type (iv) concern eight sentences with two stylistically marked specifier-like adverbs (*unicamente,*

TABLE 2
Performance of the Three Subjects on the Constituent Ordering Task

Subject	Word order errors		Marked w.o.	Class switch	Correct ordering
	(i)	(ii)	(iii)	(iv)	
AD	2	–	1	5/8	67 (89%)
EB	3	2	2	5/8	63 (84%)
CM	2	1	1	8/8	63 (84%)
C (mean) (n = 8)	0.13	0.25	0	2.75	72 (96%)

Note. (i) Number of unacceptable sentences; (ii) number of violations of the reciprocal order verb–adverb; (iii) number of sentences with a reciprocal order verb–adverb pragmatically marked; (iv) number of errors compatible with a switch from one class to another.

"uniquely" and *puramente,* "purely") that are treated as common manner adverbs (see footnote 6).

The patients show a pattern of performance relatively comparable to that of the control group. The rate of errors is 3% for AD, 7% for EB, and 4% for CM. Sentences presenting a marked order of the constituents, while preserving the correct order of the verb and the adverb, have been accepted as correct, whereas the marked solutions involving the adverbs have not been included in the number of correct responses. It must be noted that the three patients, following a well-known pattern of sensitivity to every source of linguistic "difficulty," did not recognize the two stylistically marked adverbial forms and treated them as manner adverbs, generalizing the value of their *-mente* ending (parallel to the *-ly* ending of English).[6]

Complement-like adverbs always follow the verb, both in the patients' and in the control group's responses. This means that the head-complement order is preserved, and, therefore—according to the proponents of the hypothesis of the loss of functional projections (see Introduction)—that Infl is also preserved. We will, however, pursue the logic of our experiment and focus our attention on specifier-like adverbs. The relevant results may be seen in Table 3.

In the control group's responses, the specifier-like adverb position in infinitival sentences is distributed before and after the verb, whereas, as expected, no adverb precedes the finite form (whether a lexical or an auxiliary verb). The same pattern was found in agrammatic patients.

DISCUSSION

Our experiment shows that agrammatic patients do have access to the system of rules that govern the distribution of various adverbs; i.e., in particular, head-complement directionality and, crucially, Verb Movement to Infl.

As predicted, if there were no functional categories, any order could have been possible, or specifier-like adverbs could have preceded the verb independently from its tense. This is not what the findings show. Confronted with the absence of the forbidden sequence *finite verb + adverb,* and with the sequence *adverb + infinitival verb* using only those adverbs that may actually precede it, we must conclude that the functional projection(s) of Infl is present in the grammar of aphasics. Our

---

[6] This class switch must be included in the table, for these adverbs do not allow freedom of position with nontensed verbs, and the relevant responses are (although irrelevantly) not correct. Furthermore, whereas controls may opt (hesitatingly) for this "error," and systematically abandon it when the typical "higher adverb" position between Aux and PstPrt is available, aphasics more consistently make errors in both the infinitival and the Aux + Prt sentences.

TABLE 3
Results of the Constituent Ordering Task (Specifier-like Adverbs)
According to the Opposition ± Finite Tense

V.form	Adv.posit.	AD	EB	CM	Controls ($n = 8$)
Finite	Precede	—	—	—	—
	Follow	15 (83)	17 (94)	13 (72)	16 (89)
	Other	3 (17)	1 (5)	5 (28)	2 (11)
Infinitival	Precede	3 (23)	6 (46)	5 (38)	6.9 (52)
	Follow	7 (54)	6 (46)	7 (54)	5.3 (40)
	Other	3 (23)	1 (8)	1 (8)	0.8 (8)

Note. Figures in parentheses give % of responses.

results disprove the hypothesis of an impoverished sentential structure in agrammatism due to the lack of functional projections, since the nonoccurrence of the sequence *specifier-like adverb − verb(+finite)* is only a by-product of Verb Movement to Infl.

Our conclusion, then, is that functional categories are preserved in our patients, and there is Verb Movement to the highest projection of Infl (i.e., F1). Within the theory from which this hypothesis originated, we do not see any other available explanation for the results obtained: what has been used as linguistic evidence of Verb Movement to Infl for languages like Italian or French must be used as linguistic evidence of the presence of Infl in agrammatic patients.

APPENDIX 1

Examples of adverbial occurrences in the spontaneous speech of AD, EB, and CM.[7] In the Italian transcriptions, the omitted obligatory morphemes are given within round brackets. In the glossae, square brackets are used for grammatical comments.

AD

V + Adv

Complement-like: camminato parecchio: no, eh . . parecchio no! . . . (in) fretta e furia "walked [pstprt] a lot: no, uh . . a lot no! . . . in a hurry"; *mangi meglio* "eat [2ndP instead of 3rdP] better"; *correre in fretta e furia* "to run in a hurry"; *s- studiare . . a lungo, a lungo* "to study . . for a long, long time."

---

[7] The speech of the patients is given with the necessary integrations in brackets; SAdv stands for "sentence adverbs"; and Holophr. for "holophrastic use" (essentially the omission of the verb). It must be kept in mind that Italian is a null-subject language.

SAdv

Lontano, lontano "very far away"; *forse* "maybe"; *un giorno* "one day"; *tempo fa* "time ago"; *una volta* "once upon a time."

Stereot.

Allora "then"; *di nuovo* "again"; *però* "however"; *insomma* "in sum."

Holophr.

Perché, tardi "because, late"; *però. meno, no, di più . .* "however. less, no, more . . ."

EB

For reasons of space, we omit five V + Adv examples, with: V(+fin)-"better" (1), Neg-V(+fin)-"anymore" (3), Neg-V(+fin)-"always" (1).

V + Adv

Complement-like: andare sotto "to go downstairs"; *portare sotto* "to bring downstairs"; *mi sento male qua* "I feel badly here"; *il braccio, eh,(lo) muovevo poco* "the arm, uh, it [Cl] moved [1stP] little"; *mangiarti meglio* "to eat you [Cl] better."

Specifier-like: parlare ancora "to speak still"; *no sentire più, eh, le gambe* "no to feel anymore, uh, the legs"; *no trova più* "no finds anymore"; *non sa più cosa dirle* "doesn't know anymore what to say to-her [Cl]"; *dorme sempre* "sleeps always"; *non (si) avvicinarono mai* "didn't [ReflCl] approach [3rdPP] ever."

Adv + V

Specifier-like: ancora andare "still to go."

SAdv

Poi "afterwards"; *(per) un po'* "for a while"; *quindi* "hence"; *veramente* "actually"; *adesso* "now"; *subito* "immediately"; *però* "however"; *prima di tutto* "first of all"; *di nuovo* "again"; *domani* "tomorrow."

Stereot.

Allora "then"; *e poi* "and then"; *così* "thus."

Holophr.

Pasta, eh, eh (è) cuotta, [8]*eh, eh, fuori* "pasta, uh, uh, is cooked, uh, uh, out"; *TAC eh, eh, poi bene, no?* "CAT, uh, uh, afterwards well, isn't it?"; *eh, avanti, sino a cinquanta punti* "uh, ahead, up to fifty points"; *allora, avanti avanti* "then, very much ahead."

CM

V + Adv

Complement-like: non molla-sse non, eh, l'in tempo "wouldn't let [3rdP] wouldn't, uh, it in time"; *sono andato . . . una volta* "have [1stP] gone once"; *era (ar)rabbiato molto* "was enraged a lot"; *picchiavo tanto (l')av-versario* "hit [1stP] so much the adversary"; *venuto, eh, (la) prima volta;* "come [pstprt] the first time."

Specifier-like: è quasi ingegnere "is nearly engineer"; *lavora sempre* "works always"; *invita sempre* "invites always"; *non esce mai* "doesn't go out ever"; *parla solo; solo: quasi solo /dea/ eh, del lavoro* "speaks only; only: nearly only, uh, of the work"; *parlo solo, quasi solo di* "speak [1stP] only, nearly only of"; *andavo sempre sulla pista* "went[1stP] always on the track."

Specifier-like + complement-like: (non) parlo più bene "don't speak [1stP] anymore well."

Adv + V

Specifier-like: non (ho) mai perso conoscenza "don't have ever lost consciousness."

SAdv

Ora "now"; *poi* "afterwards"; *allora* "then."

Holophr.

(Per) poco "for little"; *quando (sono) venuto, eh, (la) pri-prima volta: male;* "when have come, uh, the first time: badly."

APPENDIX 2

Adverbs Used in the Experiment

Complement-like Adverbs

completamente (completely), *smodatamente* (immoderately), *eccessivamente* (eccessively), *definitivamente* (definitively), *facilmente* (easily),

---

[8] *"cuotta":* regularization, instead of the pstprt *cotta* "cooked" (from *cuocere:* "to cook").

malamente (badly); *bene* (well), *meglio* (better); *molto* (very much); *presto* (soon); *distrattamente* (inattentively), *attentamente* (attentively), *generosamente* (generously), *umilmente* (humbly), *egoisticamente* (egoistically), *prontamente* (readily), *amorevolmente* (lovingly).

Specifier-like Adverbs

puramente (purely), *unicamente* (uniquely), *anche* (also), *quasi* (nearly); *sempre* (always), *solamente* (only), *proprio* (really), *già* (already), *ancora* (further).

REFERENCES

Belletti, A. 1990. *Generalized verb movement*. Torino: Rosenberg & Sellier.

Caplan, D., & Futter, C. 1986. Assignment of thematic roles by an agrammatic aphasic patient. *Brain and Language, 27*, 117–135.

Caramazza, A., & Zurif, E. B. 1976. Dissociation of algorithmic and heuristic processes in sentence comprehension: Evidence from aphasia. *Brain and Language, 3*, 572–582.

Chomsky, N. 1992. *A minimalist program for linguistic theory*. MIT Occasional Papers in Linguistics. Number 1.

Grewendorf, G. 1991. *Parametrisierung der Syntax: Zur 'kognitiven Revolution' in der Linguistik. Sprachwissenschaft in Frankfurt*, Arbeitspapier Nr1., J. W. Goethe Universität Frankfurt a. M.

Grodzinsky, Y. 1990. *Theoretical perspectives on language deficits*. Cambridge, MA: MIT Press.

Larson, R. K. 1988. On the double object construction. *Linguistic Inquiry, 19*, 335–391.

Lonzi, L. 1990. Which adverbs in Spec,VP?. *Rivista di Grammatica Generativa, 15*, 141–160.

Lonzi, L. 1991. Il sintagma avverbiale. In L. Renzi & G. Salvi (Eds.), *Grande grammatica italiana di consultazione*. Bologna: Il Mulino.

Lonzi, L. 1992. Adverb dislocation vs. preposing vs. semiquotation. In E. Fava (Ed.), *Proceedings of the XVII Meeting of Generative Grammar*, Trieste, 22-24 February, 1991. Torino: Rosenberg & Sellier.

Miceli, G., & Mazzucchi, A. 1990. Agrammatism in Italian: Two case studies. In L. Menn & L. K. Obler (Eds.), *Agrammatic aphasia—A cross-language narrative sourcebook*. Amsterdam: Benjamins.

Miceli, G., Mazzucchi, A., Menn, L., & Goodglass, H. 1983. Contrasting cases of Italian agrammatic aphasia without comprehension disorder. *Brain and Language, 19*, 65–97.

Nespoulous, J.L., Dordain, M., Perron, C., Jarema, G., & Chazal, M. 1990. Agrammatism in Italian: Two case studies. In L. Menn & L. K. Obler (Eds.), *Agrammatic aphasia— A cross-language narrative sourcebook*. Amsterdam: Benjamins.

Ouhalla, J. 1990. *Functional categories, agrammatism and language acquisition*. Manuscript. Queen Mary and Westfield College, London University.

Ouhalla, J. 1992. Agrammatism and linguistic theory: A review of Grodzinsky's Theoretical Perspectives of Language Deficits. *Linguistische Berichte, 139*, 182–196.

Pollock, J. Y. 1989. Verb movement, universal grammar and the structure of IP. *Linguistic Inquiry, 20*, 365–424.

Saffran, E., Schwartz, M., & Marin, O. 1980. The word-order problem in agrammatism. II. Production. *Brain and Language, 10*, 263–280.

Tissot, R. J., Mounin, G., & Lhermitte, F. 1973. *L'Agrammatisme*. Bruxelles: Dessart.

BRAIN AND LANGUAGE **45,** 340–370 (1993)

Comprehension and Acceptability Judgments in Agrammatism: Disruptions in the Syntax of Referential Dependency

GAIL MAUNER,* VICTORIA A. FROMKIN,† AND THOMAS L. CORNELL‡

*University of Rochester; †Linguistics Department, University of California at Los Angeles; and ‡Cognitive Science Program, University of Arizona

The link between brain damage and language impairment has been documented as far back as the papyrus records of Egyptian surgeons of 1700 BCE. However, it has been only in the last two decades that the characterization of disordered language resulting from focal brain damage has focused on aspects of language impairment relevant to questions of linguistic theory and normal language processing. Theoretical interest in aphasia is due, in part, to the fact that focal brain injuries not only result in selective cognitive disorders, but also may lead to specific impairments in either the construction of linguistic representations or specific language processing mechanisms. Aphasic deficits following brain damage may thus serve as a testing ground for theoretical models of the normal mental grammar. But in addition, theories of grammar may help to provide an explanation for language deficits, if one takes the view that aphasic language can only be understood in relation to the normal, intact brain and mental grammar.

Language impairments associated with damage to Broca's area have been the focus of a great deal of research, in part because the intriguing pattern of spared versus impaired comprehension that has been repeatedly observed has suggested to many the presence of a specifically linguistic deficit. Oddly, this pattern of comprehension behavior (termed "asyntactic comprehension" in Caramazza and Berndt, 1985) coexists with a pattern of remarkably normal behavior on acceptability judgment

Authors are listed in reverse alphabetical order. The preparation of this manuscript was a collaborative effort and the order of authors is not intended to reflect the magnitude of individual contributions. Special thanks to Yosef Grodzinsky, Greg Hickok, Marcia Linebarger, and Edgar Zurif for helpful discussion. During the preparation of this manuscript Cornell was supported by grants from the Cognitive Science Program and the McDonell-Pew Cognitive Neurosciences Program at the University of Arizona. Address requests for reprints to Gail Mauner, Department of Psychology, Meliora Hall, University of Rochester, Rochester, NY 14627.

21

tasks. Oversimplifying somewhat, subjects can accurately judge the grammaticality of constructions which they cannot comprehend, despite the fact that the inability to comprehend these structures is based in syntactic processing. The purpose of the first section of this paper is to present the data which needs to be accounted for. We shall discuss various attempts to fix the locus of asyntactic comprehension in some component of the grammar in order to provide both the conceptual and the empirical contexts for our own model, which accounts for both agrammatic comprehension and departures from normal sensitivity to deformations in grammaticality. In the second and third sections we present and defend our model in formal detail.

1. THE DATA AND PREVIOUS ACCOUNTS

1.1. Comprehension

Initially, the term agrammatism was coined to characterize a disorder of speech production in brain-damaged patients whose verbal output was sparse, disfluent, and marked by the omission of many grammatical formatives such as auxiliaries, inflectional affixes, pronouns, determiners, and some prepositions. Comprehension was thought to be spared. Beginning in the 1970s, several studies revealed that Broca's aphasics had difficulty comprehending sentences when the crucial cues for comprehension were purely syntactic (e.g., Caramazza & Zurif, 1976; Heilman & Scholes, 1976; Schwartz, Saffran, & Marin, 1980). For instance, agrammatics had no difficulty assigning the correct *thematic roles* to the participants in the event denoted by the verb in active declaratives such as (1) or (2), or in nonreversible passives such as (3).[1] However, assignment of the roles of chaser and chased in reversible passives such as (4) was at chance—roughly half the time the subject was interpreted as the chaser, half the time as the chased.

(1) The boy ate the tomato.
(2) The boy chased the girl.
(3) The tomato was eaten by the boy.
(4) The girl was chased by the boy.

A similar dissociation was found in agrammatic patients' comprehension of relative clauses and cleft sentences. Their ability to determine who did what to whom in semantically reversible subject-relativized (5) and subject-cleft sentences (6) was relatively unimpaired, but with semantically reversible object-relativized and object-cleft sentence (7–8), they performed at chance in determining the roles of chaser and chased (Caramazza & Zurif, 1976; Grodzinsky, 1984; Caplan & Futter, 1986).

[1] 'Thematic roles' encode the basic idea of "who did what to whom." Thus, in a sentence like *the boy is chasing the girl*, the verb *chase* assigns *the boy* a thematic role of *agent*, referring to the chaser in this scenario, and assigns to *the girl* the role of *patient*.

(5) The boy who chased the girl is fast.
(6) It was the boy who chased the girl.
(7) The boy who the girl chased is fast.
(8) It was the boy who the girl chased.

1.1.1. Nonsyntactic accounts. The first account of agrammatic comprehension difficulties proposed in terms of formal properties of language focused on difficulties with comprehension and production of closed-class lexical items and placed the locus of deficit in the phonological component of the grammar (Kean, 1977; see Lapointe, 1983, and Bradley, Garrett, & Zurif, 1980, for proposals that place the locus of impairment at other lower level components of the grammar such as morphology or in processing differences related to open- and closed-class lexical items). In Kean's account, components of the language processor were organized hierarchically with information flowing from lower components to higher ones. She argued that impairments at lower levels of the system (e.g., the phonological component) could result in what looked like impairments at higher levels. Kean's proposal is an elegant attempt to explain both the production and the comprehension deficits seen in agrammatism; however, this account runs into difficulties in the face of evidence that (1) comprehension deficits and nonfluent output are sometimes dissociable (Caramazza, Berndt, Basili, & Koller, 1981; Caramazza & Zurif, 1976; Heilman & Scholes, 1976; Kolk, van Grunsven, & Keyser, 1985; Miceli, Mazzucchi, Menn, & Goodglass, 1983; Saffran & Marin, 1975) and (2) agrammatic patients show sensitivity to the meanings (Lukatela, Crain, & Shankweiler, 1988) and presence or absence (Linebarger, Schwartz, & Saffran, 1983a) of many function words. As a consequence of these findings, current models of these behaviors are typically restricted to accounting for asyntactic comprehension specifically and not the whole collection of symptoms classically termed "agrammatism."

1.1.2. "Global" asyntactic accounts. Another class of formal explanations has characterized agrammatic comprehension as reflecting complete or partial loss of syntactic competence. The earliest of these accounts characterized agrammatic comprehension as completely asyntactic, that is, the ability to appropriately constrain the meaning of a sentence by grammatical means was lost. As a result, sentence meaning was determined by combining the meanings of lexical items in accordance with real-world plausibility (Caramazza & Zurif, 1976). Another asyntactic account was proposed by Caplan and Futter (1986), who suggested that chance performance on passives and object clefts as well as verb phrase-conjoined sentences, subject–subject relatives, and object–object relatives (examples in (9)) is the result of sensitivity to linear ordering of nouns and verbs and the application of an interpretive rule assigning thematic roles in an Agent–Theme–Goal order.

(9) (a) The frog chased the monkey and bumped the bear.
    (b) The frog that chased the monkey bumped the bear.
    (c) The frog that the monkey chased bumped the bear.
    (d) The frog chased the monkey that bumped the bear.
    (e) The frog chased the monkey that the bear bumped.

In essence, this proposal attributes only very limited linguistic knowledge to the agrammatic comprehender and suggests that the correct level of representation for analysis of agrammatic comprehension is the level of lexical categories, not phrasal nodes. However, agrammatic comprehenders are able to make many well-formedness judgments with a high level of accuracy in an off-line task, when those judgments depend on phrase level relationships. Moreover, in an on-line processing task, it has been demonstrated that agrammatics, like unimpaired adults, evince a word position effect (Shankweiler, Crain, Gorrell, & Tuller, 1989). That is, they are faster to recognize grammatical deformations when they occur later, as opposed to earlier, in a sentence. With unimpaired adults, this result has been taken as an indication that listeners begin to construct a structural representation immediately. The effect arises because, as the sentence unfolds, the number of structural possibilities that need to be considered narrows considerably, thereby leaving more processing resources available for the detection of anomalies. If this interpretation is correct, then agrammatics must be computing structures at a phrasal level on-line.

1.1.3. Partial loss—refining asyntactic accounts. Less global accounts of agrammatic comprehension, focussing on some particular aspect of syntactic processing as the locus of difficulty, have also been proposed. Grodzinsky (1986, 1990) takes as his starting point a model of grammar in which the structural representations reflecting the thematic relationships of noun phrase arguments to predicates are often mediated by abstract markers called traces (Grodzinsky assumes as a background the syntactic theory of Chomsky, 1981). In this grammatical framework, verbs assign thematic roles to elements in structurally defined positions. However, sometimes, due to the operation of other grammatical principles, a noun phrase that would normally occupy a thematic position and receive a thematic role directly, *moves* to a nonthematic position, leaving an abstract marker, called a *trace,* in its original position. The result of this movement is the formation of an *argument chain,* linking the moved noun phrase to its trace. This linkage is often represented by labeling the trace and its noun phrase antecedent with identical subscripted indices. The verb transmits a thematic role to this trace–argument complex. The passive sentence in (10) illustrates an argument chain with the noun phrase *the boy* coindexed with its trace (*t*) in the postverbal position.

(10) The boy$_i$ was hit t_i.

Grodzinsky (1986, 1990) hypothesizes that the pattern of spared and impaired comprehension in (1–8) arises as a consequence of an inability to support traces in syntactic representations. Thematic role assignment proceeds normally for noun phrases that remain in thematic positions. For noun phrases that have moved, Grodzinsky (1990) proposes that thematic assignment is accomplished by applying a Default Principle that assigns the role of *agent* to NPs in subject position unless this assignment conflicts with the semantic properties of the noun phrase (e.g., sandwiches cannot be agents). In such cases the Default Principle picks a role that matches the semantic properties of the NP from the next lower level of a Thematic Hierarchy. For passives, thematic role assignment proceeds first with the formation of a structural representation in which there is no trace linking the subject *the boy* to a thematic position, as in (11a) (for illustrative purposes, an asterisk is used to represent the undetected gap or deleted trace). The argument of the *by*-phrase *the girl* is assigned the thematic role of agent via normal grammatical processes. The subject *the boy* receives no thematic role because it is not in a thematic position and is not linked to a trace in a thematic position. The Default Principle is applied assigning *agent* to *the boy,* as illustrated in (11b). Now the asyntactic comprehender, faced with a "double agent" problem, resolves it by guessing which noun phrase should be assigned *agent* and which *patient*. The double agent problem never arises in active declaratives because thematic role assignment in actives is not mediated by a trace.

(11) (a) The boy was hit * by the girl.
      ?   Agent
    (b) The boy was hit * by the girl.
      Agent   Agent

A similar explanation for comprehension performance on subject and object relatives is given.

There are some technical difficulties with Grodzinsky's account. For example, the Default Principle is meant to apply to "lexical" noun phrases. However, as Caplan and Hildebrandt (1986) point out, in the grammatical framework assumed by Grodzinsky, there is no overt noun phrase within the relative clause that is without a thematic role to trigger the application of the Default Principle.[2] A more general concern about heuristic strategies also arises. Given the fact that a compensatory heuristic is outside general principles of linguistic organization, what constrains

---

[2] The NP modified by the relative clause in, e.g., the object relative in (9c), is not actually *in* the relative clause—it receives its thematic role from the matrix verb *bump*. According to the theory Grodzinsky assumes, the head of the relative clause would be construed with a nonovert relative pronoun which is itself coindexed with the trace in subject position.

different individuals to formulate the same heuristic following brain damage? Grodzinsky's (1990) answer to this question is that the Default Principle, on first application, reflects the nonlinguistic knowledge that the role of agent is associated with great regularity with subject position. This implies that what conditions the application of agent assignment is the presence of an NP without a thematic role in subject position. However, if this is the case, then we have no explanation for the at-chance assignment of thematic roles in object–object relatives such as (9e) in which there are no overt NPs that are not assigned thematic roles directly, without the mediation of traces.

To some degree this is a technical, perhaps strictly theory-internal problem over the "lexical" status of the missing relative pronoun—one could imagine an appeal to principles of grammar which Grodzinsky apparently assumes which would avoid this problem. But here we encounter another and perhaps more serious problem with Grodzinsky's trace-deletion account: namely, the extent to which that model can appeal to principles of grammar. A number of principles of grammar conspire to assure the existence of traces in the representation of normal syntactic structure. These same principles are also involved in fixing the properties of other constructions. As Sproat (1986) notes, there is evidence from grammaticality judgment studies that agrammatics must be forming these other constructions correctly (Linebarger et al., 1983a). Therefore, Sproat concludes, these subjects must retain the grammatical competence necessary to establish traces in the contexts where they are required.[3] Consequently, the trace deletion hypothesis must be a hypothesis about the nature of the data structures which the agrammatic's processor is able to employ, rather than a hypothesis about their grammatical competence. Grodzinsky (1990) adopts just this position. This move is problematic due to the lack of a clear grammar–parser relation underlying the representational account. Of course, there is no reason to reject, a priori, the possibility of a truly explanatory link between a grammatical competence within which traces are for the most part just like any other NP and a

---

[3] More direct evidence, bearing specifically on traces, is harder to come by. Linebarger et al. (1983a) argue that agrammatic individuals are sensitive to gap violations, but only some of their stimuli, like (i), clearly bear on movement constructions. Other gap violations either are not the result of movement (PRO-gaps) or involve additional violations (e.g., case marking or Theta Criterion). Thus, although their subjects' error rates are low, it is difficult to tell from their summary data what part sentences like (i) play in the errors that do occur.

(i) * The boy was expected would pick up his toys before napping.

One prediction that the trace-deletion hypothesis would appear to make, relevant to a grammaticality judgment task, is as follows. Agrammatic individuals should have difficulty rejecting as ungrammatical sentences containing *wanna* contractions across gaps, as in (ii).

(ii) * Who do you wanna win the race tomorrow.

Sentences like (ii) have never been tested, to the best of our knowledge.

parser with resources specially assigned to the maintenance of traces. Nonetheless, it is important to note that this account does incur an explanatory debt here; at some point it must be made clear why elements which are epiphenomenal in linguistic competence should be phenomenal in linguistic performance.

While it would be unfair to saddle Grodzinsky with the task of explaining the grammar–parser relation, this problem does have concrete ramifications in the study of agrammatism because of the problems which grammaticality judgment studies have introduced into this field. In fact, several researchers have argued that there is a close relationship between parsing and judgment (Linebarger, Schwartz, & Saffran, 1983b; Shankweiler et al., 1989). If this link is real, then a reasonable criterion for any account of agrammatic comprehension is that it also accommodate agrammatics' judgments. In addition, in general, the farther the parser gets from the grammar the harder it gets to account for deficits to grammaticality judgment performance.

1.2. Well-Formedness Judgments

The characterization of asyntactic comprehension has been complicated by a number of studies by Linebarger and her colleagues (Linebarger, Schwartz, & Saffran, 1983a; Schwartz, Linebarger, Saffran, & Pate 1987; Linebarger, 1989, 1990), who have found that subjects with attested dissociations in comprehension between activities and passives, and between subject and object relatives, are able to discriminate grammatical from ungrammatical sentences in the very constructions they find difficult to interpret.[4] For instance, Linebarger (1989, 1990) reports that agrammatic individuals could distinguish ill-formed passive sentences from well-formed passives and actives, as illustrated in (12).

(12) (a) *John was finally kissed Louise.
     (b) The boy was followed by the girl.
     (c) *The boy was followed the girl.
     (d) The boy was following the girl.

Additionally, their agrammatic subjects showed considerable sensitivity to a wide variety of other grammatical deformations. On the face of it, this would suggest that syntactic abilities have been spared. However, the grammaticality judgment picture is not entirely straightforward. There were some conditions which elicited relatively high error rates. One subset of the difficult conditions involves tag questions when the subject of the tag does not agree in person, number, or gender with the host sen-

---

[4] Other studies showing remarkably preserved judgment abilities include Lukatela, Crain, and Shankweiler (1988) and Shankweiler, Crain, Gorrell, and Tuller (1989).

tence's subject or when the tag's auxiliary verb selection does not agree in tense, modality, or aspect with the host sentence's verb, illustrated in (13). Both types of grammatical deformations were frequently accepted as grammatical.

(13) (a) *The woman is outside, isn't it?
     (b) *John is tall, doesn't he?

Agrammatic subjects also had difficulty in judgment tasks involving other kinds of agreement as well. Specifically, violations involving gender, number, and animacy in pronouns and reflexives (14 a–14c) or violations involving misselection of auxiliaries (14d) elicited high error rates.

(14) (a) *The man itself came.
     (b) *The girl fixed themselves a sandwich.
     (c) *The pencil who he bought is sharp.
     (d) *John was happy and so did George.

Linebarger and her colleagues suggest that these problematic judgment cases and the active/passive and subject relative/object relative comprehension dissociations are related, but that they are not the result of a specifically syntactic impairment. The overall sensitivity to grammatical deformations, they argue, should be taken as strong evidence for preserved ability to recover (all) syntactic structure. Linebarger (1989) observes that the cases in which agrammatic individuals evince difficulty detecting ungrammaticalities all involve noncategorial feature clashes between anaphorically linked elements. She suggests that, in both the difficult cases of comprehension and grammaticality judgment, although agrammatic individuals may correctly parse an input sentence, they fail to map from syntactic structure to semantic interpretation. Thus, their comprehension problems arise because they are unable to make the mapping from grammatical functions to thematic roles. As Linebarger herself notes, a strong version of the semantic mapping hypothesis cannot be maintained. Agrammatic individuals are able to map thematic roles onto grammatical functions in actives and subject relatives with great consistency and experience little difficulty in interpreting sentences involving subject-raising (Schwartz et al., 1987). A semantic mapping deficit can be maintained only if the hypothesis is complicated by some factor that will distinguish sentences that are easy to interpret or judge from those that are more difficult. Linebarger (1989) suggests that the hard cases of grammaticality judgment, which all involve coindexed anaphoric elements, arise because "the language processor does not immediately evaluate the semantic consequences of the coindexations" (p. 226). A similar explanation is offered for problems with thematic role assignment. As many have observed, thematic role assignment is difficult when it is mediated by a trace (Grodzinsky, 1990; Hildebrandt, Caplan, & Evans, 1987; Cornell, Fromkin, & Mauner 1989; Mauner, Cornell, & Fromkin, 1990). Linebarger suggests that although agrammatics do link NPs with their traces, they are unable to utilize this structural information for mapping thematic roles. However, we still have to explain why, under this hypothesis, there should be any differences in the comprehension of subject and object relatives. While passives differ from actives in that only passives have a moved element, both subject and object relatives involve assigning thematic roles to moved elements and thus, under this hypothesis, should pose equivalently severe difficulties for agrammatic comprehenders.

1.3. The Double Dependency Model

The analysis we will propose (like Grodzinsky's) rests on the fundamental observation that subjects' chance performance in comprehension tasks suggests that they are faced with an ambiguity of some kind arising from the process of forming and evaluating syntactic chains. It also preserves the intuitions underlying Linebarger et al.'s Mapping Hypothesis, namely that the syntax is underconstraining the process of semantic interpretation, although we identify the problem as a defect in the construction of the syntactic structure itself rather than in the interpretive mechanisms which bring it to bear on the semantic construal. We turn first to the comprehension problem.

To explain the chance assignment of thematic roles in some constructions but not others, it is necessary to posit a deficit strong enough to present the agrammatic with at least two alternative interpretations where the normal has only one. Obviously, the deficit must be such that only passives and object-extracted relatives induce this ambiguity. The core of this analysis is the observation that, given certain assumptions common in very recent versions of syntactic theory, particularly Government Binding Theory (GB), there is a principled grammatical distinction between active declarative and subject-extracted relative clauses on the one hand, and passive declarative and object-extracted relative clauses on the other. We will present the relevant theoretical apparatus in detail in the next section, but the essence of our proposal is this: syntactic structures contain structures which instantiate and record certain grammatical dependencies; actives and subject relatives contain only a single instance of this kind of dependency, passives and object relatives contain two. The correlation of chance performance with "double dependency" structures leads us to the what we now refer to as the Double Dependency Hypothesis (cf. Mauner 1989; Cornell et al., 1989, 1990; Mauner et al., 1990).

The Double Dependency Hypothesis

(1) the deficit underlying asyntactic comprehension affects the processing of syntactic referential dependencies, and

(2) when there is only one such dependency the resulting syntactic representation, although abnormal, is not ambiguous, but when there are two such dependencies the resulting representation is semantically ambiguous.

This hypothesis underlies our model. In the next two sections we will show that, within syntactic theory, there is a mechanism that will undermine thematic interpretation in accordance with this hypothesis and which, moreover, bears a principled relation to the agreement difficulties subjects experience in acceptability judgment experiments, but which does not affect their abilities to judge, e.g., deformed passives like (12a and 12c).

The analysis we will present here differs in a number of respects from our past proposals (Cornell et al., 1990; Mauner et al., 1990). Cornell et al. (1990) combined the Double Dependency Hypothesis with a hypothesized insensitivity to passive-voice morphology. However, as noted above, the results in Linebarger (1989), dealing with judgments of passive and active voice morphology in sentences like (12), rule out this possibility—clearly, subjects *are* sensitive to details of voice morphology. The analysis presented in Mauner et al. (1990) is much more in line with the present analysis; however, it treats thematic roles as features on a par with person or gender features and hypothesizes that none of these features are transmitted along syntactic chains. This accounts for the data, but fails to establish an explanatory link between thematic roles and agreement features. In addition, the treatment of thematic roles as features is somewhat suspect on conceptual grounds. If an NP bears the thematic role of *agent,* this does not establish a simple property of the NP, but rather establishes a *relation* between the NP and a predicate. In a sentence like *John hugged Mary,* it is not just that *John* is an agent, but that *John* is the agent of *hug.* This distinction was noted, for example, by Stowell (1981), who proposes that thematic role assignment involves the coindexation of a slot in a verb's "thematic grid," i.e., its argument structure, with the argument which is to bear the role associated with that slot. When we examine the semantic interpretation of thematic roles in the next section, we will see that this analysis is much closer to the actual logical representation of a sentence's meaning than an analysis where thematic roles are simply features borne by an NP, on a par with number or person. When we confront these subtleties of thematic role assignment head on we find a more explanatory connection between agrammatics' problems with judging agreement violations and their problems assigning the correct thematic interpretation to a sentence.

2. THEORETICAL UNDERPINNINGS

In this section we will outline the basic linguistic concepts needed to present our model. First, we distinguish the semantic notions of *thematic role* and *thematic interpretation* from the syntactic notions of θ-*role assignment* and the *Theta Criterion*. The notions commonly termed "theme" and "θ" are related, as the names suggest, but also distinguishable. This distinction is crucial to understanding the relation between agrammatics' comprehension and grammaticality judgment performance. We also distinguish the process of chain formation, or "movement," from the process of coindexation. These rather subtle distinctions are implicit in standard versions of GB theory, but not much employed there. However, in the study of abnormal language they become crucial. Finally, we will describe two recent linguistic proposals, which we will adopt essentially unchanged from their formulation in the syntax literature—the "VP-Internal Subject Hypothesis," which argues that all NPs in a clause originate inside the verb phrase, and the theory of Passive developed in Jaeggli (1986) and Baker, Johnson, and Roberts (1989), which suggests that passives are like object-relatives in that both thematic roles assigned by the verb are assigned indirectly.

2.1. Reference, "Referential Indices," and Agreement

In syntax, the problem of reference is much simpler than it is in semantics. We are much less concerned with what a noun phrase like *every bear* "refers to" than we are in which linguistic expressions in a sentence depend on another noun phrase for their reference. That is, we divide the universe of syntactic expressions into those which are referentially dependent and those which are not. The property of being referentially independent is then referred to as "having reference" or "being referential." The referential expressions, or "R-expressions," then become the constants around which a very complex syntactic calculus for determining what may refer to what unwinds itself.

Referential dependence (which we will abbreviate as *R-dependence*) is customarily marked by syntacticians with the device of shared indices, written as subscripts on the relevant elements, as in (15).

(15) [Every bear]$_i$ is pointing at herself$_i$.

We think of the index as being assigned to the R-expression *every bear* when it is introduced into the syntactic structure and then assigned to the reflexive that is linked to it. These indices are often referred to as "referential indices." To avoid the many conceptual problems involving what we pretheoretically mean by "reference," we will follow Bouchard (1984) in terming them simply R-indices. It will become clear that the correct distribution of R-indices is crucial to establishing an appropriately constrained thematic interpretation of a sentence. In addition, agreement between phrasal elements is closely tied to R-dependence (see Bouchard, 1984, for a detailed examination)—shared R-indices evidently entail shared agreement features. We will assume here a theory in which this consequence is explicit: coindexation will always be taken to involve agreement.[5]

2.2. Theta Theory and Chain Formation

2.2.1. Theta Theory.
The syntax behind thematic interpretation involves the assignment of θ-*roles* and the formation of *chains*. It is crucial to distinguish the syntactic operation of θ-role assignment from the semantic notion of thematic interpretation. The syntax is much more concerned with the number of arguments a predicate requires than in particular conceptual labels like *agent* or *patient*. Thus sentences like *John hit* or *Mary sneezed Jane* are ruled out because they do not have the appropriate number of arguments to satisfy the verb's θ-requirements. In addition, and most crucially for our purposes, θ-assignment is a condition on movement chains, in particular on the structurally lowest trace of movement. Distinguishing "θ well-formedness" from "thematic interpretation" amounts to determining, respectively, whether the most deeply embedded element of a chain is found in a θ-marked position and how predicate-variables are bound in the semantics.

Theta Theory (Chomsky, 1981) consists largely of a single principle regulating the relation of θ-roles to argument-type categories (noun phrases in particular). The *Theta Criterion* states, essentially, that (a) every NP must have a single, unique θ-role, and (b) every θ-role must be assigned to a single, unique NP. *John hit* violates clause (b) because *hit* has two roles to give away, but only one of them is actually assigned, and *Mary sneezed Jane* violates clause (a), in that *sneeze* assigns only a single θ-role, so *Jane* must go without.

The mechanism of θ-role assignment involves the identification of an argument phrase with a position in a predicate's argument structure, or θ-*grid*. This identification entails that all the properties of the grid position become properties of the argument, and all the properties of the argument become properties of the grid position. In particular, if the argument bears an R-index, then its grid position must bear the same index.[6] This approach thus implements the theory of Stowell (1981) (and see also Higginbotham, 1985; Williams, 1989), according to which an argument in a structural θ-position is assigned a particular θ-role by virtue of being *coindexed* with a particular slot in the θ-grid.

---

[5] Cornell (1992) presents in more formal terms the theory of θ-assignment, chain formation, and agreement which we assume here.

[6] See Cornell (1992) for formal details.

2.2.2. Chain formation. Within the framework of GB syntax, it is assumed that predicates assign their θ-roles locally, within the phrase that they head. In particular, a verb is assumed to assign all of its θ-roles within the verb phrase. When an element appears displaced from the position in which it would normally receive its θ-role, some mechanism must be invoked to assure that the displaced element remains somehow connected with that role. In GB theory that mechanism is syntactic movement or chain formation. Consider a sentence like (16), in which *John* gets its θ-role from *left,* not from *appears.*

(16) John appears to have left already.

It is standardly argued that the NP *John* has *moved* from the position in which it is assigned its θ-role by *left* and into the surface subject position of *appears.* In doing so it has left an empty, unpronounced syntactic placeholder, called a *trace,* in its place. Traces are R-dependent elements, whose dependence on their antecedent is marked in the usual way with a shared index, as in (17).

(17) John$_i$ appears t_i to have left already.

The set comprising an overt NP (e.g., *John*) and the traces that are linked to it (that it "binds") is referred to as a *chain.* Various conditions must be satisfied in order for a chain to be well-formed. Each separate link of the chain is subject to locality conditions which express how much structure can intervene between one chain element and the next (between a trace and its antecedent). In addition, all the elements of a chain are assumed to be coindexed, that is, they all bear the same R-index. They get that index from their structurally highest element, which must either be an R-expression or an R-dependent NP which is bound to some previously established R-index. Consider a fairly complex example like (18), where we have two chains, ⟨*everybody, t*⟩ and ⟨*he, t'*⟩, which share the same R-index (*i*). The index is introduced by the R-expression *everybody.* The second chain gets its R-index from the first in the process of fixing the reference of the pronoun *he.*

(18) Everybody$_i$ appears t_i to think he$_i$ has been gypped t'_i.

A final condition on chains is that the bottom-most element, or *foot,* of a chain must be in a θ-marked position. If we think of chains as providing, within the syntax, a calculus for correctly associating NPs with θ-roles, then the condition is unsurprising and follows quite naturally from this explanation.

The establishment of chain links and the coindexing of chain elements are not generally dIstinguished in the syntactic literature. In approaching the problems posed by agrammatics' comprehension and grammaticality judgment performance, however, it is crucial to distinguish the two. We will denote chains and other R-dependencies using angle-bracket notation and use subscripts to denote R-indices. It now becomes possible in principle to have a chain $\langle \alpha_i, \beta_j \rangle$, where the two elements of the chain have distinct subscripts. We rule this out with the following condition.

Coindexation Condition

If α is R-dependent on β, then they must bear the same R-index.

There is an important contrast that must be borne in mind between the way in which a trace and its antecedent satisfy the Coindexation Condition, and the way in which a θ-grid position and its argument satisfy it. The coindexing of a trace with its antecedent is actually effected by the Coindexation Condition—nothing else in the grammar requires it. The coindexation of the grid position with its argument is effected by the Theta Criterion. As a result of the identification of an argument with its grid position, the argument and grid position would be coindexed whether or not the Coindexation Condition was part of the grammar. This distinction will become important in our account of the comprehension data.

It is worth taking a moment to justify this distinction between chain formation and coindexation, since we are making distinctions that will appear unfamiliar to many linguists. The locality conditions which the grammar places on traces and their antecedents all refer to individual chain links and make no reference to the R-index which the two elements share. Once the movement step is complete the conditions have done their work. Even in a chain formation variant of the theory no crucial reference is made to R-indices, but rather to an extremely local "antecedent-of" or "chain-link" relation. We can thus take the chain-link relation as primary and treat coindexation as a condition on chains formed in this way.

In addition, the Theta Criterion requires that chains be distinct from each other. In (18), the chain formed by *everyone* and *t* receives its θ-role from *think,* while the chain formed by *he* and *t′* is assigned its role by *gyp.* From this, we can see that R-indices cannot be used to distinguish chains from each other. If we were to identify chains with their R-indices, there would be a single chain in (18), despite the fact that the sentence contains two distinct thematic roles.

2.2.3. Thematic interpretation. Following the interpretive scheme outlined in Higginbotham (1985) (cf. Williams, 1989, and references therein), as well as recent work on argument structure (e.g., Grimshaw, 1990), we assume that θ-grid positions are linked to variable occurrences in the representation of a predicate's meaning. Coindexation in the syntax has the semantic consequence of identifying occurrences of formal variables in the semantics; roughly, indices are interpreted as variables. For example, the θ-grid for the verb *admire* in example (19) takes two arguments. Let us denote the admirer as role 1 and the object of admiration as role 2 (these θ-roles are generally referred to as the external argument (1) and the internal argument (2)). These grid slots are identified with their respective arguments in the sentence via coindexation, as above.

(19) The man$_i$ is admiring a woman$_j$.
$$\langle 1_i, 2_j \rangle$$

Translating into a rather informal representation of the meaning of (19), we get (20).

(20) x is the man and y is a woman and x admires y

With a moved element, such as the subject of a passive, as in (21), the relevant aspects of interpretation proceed roughly as follows.

(21) The woman$_i$ was much admired t_i.
$$\langle 1, 2_i \rangle$$

The trace t is coindexed with the internal argument slot of *admire* by virtue of θ-assignment, and with *the woman*, by virtue of chain formation. We now get a meaning wherein the variable introduced by *the woman*— let us suppose it is still y—is equated with the variable associated with slot 2.

(22) y is the woman and (for some x) x admires y

This admittedly rather informal treatment of thematic interpretation should make it clear that the distribution of R-indices in the syntactic structure is crucial to determining who winds up doing what to whom in the semantic structure. In (19) the grammatical subject is interpreted as the admirer, while in (21) it is interpreted as the admiree, solely as a result of which grid position the subject's R-index binds.

We now see that thematic interpretation is related to agreement phenomena in that they both crucially involve R-dependencies. However, while traces are R-dependent elements, and movement chains are instances of R-dependencies, there is an important difference between this sort of R-dependency and the one which exists between a reflexive pronoun and its antecedent. In a sentence like *John admires himself*, the interpretation of *himself* depends on the interpretation of an antecedent, but the two terms of that dependency each have their own θ-role. Chains differ in that the R-dependency between a trace and its antecedent has only a single θ-role. We will refer to this sort of dependency as a *thematic* R-dependency and to anaphor-antecedent dependencies as *nonthematic* R-dependencies. We now have the beginnings of an explanation for why asyntactic comprehension should co-occur with difficulties in judging agreement violations—there is a deficit affecting R-dependencies. While we argue that this deficit affects all R-dependencies, we will also show that, for independent reasons, only disruptions to thematic R-dependencies lead to a disruption in thematic interpretation.

2.3. Some Recent Developments in Syntactic Theory

2.3.1. The VP-Internal Subject Hypothesis. We noted above that θ-role assignment is an extremely local phenomenon, with θ-roles all being assigned within the phrase which the assigner heads. In particular, a verb will assign all of its θ-roles within the VP. There is, however, one striking apparent exception to this generalization. If we consider a sentence like (23), we note that the subject *such activities* is quite far removed from the VP headed by *taking place*.

(23) [Such activities] may have been [$_{VP}$ taking place here] for centuries.

This odd fact about θ-role assignment is striking enough to have received considerable attention in recent syntactic literature. A number of researchers reached the conclusion, more or less independently around 1985 and 1986, that subjects bind a trace in the VP; thus, through the mediation of a chain, they are assigned their θ-roles locally, like any other argument (Koopman & Sportiche, 1988; Kitagawa, 1986; Speas & Fukui, 1986; Kuroda, 1986).[7] According to this analysis, (23) is much like the passive in (24), where the noun phrase *such songs,* which receives its θ-role in the postverbal direct object position, raises to the surface subject position.

(24) As of next Monday, [such songs]$_i$ will have been [sung t_i on this occasion] for seven centuries.

Of course, this theory entails that even in such simple sentences as *Matter exists*, the subject binds a trace in the VP headed by *exists*. And the simple active declarative sentence in (25a) has the analysis in (25b).

(25) (a) A boy is chasing a girl.
     (b) [A boy]$_i$ is [t_i chasing a girl].

Given our previous discussion of R-dependencies, the VP-Internal Subject Hypothesis clearly has consequences for the analysis of asyntactic comprehension. Indeed it is the key to the Double Dependency Deficit Model (cf. Mauner, 1989; Cornell et al., 1989, 1990; Mauner et al., 1990), and also to Hickok's (1992) trace-deletion analysis. Under the VP-Internal Subject Hypothesis, one striking similarity between active declaratives such as (25) and subject-extracted relative clauses as in (26a) emerges—they both contain a single thematic R-dependency, in this case the chain ⟨[*the frog*],*t*,*t*′⟩.

(26) (a) [The frog]$_i$ which$_i$ t_i is t'_i chasing [the lion]$_j$ is fast.
     (b) [The frog]$_i$ which$_i$ [the lion]$_j$ is t_j chasing t_i is fast.

---

[7] See also Fillmore (1968) for an earlier analysis along these lines.

Object-extracted relatives like (26b), on the other hand, contain two thematic R-dependencies, the chains $\langle which_i, t_i \rangle$ and $\langle [the\ lion]_j, t_j \rangle$. As we shall see in the next section, passives also contain two thematic R-dependencies, although only one of them is a chain.

2.3.2. The distribution of R-indices in passives. One striking fact about passives is that a verb which is normally transitive, when passivized, no longer requires that its external argument (its "logical subject") be realized. Thus sentence (27) is as acceptable as (28).

(27) John was hit on the arm.
(28) John was hit on the arm by his older brother.

Given the Theta Criterion, (27) is problematic because there are more thematic roles in the verb's θ-grid than there are arguments to which those roles can be assigned (contrast (27) with the unacceptable *John hit on the arm*). A solution to this problem is suggested by Jaeggli (1986) and Baker et al. (1989). They propose that the passive participial morpheme (usually written -*en*) is introduced into the syntax separately from the verb with which it later combines. This combination results in assigning the external argument either directly to the passive morpheme -*en* or to a null element which the presence of -*en* licenses.

This theory attempts to account for the nature of the passive by assuming that (a) θ-assignment is still obligatory for the external argument role, just as in all active clauses, and (b) θ-assignment proceeds normally, except that either -*en* or an element licensed by -*en* is in the position to which that role is assigned. Since the *by*-phrase is optional it cannot be the direct recipient of the obligatory external θ-role. If it is present, it is coindexed with an element which is itself always present in a passive. The NP in the *by*-phrase receives its θ-role indirectly, just like a moved element. Thus sentence (29) may have either of the two analyses in (30), depending on one's particular theory of passive, but in both cases there are two thematic R-dependencies.

(29) A boy is being chased by a girl.
(30) (a) [A boy]$_i$ is being chase + en$_j$ t_i by [a girl]$_j$.
    (b) [A boy]$_i$ is being e$_j$ chase + en t_i by [a girl]$_j$.

Note that no one is arguing that the *by*-phrase *is* a moved element. Nonetheless, the structure which is created to assign it its θ-role has most or all of the crucial properties of a chain. In particular, it is a set of coindexed elements sharing a single θ-role. As a consequence of this analysis, passives, like object-relatives, contain two thematic R-dependencies, where actives and subject-relatives contain only one.

3. ASYNTACTIC COMPREHENSION WITH PRESERVED GRAMMATICAL SENSITIVITY

Given the framework of the previous section, we can state our claims succinctly. Recall that we are working within the more general framework of the Double Dependency Model, repeated below.

The Double Dependency Hypothesis

1) the deficit underlying asyntactic comprehension affects the processing of syntactic R-dependencies, and
2) when there is only one such dependency the resulting syntactic representation, although abnormal, is not ambiguous, but when there are two such dependencies the resulting representation is semantically ambiguous.

We can explain why this generalization should hold if we assume the following model of the deficit.

Coindexation Condition

If α is R-dependent on β, then they must bear the same R-index.

Deficit Model

Asyntactic comprehension with spared grammaticality judgment arises when subjects do not have, or can make no use of, the Coindexation Condition.

That is, the observed comprehension performance appears when referential dependencies fail to be marked with shared R-indices.

In this section we will show how this hypothesis accounts for both the comprehension data (i.e., spared comprehension of active clauses and subject-extracted relative clauses and impaired comprehension of passive and object-relative clauses) and the grammaticality judgment data (i.e., spared judgments of passive and other movement-based constructions with impaired judgments of agreement among referentially dependent elements).

3.1. Deriving the Comprehension Data

Let us then consider the consequences of our hypothetical deficit model for otherwise normal syntactic processing. GB is a constraint-based theory of grammar—any syntactic structure can be entertained as the analysis of a given expression, as long as it satisfies the well-formedness constraints in a listener's grammar. For any given utterance, the number of structural descriptions that can simultaneously satisfy all these constraints is, in fact, quite small. The effect of removing a constraint from the grammar is to increase the number of structural descriptions consistent with the constraints of the listener's grammar. In the following discussion we need not assume that the human processor behaves in exactly this way, freely generating arbitrary syntactic structures until one of them satisfies the conditions of the grammar. But we will assume that the processor, within the limits of memory and processing resources, is *correct with respect to the grammar*—it is able to construct any syntactic structure which the grammar makes available for the input expression.[8]

We will demonstrate first that the inability to use the Coindexation Condition allows syntactic structures with the interpretations we see in comprehension experiments. Then we will tackle the harder problem of ruling out structures whose interpretations do not appear in our corpus of evidence.

Consider the structures of the passive in (31) and the object-extracted relative clause in (32), under the VP-Internal Subject Hypothesis. (*Op* here represents a null Wh-operator, which takes the place of the overt relative pronoun.)

(31) [The boy] was chase + en *t* by [the girl].
(32) [The boy] [Op that [the girl] is *t1* chasing *t2*] is tall.

In each of these examples there are two (thematic) R-dependencies—in (31) $\langle$[*the boy*], *t*$\rangle$ and $\langle$[*the girl*], -*en*$\rangle$, and in (32) $\langle Op, t2 \rangle$ and $\langle$[*the girl*], *t1*$\rangle$. Taking the passive first, assume that the R-expression *the boy* is marked with R-index *i*, and *the girl* with R-index *j*. Two possible assignments of indices to dependent elements are given in (33).

(33) (a) $\langle$[the boy]$_i$, $t_i$$\rangle$, $\langle$[the girl]$_j$, -en$_j$$\rangle$
     (b) $\langle$[the boy]$_i$, $t_j$$\rangle$, $\langle$[the girl]$_j$, -en$_i$$\rangle$

For normals, (33b) is ruled out by the Coindexation Condition. However, the agrammatic parser is released from this constraint and thus permits this assignment. The R-indices assigned to the trace and the passive morpheme will then mark the patient and agent θ-grid slots, respectively, yielding an interpretation like:

$$x \text{ is the boy, } y \text{ is the girl and } x \text{ chased } y$$

This is the interpretation a normal speaker would only assign to an active clause. Of course, the correct analysis, with index assignments as in (33a), is compatible with the grammar of both the normal and, a fortiori, the agrammatic, yielding the correct interpretation:

---

[8] Note that the parser·must construct descriptions of sentences like (i) since such sentences are still interpretable.

(i) * The child seems sleeping.

However, the structure it assigns must be detectably "subpar," since we invariably judge such sentences as deviant. Thus we understand "correct" to mean "assigns a fully well-formed structure to all and only grammatical sentences."

x is the boy, y is the girl and y chased x

Object-extracted relative clauses are treated similarly. Without the Coindexation Condition it is possible to assign indices arbitrarily to the θ-
positions occupied by the two traces. Accordingly, the two assignments
in (34) are possible.

(34) (a) $\langle Op_i, t2_i \rangle, \langle [\text{the girl}]_j, t1_j \rangle$
     (b) $\langle Op_i, t2_j \rangle, \langle [\text{the girl}]_j, t1_i \rangle$

The distribution of indices to dependent elements in (34a) is the correct
assignment, yielding the normal interpretation. The indexing in (34b)
leads to the backward interpretation which agrammatics select half of the
time.

Active declaratives and subject-extracted relative clauses differ from
passives and object-extracted relative clauses in that their direct objects
do not move, but instead are assigned θ-roles directly. Direct objects are
inserted into the phrase marker already bearing unique R-indices, and
they mark the verb's argument slot with those R-indices, unaffected by
the loss of the Coindexation Condition.[9] The examples in (35) and (36)
provide the structures for an active and a subject-extracted relative clause
under the VP-Internal Subject Hypothesis.

(35) [The boy] is t chasing [the girl].
(36) [The boy] [Op that $t1$ is $t2$ chasing [the girl]] is tall.

The active in (35) includes a single thematic R-dependency—the chain
$\langle [\textit{the boy}], t \rangle$—as does the subject-extracted relative with the chain $\langle Op,$
$t1, t2 \rangle$. Assume that the R-index of *the boy* is i and that of *the girl* is j.
The problem at hand is to ensure that the trace(s) are assigned the correct
index i, as in (37a).

(37) (a) $\langle [\text{the boy}]_i, t_i \rangle, \langle [\text{the girl}]_j \rangle$
     (b) $\langle [\text{the boy}]_i, t_j \rangle, \langle [\text{the girl}]_j \rangle$

We will begin by discussing the active case (35). Under a coindexation
deficit, t is not necessarily coindexed with *the boy*—it may be assigned
an index arbitrarily. Suppose that we freely choose to assign the index j
to the trace t, as in (37b). As a result, *the girl* is associated with both
θ-roles assigned by *chase*, while *the boy* has no role at all. Note that this
is true despite the fact that the chain headed by *the boy* has its foot in a
θ-position, as required by our version of the Theta Criterion.

The resulting structure, including the indexing in (37b), is allowed by
the agrammatic's syntax, but, if it has any interpretation at all, that interpretation is quite deviant. Since *the girl* binds both thematic roles, the
intended meaning must include (38).

(38) x is the girl and x chases x

[9] Recall the discussion in Sections 2.2.1 and 2.2.2.

This interpretation is not nonsensical; however, it is problematic because no interpretation is assigned to the orphaned NP *the boy*. Suppose that declarative clauses denote propositions or closed sentences (formulae with no free variables). The meaning fragment in (38) is just such an object. *The boy,* on the other hand, denotes an individual. There is no way to combine an individual with a closed sentence to yield another closed sentence. Hence, under widely shared assumptions about natural language semantics, the interpretation of (35) required by the syntactic structure in (37b) is deviant on semantic grounds. In fact, any indexing other than that of (37a) is subject to this problem. Thus, the requirement that syntactic clauses be interpretable assures the correct indexing in active declaratives.

The correct indexing is also assured in subject-extracted relatives, although the semantics is more complex. Consider the two possible assignments of indices shown in (39). (To simplify discussion we will disregard $t1$, the higher trace in (36) since the index assigned to it plays no role in the thematic interpretation of the sentence.)

(39) (a) $\langle \text{Op}_i, t2_i \rangle, \langle [\text{the girl}]_j \rangle$
    (b) $\langle \text{Op}_i, t2_j \rangle, \langle [\text{the girl}]_j \rangle$

A relative clause is interpreted as an open sentence, a sentence containing a single free variable identified by the Wh-operator *Op*. Intuitively, it is interpreted as the set of all individuals which can truthfully stand in the position of the extracted variable. Thus the meaning of the NP *the boy that is chasing the girl* involves the intersection of the set of boys with the set of things that are chasing girls. In (39b), however, with the NP *the girl* binding both θ-grid positions, we once again have an expression that has, in part, an interpretation as a closed sentence:

$$x \text{ is the girl and } x \text{ chases } x$$

There is no free variable for the Wh-operator to bind in this expression and thus it is a case of "vacuous quantification," and is ruled out as such (see, e.g., Chomsky, 1989, 1992). Once again, the deviant indexing is allowed by the agrammatic's grammar, but leads to a deviant interpretation and is accordingly rejected. As with active declaratives, the only assignment of indices that will yield a well-formed semantic interpretation is the correct one.[10]

Since we are making an appeal to higher level processes, it is worth

---

[10] Note in passing that there are similarly deviant indexings that could be assigned to the double dependency cases in (31) and (32), as illustrated in (i). In (i), both θ-positions are assigned the R-index of *the girl*, leaving *the boy* stranded outside the proposition.

    (i) $\langle [\text{the boy}]_i, t_j \rangle, \langle [\text{the girl}]_j, \text{-en}_j \rangle$.

As before, this assignment of indices would be rejected by appeal to higher level interpretive processes.

taking a moment to consider the relation of this approach to the kind of
higher level strategy that Grodzinsky (1990) assumes. Grodzinsky's Default Principle takes as input an underspecified syntactic representation
with an NP lacking a θ-role and outputs an "over-specified" representation in which two NPs have the same θ-role. The resulting representation
is still uninterpretable and must be subjected to a further process, which
suppresses one or the other of the agent roles in favor of some other
nonagentive role, to yield an active or passive interpretation. In contrast,
our approach assumes a fully specified syntactic structure which has one
or more perfectly acceptable interpretations. In Grodzinsky's approach,
agrammatic comprehension performance results from struggling to adapt
to uninterpretable representations. In contrast, we assume that subjects
actively avoid deviant interpretations. To the best of our knowledge,
none of our assumptions about semantic interpretation extend beyond
what is currently assumed in various semantic frameworks. Our assumption that the parser can (within the limits of memory and its computational
resources) assign any of the structures which the grammar allows is a
reasonable one, in particular as we are assuming a fairly minor impairment of the knowledge base at its command. Arguably, then, our
approach is simpler and makes fewer novel assumptions than Grodzinsky's—the pattern of asyntactic comprehension follows straightforwardly if we inhibit the Coindexation Condition and do nothing else.[11]

3.2. Accounting for the Preserved Acceptability Judgments

Grammaticality judgment, given a GB-based model of the grammar,
involves simultaneously satisfying a number of independent constraints
on what counts as a fully well-formed syntactic structure. Individually,
constraints rule out only a small portion of the structures which could be
posited for an input sentence. That is, each principle of grammar *overgen-
erates* syntactic structures, and it is only when the constraints are applied

---

[11] There are results that this approach could not in principle account for. Chance performance is the absolute floor for this approach. Below chance performance is anomalous.
Grodzinsky (1990) refers to unpublished data which show that passives of psych predicates
like *admire* and *understand* are interpreted incorrectly most of the time—they yield below-
chance performance. Such performance necessarily entails the addition of some new piece
of processing machinery—pure loss accounts cannot in principle account for below chance
performance. In fact, these data are a problem for everybody. They force Grodzinsky away
from a more appealing version of his Default Principle, according to which the θ-roles
assigned by default must come from among the roles associated with the verb in question,
to a much less appealing version, according to which subjects are assigned *agent* regardless
of the semantics of the verb. In a footnote, Grodzinsky argues that this is a modularity
effect, but this does not seem possible. Given that the nature of a particular thematic role
is a fact about a predicate's lexical semantics, one would assume that detailed thematic
information would be available at the level of interpretation if anywhere.

collectively that all but the correct structural analyses are ruled out. We have proposed that one constraint, the Coindexation Condition, is compromised in agrammatism. The inability to bring this constraint to bear on the selection of a syntactic analysis results in a greater number of analyses of a particular sentence being entertained. In this section we will discuss how the loss of this constraint affects acceptability judgments.

3.2.1. Passives. Accurate grammaticality judgments of passive sentences and sentences containing the kind of movement found in relative clauses seem most paradoxical in light of comprehension performance. Accordingly, we will first reexamine the data from Linebarger (1989) where subjects' sensitivity to details of the passive construction was tested.

(40) (a)   John has finally kissed Louise.
    (b) *John was finally kissed Louise.
    (c)   The boy was followed by the girl.
    (d) *The boy was followed the girl.
    (e)   The boy was following the girl.

Descriptively, the problem with both (40b and 40d) is that a passive participle cannot be followed by a direct object. Example (40a) demonstrates that the participial form itself is not enough to support the relevant distinction. Therefore the identification of a passive voice clause cannot depend only on the local relation between the passive participle and the expression that follows it. Nor is it enough to identify the relevant auxiliary verb, *be,* as it is used both in passive (40c) and in progressive constructions (40e). In order to identify the clause as being in the passive voice, subjects must correctly identify the auxiliary verb as a form of *be,* and the participial form as the *-en* form.

According to Linebarger (1989), subjects scored 89.1% correct on sentences like those in (40), indicating not only that they can put *be* and *-en* together to identify occurrences of passive voice, but also that they know that passive constructions cannot support direct objects. According to GB theory the essence of the passive construction is the formation of a chain connecting the surface subject to the direct object θ-position, and that this instance of chain formation is motivated by precisely the property which these stimuli test, namely by the inability of the passive participle to support an overt direct object. Evidently subjects know everything they need to build the necessary chains, although they cannot bind the traces involved in a way that would force the correct interpretation. Thus their analyses of the acceptable stimuli are going to be normal in every respect but the R-indices assigned to the dependent elements.

For grammatical cases (40a, 40c, and 40d), the agrammatic's grammar still allows any reading that the normal's does, so these should be acceptable to agrammatic subjects. As for the ungrammatical cases (40b and 40d), we have not suggested anything that would compromise subjects' sensitivity to passive morphology or their recognition that a passive participle cannot properly license an overt NP in direct object position. These properties do not depend on R-indices in any way. Their ability to reject these stimuli, which both contain overt NPs in direct object position, is thus unsurprising.

3.2.2. Relative clauses. Linebarger (1989) claims that chain formation is intact in agrammatics. Thus preserved ability to correctly judge constructions involving ''Wh-movement'' is just as paradoxical as their ability to judge passives correctly. Linebarger cites two conditions as evidence for her claim that asyntactic comprehenders construct chains: the empty elements and Wh-moved subcategorization conditions, exemplified in (41) and (42) together with the percentage of correct responses.

(41) Empty elements (83.7% correct)
    (a) Frank thought he was going to get the job.
    (b) *Frank thought __ was going to get the job.
    (c) That's who Frank thought __ was going to get the job.
    (d) *Who __ thought __ was going to get the job?

(42) Wh-moved subcategorization (83.1% correct)
    (a) *The principal frowned the boy.
    (b) *Who did the principal frown?
    (c) Why did the principal frown?

In (41b), there is a gap where a pronoun should be. Construing the empty element as a trace bound by *Frank* would violate the Theta Criterion, at least, since *Frank* would then be part of a chain containing two θ-positions. In addition, it would violate various locality conditions on chain formation, which we assume are intact. Crucially, the judgment of (41b) does not depend on any particular assignment of an R-index or agreement features to the empty position. The same argument applies to (41d). *Who* can bind one of the gaps in (41d), but it would fall victim to the Theta Criterion if it bound both.

Example (42) also involves a Theta Criterion violation, as long as subjects retain the ability to tell that *who* is a noun phrase while *why* is an adverbial. That is, *who* is subject to the Theta Criterion, so the intransitive verb *frown* cannot license both it and *the principal. Why,* on the other hand, stands for a modifier, and does not need a θ-role. As long as subjects retain the ability to construct chains, they can detect whether the foot of the chain is (and needs to be) in a θ-marked position. Therefore they can judge sentences like those in (42) accurately.

The only condition involving movement which appears in Linebarger

(1989) and which clearly involves R-indices is the Wh-head agreement condition (43). Significantly, subjects *did* have trouble with this condition.

(43) Wh-head agreement (63.1% correct)
   (a) *The pencil who he brought was nice.
   (b) The pencil which he brought was nice.

This example has no bearing on the issue of chain formation in asyntactic comprehenders since what is at issue is the quasi-pronominal relation between the relative pronoun and the noun phrase which the relative clause modifies. Under our assumptions, there is no sharing of an R-index in this construction, and therefore the humanness of the antecedent ought not to be expected to constrain the choice of relative pronoun. Hence subjects cannot be expected to know for sure whether the sentence is grammatical or not. Thus, although this condition does not bear on movement in any direct sense, nonetheless it does supply us with more evidence that whenever we can see the effects of R-index sharing (or lack thereof), we find that they are not in fact being shared. In sum, our analysis, which permits passives to be judged accurately (even though we must concede the ability to construct chains) will also permit Wh-movement constructions to be judged correctly (given, once again, the restrictive assumption that these subjects can form chains).

3.3. Accounting for the Difficult Acceptability Judgments

3.3.1. Reflexives. Grodzinsky, Wexler, Chien, and Marakovitz (1989) argue that agrammatics respect the conditions of the Binding Theory. In particular, their responses to a picture-judgment task indicate that they know that the reflexive in (44) must refer to Mama Bear and cannot have reference outside the sentence, as it could if it were a pronoun.

(44) Is Mama Bear washing herself?

The situation here is thus very close to the data involving movement constructions discussed in the previous section. Evidently subjects can construct the relevant link between *herself* and *Mama Bear* in (44) and are sensitive to the kinds of locality conditions which obtain in such cases.

    However, as with Wh-animacy agreement (43), they are unable to impose feature agreement conditions on reflexives. As Linebarger et al. (1983) show (and see also Linebarger, 1989), sentences like (45) are acceptable to agrammatics.

(45) *The girl fixed himself a sandwich.

Given our hypothetical deficit it is not surprising that subjects can link anaphors to their antecedents without having coindexation as a consequence, as it should be for normals. As reflexives are another species of R-dependent element, we expect that the Coindexation Condition should apply to them, for normals, but not for agrammatics.

Unlike the case of chains, there has been some discussion in the syntax literature on whether or not anaphoric binding and coindexing are dissociable (cf. e.g., Higginbotham, 1983, 1985; Montalbetti & Wexler, 1985). For our purposes it is sufficient to consider a case like (46).

(46) John thought he$_i$ would buy himself$_i$ a doughnut.

In order to satisfy the locality conditions on anaphoric binding, *he*, and not *John*, must be taken as the relevant antecedent for *himself* even though both *he* and *John*, being coreferential with *himself*, are reasonably considered to be antecedents of the reflexive. We will therefore assume, following Higginbotham (1983), that there is an explicit link relation of some kind between *himself* and *he*, much like the chain-link relation underlying movement constructions. This link forms the basis of the judgments which Grodzinsky et al. (1989) observe. Since reflexives are (non-thematic) R-dependent elements, the Coindexation Condition applies to them and assures them their proper R-index. Of course, if the Coindexation Condition cannot be applied, then the index need not be assigned correctly, and therefore the correct assignment of agreement features is not entailed.

3.3.2. Head–head agreement. In addition to agreement in referentially dependent NPs these subjects also had problems with certain word level items which have to obey copying or matching conditions much like phrasal agreement. The relevant conditions involved a VP-deletion construction (47) and tag questions with auxiliary copying violations (48).

(47) *George was angry and so did Tom.
(48) *John is very tall, doesn't he?

The primary violation is the misselection of the relevant auxiliary verb in the dependent clause. At first blush, the relevant conditions here would seem to involve strict identity of the elements involved: if *was* was used in the main conjunct, as in (47), then *was* must be used in the reduced conjunct. Therefore, it is not immediately clear in what sense these data reflect the same deficit as those already discussed. Note, however, that if the initial VP or clause contains a lexical verb, then the auxiliary of the second VP or clause must be a form of the auxiliary *do*.

(49) Everyone likes John, don't they?

Further, there are cases, like (49), where the agreement features in the two clauses are permitted to differ, so simple identity of forms is descriptively insufficient.

The issue of the "reference" of word level syntactic expressions is somewhat tricky, as they are interpreted not as entities or groups of entities in the domain of discourse, but as functions or relations over that domain. However, it is fairly clear that the "referential" features relevant to auxiliary verbal elements must be verbal ones, rather than the nominal features of person, number, or gender. In particular, we expect the relevant feature sharing to involve tense, aspect, modality, and voice. If we assume that the second auxiliary in (47) and (48) is a referentially dependent verbal element that must be bound by a verb with "inherent verbal reference" (i.e., the verbal equivalent of an R-index), then it ought to inherit the features of the inflected auxiliary of the main clause. Thus, in (47), the dependent auxiliary should have inherited the properties of being past tense and copular. If it had, then there would have been only one way to realize those features, namely as a past tense form of the verb *be*.

On this account, auxiliaries in tag questions and VP-deletion constructions are referentially dependent elements that get their features from a tensed element in the main clause (the initial conjunct in the VP-deletion examples, and arguably the tag clause in tag questions—cf. Mauner, 1990). These features determine which form of the auxiliary the dependent element must be spelled out as. Although the specific content of the relevant feature bundle has changed as we move from the nominal system to the verbal, the essential identification of "referential" features of one element with those of another remains the same and so remains subject to the asyntactic comprehension deficit. No other constraint of the grammar requires that the dependent auxiliary be spelled out one way or another, so (47) and its grammatical counterpart are equally well-formed to an agrammatic.

4. CONCLUSIONS

No theory of language *use* is likely to be successful in ignorance of a theory of *language*. Linguists have long realized that the theory of language is far from trivial and very often defies our pretheoretical, "common-sense" notions of what language "must" be like. Therefore the attempt to construct a jury-rigged theory of language to deal with some behavioral data is a very dangerous enterprise, especially when highly articulated theories exist ready-made. Even the study of abnormal language cannot proceed without reference to a theory of normal language—as we see, such a theory can provide the required explanatory links which tie together superficially diverse behaviors. It is only once we have a well worked out theory of grammar that we discover that judgment and comprehension of passive constructions are two very different things, but judgment of agreement and comprehension of passive are closely related.

On the other hand, no theory of language is likely to be successful in

ignorance of data which might bear on it. There are many issues that
cannot be resolved, many details which cannot be filled in, solely by
reference to the linguistic intuitions of adult native speakers. Even in the
restricted context of this article, we have found it necessary to refine
standard conceptions of chain formation, the relation of thematic interpretation to θ-role assignment, and the interpretive process in order to
account for the data examined here. The use of abnormal language data
is not just a question of adding extra support to existing theories (although
we believe that the utility of the VP-Internal Subject Hypothesis, both in
our work and in Hickok's (1992), does in fact add additional support to
that proposal). It can also be used, as we have seen, to refine such core
notions of syntax as chain formation and θ-well-formedness.

In conclusion, then, we find that the acceptability judgment data presented in Linebarger et al. (1983a) and subsequent work is not as paradoxical as it must at first have appeared. Pursuing the lines of approach
opened up by Grodzinsky, on the one hand, and by Linebarger,
Schwartz, and Saffran on the other, and working within a well-developed
theory of the normal grammar, we are able to shed light on the deeper
connections between subjects' superficially divergent performance on
judgment and comprehension tasks. We find that the syntax of referential
dependency is critically impaired in these subjects, which is revealed
both in their difficulties in handling grammatical features associated with
the referential properties of noun phrases and in their difficulties with
variable binding and thematic interpretation. The disruption of this "referential calculus" within general syntactic processing leads to guessing
behavior on a picture-selection task, and to overacceptance of ungrammatical stimuli in an acceptability judgment task.

Note, however, that this deficit model leaves open several possible
refinements, which it would be beyond the scope of this article to address.
First, although we argue that this deficit reflects the failure of the processor to act in accordance with a principle of (normal) grammar, we cannot
satisfactorily address the question of whether this is due to a fundamental
loss of grammatical *competence* in the asyntactic comprehender or to a
deficit to *processing,* according to which the knowledge is still present,
but cannot be used in these tasks. Second, if the deficit is determined to
be a processing deficit, the question arises as to whether there is a focal
disruption of the processor, according to which there is a progressing
submodule dedicated to marking coreference relations, and this module
is compromised by a brain injury, or, on the other hand, whether there is
a general disruption of processing which shows up in these constructions
because they are more complex and expensive to compute. Even in this
latter case, the observed correspondence of particularly expensive constructions to certain distinctions clearly evident in the theory of syntax
would argue that the correct measure of complexity must be one which

respects the structure of the grammar. We believe, then, that all these scenarios involve applications and refinements of the theory presented here and do not bear on its ability to make the distinctions we find in the data and to connect them to well-understood aspects of normal linguistic competence.

REFERENCES

Baker, M., Johnson, K., & Roberts, I. 1989. Passive arguments raised. *Linguistic Inquiry,* **20** (2) 219–252.

Bouchard, D. 1984. *On the content of empty categories.* Dordrecht: Foris.

Bradley, D. C., Garret, M. E. & Zurif, E. B. 1980. Syntactic deficits in Broca's aphasia. In D. Caplan (Ed.), *Biological studies of mental processes.* Cambridge, MA: MIT Press.

Caplan, D., & Futter, C. 1986. Assignment of thematic roles by an agrammatic aphasic patient. *Brain and Language,* 27, 111–134.

Caplan, D., & Hildebrandt, N. 1986, Language deficits and the theory of syntax: A reply to Grodzinsky. *Brain and Language,* **27**, 168–177.

Caramazza, A., & Berndt, R. S. 1985. A multicomponent deficit view of agrammatic Broca's aphasia. In M.-L. Kean (Ed.) *Agrammatism.* New York: Academic Press.

Caramazza, A., & Zurif, E. B. 1976. Dissociation of algorithmic and heuristic processes in language comprehension: Evidence from aphasia. *Brain and Language,* 3, 572–82.

Caramazza, A., Berndt, R. S., Basili, A., & Koller, J. 1981. Syntactic processing deficits in aphasia. *Cortex,* 17, 333–348.

Chomsky, N. 1981. *Lectures on government & binding.* Dordrecht: Foris.

Chomsky, N. 1989. Some notes on economy of derivation and representation. *MIT Working Papers in Linguistics,* **10,** 43–74.

Chomsky, N. 1992. A minimalist program for linguistic theory. *MIT Occasional Papers in Linguistics,* **1.**

Cornell, T. L. 1992. *Description theory, licensing theory and principle-based grammars and parsers.* Ph.D. dissertation, Univ. of California, Los Angeles.

Cornell, T. L., Fromkin, V. A., & Mauner, G. 1989. *A computational model of linguistic processing: Evidence from aphasia.* Paper presented at the Academy of Aphasia, Santa Fe, NM.

Cornell, T. L., Fromkin, V. A., & Mauner, G. 1990. A formal model of linguistic processing: Evidence from aphasia. In *Proceedings of the West Coast Conference on Formal Linguistics (WCCFL).* Stanford, CA.

Fillmore, C. J. 1968. The case for case. In E. Bach & R. Harms (Eds.), *Universals in linguistic theory.* New York: Holt, Rinehart & Winston. Pp. 1–88.

Grimshaw, J. 1990. *Argument structure.* Cambridge, MA: MIT Press.

Grodzinsky, Y. 1984. The syntactic characterization of agrammatism. *Cognition,* **16,** 99–120.

Grodzinsky, Y. 1986. Language deficits and the theory of syntax. *Brain and Language,* **27,** 135–159.

Grodzinsky, Y. 1990. *Theoretical perspectives on language deficits.* Cambridge, MA: MIT Press.

Grodzinsky, Y., Wexler, K., Chien, Y.-C., & Marakovitz, S. 1989. *The breakdown of binding relations.* Poster presented at the Academy of Aphasia, Santa Fe, NM.

Heilman, K. M., & Scholes, R. J. 1976. The nature of comprehension errors in Broca's, Conduction, and Wernicke's aphasias. *Cortex,* **12,** 258–265.

Hickok, G. 1992. *Agrammatic comprehension and the trace-deletion hypothesis.* MIT Department of Brain & Cognitive Sciences Occasional Paper, **45.**

Hickok, G., Canseco-Gonzalez, E., & Zurif, E. 1992. *Traces in the explanation of Broca's aphasia*. Paper presented at TENNET III, Montreal.

Higginbotham, J. 1983. Logical form, binding, and nominals. *Linguistic Inquiry*, **14**, 395–420.

Higginbotham, J. 1985. On semantics. *Linguistic Inquiry*, **16**, 547–593.

Hildebrandt, N., Caplan, D., & Evans, K. 1987. The man(i) left t(i) without a trace: A case study of aphasic processing of empty categories. *Cognitive Neuropsychology*, **4**(3), 257–302.

Jaeggli, O. A. 1986. Passive. *Linguistic Inquiry*, **17**(4), 587–621.

Kean, M.-L. 1977. The linguistic interpretation of aphasic syndromes: Agrammatism in Broca's aphasia, an example. *Cognition*, **5**, 9–46.

Kitagawa, Y. 1986. *Subject in Japanese and English*. Ph.D Dissertation. Univ. of Massachusetts.

Kolk, H. H. J., van Grunsven, M. J. F., & Keyser, A. 1985. On parallelism between production and comprehension in agrammatism. In M.-L. Kean (Ed.), *Agrammatism*. New York: Academic Press.

Koopman, H., & Sportiche, D. 1988. *Subjects*. Manuscript, Univ. of California, Los Angeles.

Kuroda, S.-Y. 1986. *Whether we agree or not*, Manuscript, Univ. of California, San Diego.

Lapointe, S. G. 1983. Some issues in the linguistic description of agrammatism. *Cognition*, **14**, 1–39.

Linebarger, M. C. 1989. Neuropsychological evidence for linguistic modularity. In G. N. Carlson & M. K. Tanenhaus (Eds.), *Linguistic structure in language processing*. Dordrecht: Kluwer. Pp. 197–238.

Linebarger, M. C. 1990. Neuropsychology of sentence parsing. In A. Caramazza (Ed.), *Cognitive neuropsychology and neurolinguistics*. Hillsdale, NJ: Erlbaum. Pp. 55–122.

Linebarger, M., Schwartz, M., & Saffran, E. 1983a. Sensitivity to grammatical structure in so-called agrammatic aphasics. *Cognition*, **13**, 361–392.

Linebarger, M., Schwartz, M., & Saffran, E. 1983b. Syntactic processing in agrammatism: A reply to Zurif and Grodzinsky. *Cognition*, **15**, 215–225.

Lukatela, K., Crain, S., & Shankweiler, D. 1988. Sensitivity to inflectional morphology in agrammatism: Investigation of a highly inflected language. *Brain and Language*, **33**, 1–15.

Mauner, G. 1989. A structural account of sentence comprehension and related phenomena in agrammatism. Manuscript, Univ. of California, Los Angeles.

Mauner, G. 1990. Getting to the root of tags. In *Proceedings of the Formal Linguistics Society of Mid-America (FLSM)*. Madison, WI.

Mauner, G., Cornell, T. L., & Fromkin, V. A. 1990. *Explanatory models of aphasia*. Paper presented at the Academy of Aphasia, Baltimore.

Miceli, G., Mazzucchi, A., Menn, L., & Goodglass, H. 1983. Contrasting cases of Italian agrammatic aphasia without comprehension disorder. *Brain and Language*, **19**, 65–97.

Montalbetti, M., & Wexler, K. 1985. Binding is linking. In *Proceedings of the West Coast Conference on Formal Linguistics* (WCCFL-4). Stanford, CA.

Saffran, E., & Marin O. S. M. 1975. Immediate memory for word lists and sentences in a patient with deficient auditory short-term memory. *Brain and Language*, **2**, 420–433.

Schwartz, M. F., Linebarger, M. C., Saffran, E. M., & Pate, D. S. 1987. Syntactic transparency and sentence interpretation in aphasia. *Language & Cognitive Processes*, **2**, 85–113.

Schwartz, M. F., Saffran, E. M., & Marin, O. S. M. 1980. The word order problem in agrammatism: I. Comprehension. *Brain and Language*, **10**, 249–262.

Shankweiler, D., Crain, S., Gorrell, P., & Tuller, B. 1989. Reception of language in Broca's aphasia. *Language & Cognitive Processes*, **4**, 1–33.

Speas, M., & Fukui, N. 1986. *Specifiers and projections*. MIT Working Papers in Linguistics.

Sproat, R. 1986. Competence, performance, and agrammatism: A reply to Grodzinsky. *Brain and Language,* **27,** 160–167.

Stowell, T. 1981. *Origins of phrase structure.* Ph.D. dissertation. MIT.

Williams, E. 1989. The Anaphoric nature of Theta-Roles. *Linguistic Inquiry,* **20,** 425–456.

Zurif, E. B., & Grodzinsky, Y. 1983. Sensitivity to grammatical structure in agrammatic aphasics: A reply to Linebarger, Schwartz, and Saffran. *Cognition,* **15,** 207–213.

BRAIN AND LANGUAGE **45,** 423–447 (1993)

Verb-Argument Structure Processing in Complex Sentences in Broca's and Wernicke's Aphasia

L. P. Shapiro, B. Gordon, N. Hack, and J. Killackey

Florida Atlantic University

We describe three experiments that explore the real-time access of verb-argument structures in a group of normal control subjects, a group of Broca's aphasic patients, and a group of Wernicke's aphasic patients. Specifically, we examine whether our subjects exhaustively access the thematic representations of verbs in active, passive, cleft-subject, and cleft-object sentences. We find that our normal control subjects and Broca's aphasic patients are sensitive to the thematic properties of verbs, regardless of sentence type. Our Wernicke's aphasic patients do not show on-line sensitivity to this lexical property. We discuss these results in terms of multiple resources dedicated to specific sentence processing devices, a possible semantic deficit in Wernicke's aphasia, and a double-dissociation between the operation of accessing a verb's thematic properties and the operation of computing the trace–antecedent relation. © 1993 Academic Press, Inc.

INTRODUCTION

A verb's contribution to the analysis of sentence structure and interpretation has recently been cast in terms of its argument structure properties or sets of thematic roles (i.e., thematic grids). As a simple example, consider that when we acquire the verb *hit,* we likely gain the real-world fact that *hit* requires both a "hitter" and an affected object—the "hittee." In terms of linguistic information we know that *hit* has a two-place argument structure; it needs an argument playing the role of Agent and an argument playing the role of Theme in order to satisfy the verb's thematic structure. What we acquire in this instance, then, is a phonological form (that varies across languages) and the entailments to which the phonological form refers (that likely do not vary significantly across lan-

We thank Margaret O'Grady and Tracy Love of the Aphasia Research Center in Boston, Dr. Cynthia Thompson of Northwestern University, and Dr. Nancy Spence of Bethesda Memorial Hospital for their help in the recruitment and running of subjects. The work reported here was supported by NIH Grants DC00494, DC01948, and AG10496.

52

guages). The verb thus contributes to structure and meaning by determining the number of logical arguments in a sentence and by detailing the thematic roles the arguments play in the sentence.

In terms of sentence processing, the verb and its properties could, in principle, provide information that goes beyond the lexical item's category. Indeed, our previous work (Shapiro, Zurif, & Grimshaw, 1987, 1989; Shapiro, Brookins, Gordon, & Nagel, 1991) has shown that when the verb is encountered in a sentence, all thematic information about the verb is activated, subsequently allowing the arguments in the sentence to receive their proper thematic assignments (see also Boland, 1990; Ferreira & Henderson, 1990; Stowe, 1989; Tanenhaus, Carlson, & Trueswell, 1989). More recently we have shown that, given a verb with multiple argument structure possibilities (or thematic grids), a subject's preferred argument structure may be used as the initial parse once the verb is encountered (Shapiro, Nagel, & Levine, 1993; see also Trueswell, Tanenhaus, & Kello, 1992).

Issues of thematic assignment have also entered into the description of the deficits found in Broca's aphasia. For example, it is well-established that agrammatic Broca's aphasic patients have problems interpreting sentences like passives and cleft-object sentences, yet they do not have difficulty interpreting cleft-subjects. Consider the following:

1. Joelle hit Dillon.
2. Dillon$_i$ was hit $trace_i$ by Joelle last night.
3. It was Dillon$_i$ who Joelle hit $trace_i$ last night.
4. It was Joelle$_i$ who $trace_i$ hit Dillon last night.

In the passive (2) and cleft-object (3), the post-verb direct object position is not lexically filled. Instead, the position is occupied by a *trace* (or "gap") of its antecedent, the moved NP "Dillon." The trace and its antecedent are co-indexed, representing the fact that they co-refer. Unlike the simple active sentence in (1) "Joelle hit Dillon" where "Dillon" is in the direct object argument position and receives its thematic role directly from the verb, "Dillon" in both the passive (2) the cleft-object sentence (3) receives its thematic role indirectly by virtue of its co-indexation with its trace. The role of Theme is assigned to the direct object position occupied by the trace, but because the trace is co-indexed with its antecedent, the thematic role is effectively passed on to "Joelle" via a "theta-chain" consisting of the trace and its antecedent. In the cleft-subject (4), a trace is represented in the subject position and Agent is passed on to the antecedent "Joelle." "Dillon" is in the direct object position; Theme is assigned to it directly.

In an off-line task where a listener is presented with a sentence and has to point to one of two pictures, the Broca's aphasic patient will perform at-chance when confronted with passive and cleft-object sentences, sometimes pointing to the correct picture and sometimes pointing to an incorrect picture where the referents have been reversed. When confronted with active sentences and cleft-subjects, above-chance performance is observed. Grodzinsky (1990) has offered a descriptive generalization that captures this pattern: Traces are deleted and thematic role assignment to the moved constituent cannot occur. In the passive and cleft-object cases, the moved NP is left without a proper thematic role. The Broca's aphasic patient, according to Grodzinsky, thus relies on an agent-first strategy, resulting in two "agents" and at-chance performance. In the cleft-subject case, the agent-first strategy fortuitously mimics normal grammatical assignment and above-chance performance is observed (see also Hickok, Zurif, & Canseco-Gonzalez, 1993, for an extension of this hypothesis).

Although thematic assignment may ultimately enter into a linguistic description of Broca's aphasia, Shapiro and Levine (1990) have found that these patients appear normally sensitive to the thematic representations of verbs at the point where the verb is encountered in a sentence, suggesting that the operations of access and thematic assignment can be dissociated in aphasia. For example, consider the following:

5. The old man exhibited the toy.
6. The old man sent the toy.

The verb *exhibit* allows only a single two-place (Agent Theme) argument structure as in (5), where the argument represented by "the old man" is assigned the role of Agent and the argument represented by "the toy" is assigned the role of Theme. The verb *send* also allows a two-place (Agent Theme) structure as in (6), but allows a three-place (Agent Theme Goal) structure as well, as in "The old man sent the toy to the girl," where "the girl" that falls within the prepositional phrase "to the girl" has the thematic realization of Goal of the action. In a cross-modal interference task where subjects were required both to listen to sentences for meaning and to make a lexical decision on an unrelated probe visually presented in the immediate vicinity of the verb, verbs that allowed more argument structure possibilities, like *send,* resulted in greater interference and processing load than verbs that allowed fewer possibilities, like *exhibit.* We interpreted this pattern (and similar patterns involving other verb types) as showing the exhaustive access of multiple thematic information about a verb in the verb's immediate temporal vicinity. Our fluent aphasic subjects, however, did not show this normal sensitivity to thematic information.

One limitation of the Shapiro and Levine study was that all the sentences used in the cross-modal task were ultimately interpretable by our agrammatic aphasic subjects. Perhaps more "complex" sentences would yield a different pattern. For example, sentences containing trace–

antecedent relations—sentences that agrammatic Broca's patients cannot normally interpret—might disclose a deficit in immediately accessing a verb's thematic properties. We address this issue in our present set of experiments. Before detailing these experiments, we offer one reason why such sentence structures might interact with—and disrupt—the normal access of thematic information for these patients.

Recently, a "reduced capacity" hypothesis has been proposed to account for the deficits found in Broca's aphasia (Caplan, 1992; Frazier & Friederici, 1991; Haarmann & Kolk, 1991; MacDonald, Just, & Carpenter, in press). Although there are variations on this theme, the basic premise is that processing the structure and meaning of sentences requires the availability of enough resources to complete the task, the resources stemming from a single "central processing capacity" (Frazier & Friederici, 1991), a general attentional pool (McNeil, Odell, & Tseng, 1990), or working memory (Caplan & Hildebrandt, 1988; MacDonald et al., in press). Broca's patients have a capacity reduction, according to Frazier and Friederici's account, and different sentence structures and different tasks used to assess comprehension performance place various demands on the central processor. Using this hypothesis, Frazier and Friederici attempt to explain a host of behaviors that have been associated with Broca's aphasia, including the inability of these patients to comprehend sentences involving empty categories (e.g., traces), and a so-called complexity effect where comprehension of sentences with more nodes (or a larger ratio of nonterminal to terminal nodes) is more easily disrupted relative to sentences with fewer nodes (Caplan & Hildebrandt, 1988; Haarmann & Kolk, 1991). The hypothesis also predicts that normal subjects will show the same sorts of deficits that Broca's patients show, given certain task demands and time constraints.

We have explained the activation of a verb's lexical properties in terms of processing resources as well: A verb with more argument structure possibilities in its lexical entry requires more resources than a verb allowing fewer possibilities. Yet in Shapiro and Levine (1990), both our normal control subjects and our agrammatic Broca's patients showed similar patterns. That is, although it may be computationally expensive to access a verb's thematic representations, it is surely within the capacity of the agrammatic Broca's system to do this work. Perhaps, however, processing sentences involving trace–antecedent relations might compete for the resources necessary to activate multiple thematic information. To see this more clearly, consider again the passive and cleft-object sentences:

7. Dillon*i* was hit *trace*i by Joelle last night.
8. It was Dillon*i* who Joelle hit *trace*i last night.

Note that in (7) and (8) both the verb *hit* and the trace in the direct object position occur within the same temporal vicinity during the on-line processing of the sentence. It seems reasonable, then, to suggest that the resources required to process passives and cleft-objects might compete for the resources required to compute the thematic representations of verbs—specifically since both processes are likely operating concurrently. From the reduced capacity hypothesis, we would predict that Broca's aphasic subjects will not show normal access to all of a verb's multiple thematic information in the immediate vicinity of the verb in sentences where the more complex trace–antecedent relation must also be computed.

There is another possibility, however. The lexical process that computes a verb's thematic representations could be independent from the process that computes the syntactic trace–antecedent relation. That is, perhaps there is not a *single* resource for the sentence processing system as is assumed by the capacity limitation hypothesis, but, instead, *dedicated* resources are available for specific processes (see Klapp, Marshburn, & Lester, 1983, and Monsell, 1984, for similar viewpoints involving dedicated working memory systems). Indeed, evidence suggests that sentence structure may be irrelevant to the access of a verb's multiple thematic properties. In Shapiro, Zurif, and Grimshaw (1989), we used sentences that were structurally biased, sentences that pointed to one of the verb's multiple argument structure possibilities. Even in this case we observed that normal subjects activate all of a verb's argument structures, including those not relevant to the presented sentence. We interpreted this result as evidence for the modularity of lexical (verb-argument structure) access: The operating characteristic of verb access is such that it ignores sentence context. It is of course possible that this "modularity effect" will disappear under conditions of brain damage. On this view modularity would simply be a function of a normally fast-acting access device that does not extend beyond available computational resources. A resource limitation, however, might function to "slow down" the process (Kolk & van Grunsven, 1985; Haarmann & Kolk, 1991), allowing sentence context to penetrate the system. To our knowledge there are no observations where normally modular processes have become "contextually penetrable" because of brain damage, even in the case of slowed processing (see, for example, Swinney, Zurif, & Nicol, 1989).

Nevertheless, it is with these two possibilities in mind—a single resource for sentence processing or dedicated resources—that we ran the following experiments.

THE PRESENT EXPERIMENTS

We ran three experiments. In each we compared pure transitive verbs to dative verbs, and we compared what we have called "two-complement" verbs to "four-complement" verbs. Our "pure" transitive verbs, like *fix*, allowed only a two-place (Agent Theme) argument structure and our "dative" verbs, like *send*, allowed both a two-place (Agent Theme) and three-place (Agent Theme Goal) argument structure. Our complement verbs selected from a small corpus of semantic types that are associated with complex NP's or sentential clauses (Grimshaw, 1979, 1990; Pesetsky, 1983). Our two-complement verbs allowed both an (Agent Theme) and an (Agent Proposition), the proposition associated with a *that* clause. Consider the two-complement verb *expect:*

9. [The detective] expected [the phone call].
    Agent   Theme
10. [The detective] expected [that the criminal would be freed].
     Agent   Proposition

Our four complement verbs allowed an (Agent Theme), (Agent Proposition), (Agent Exclamation), and (Agent Interrogative), the latter two associated wtih *wh*-clauses. Consider the four-complement verb *discover:*

11. [The detective] discovered [the secret].
    Agent   Theme
12. [The detective] discovered [that the man was crazy].
    Agent   Proposition
13. [The detective] discovered [what a fool he had been]!
    Agent   Exclamation
14. [The detective] discovered [why the man was crazy].
    Agent   Interrogative

We used the cross-modal lexical decision (CMLD) task, a dual task in which sentences are presented to subjects over headphones. This task has been successful in measuring the time course of sentence processing, including lexical-level effects (e.g., Shapiro et al., 1987; Boland, 1991) and integration effects (e.g., Ni, Fodor, Crain, & Shankweiler, 1993; Shapiro et al., 1991). Our use of this task involves the following: At a specific point during the temporal unfolding of the sentence, a visual lexical decision probe (word/nonword) is presented on a computer monitor. When the probe forms a word in English, *it is not related to the sentence or continues the sentence in any meaningful way.* The subject is required to both attend to the tape-recorded sentence for meaning and to make a lexical decision on the visually presented probe. The reaction times (RT's) associated with the CMLD are purportedly a measure of processing load taken from the immediate vicinity in the sentence where the probe is presented so long as certain characteristics of each probe (e.g., frequency of occurrence and number of letters and syllables) are controlled. For example, the RT's associated with the probe when presented in the immediate temporal vicinity of the verb appear to reflect the amount of argument structure information associated with the verb in its lexical entry. In our previous work our dative verbs yielded longer RT's on the CMLD than our pure transitives, and our four-complement verbs yielded longer RT's than our two-complement verbs (e.g., Shapiro et al., 1987, 1991; Shapiro & Levine, 1990).[1]

Our first experiment examined argument structure access in active and passive sentences; our second used cleft-subject and cleft-object sentences; and our third used "padded" cleft-subject and cleft-object sentences—the padding accomplished by a prepositional phrase (PP) placed before the verb—adding to the phrasal density, and complexity, of the sentences. From the reduced capacity hypothesis, we predicted that subjects—particularly our Broca's aphasic patients—would show a normal distinction between verbs that differ in terms of their thematic properties only in sentence types (actives, for example) that by hypothesis should recruit less resources. In sentences where verb access and the trace-antecedent relation compete for resources, thematic access should be disrupted. However, if the access of a verb's thematic information is independent from the snytactic processes of computing the trace-antecedent relation—if there are distinct resources dedicated to each process—then whenever a subject showed a normal distinction between verbs that differ in terms of thematic information, this sensitivity would hold regardless of the type of the sentence in which the verb was contained.

---

[1] In an effort to examine the boundaries of the argument structure effect, Shapiro et al. (1991) recently ran a series of experiments using the cross-modal lexical decision task and different types of lexical decision probes. We again observed distinctions among verbs having different argument structure configurations. However, Schmauder, Kennison, and Clifton (1991) also used different sets of probes and reported a failure to replicate the original Shapiro et al. (1987) study. We are left with the following: Shapiro and colleagues have observed argument structure effects in experiments conducted in different laboratories and with different subject populations. But Schmauder et al. could not replicate these effects in their study. We currently have no explanation for this discrepancy. We note here that regardless of this discrepancy, most sentence processing theories of which we are aware have, as one component, a thematic processor that accesses all thematic information when the verb is encountered (e.g., Boland, 1991; Ferreira & Henderson, 1990; Stowe, 1989; Tanenhaus et al., 1989; Trueswell et al., 1993). Such a claim is an empirical one, and there are considerable data to support it. For example, in a cross-modal integration task where subjects heard sentence fragments containing either transitive or intransitive verbs and had to name a visually presented word immediately following the verb, Trueswell et al. found longer naming times on probes that violated the verb's subcategorization information. These data strongly suggest that multiple subcategorization information (that can be roughly recast in terms of argument structure) is made available immediately when the verb is encountered. Similarly, using both cross-modal naming and lexical decision (integration) tasks, Boland (1991) found that the multiple argument structure configurations of a verb are accessed in parallel.

EXPERIMENT 1

Method

Subjects. Three groups of subjects were included in all of the experiments: a group of normal controls ($N = 10$) matched as closely as possible for age (range from 62 to 75 years) and educational level to the aphasic groups; a group of Broca's aphasic patients ($N = 6$; age range from 65 to 79 years); and a group of Wernicke's aphasic patients ($N = 4$; age range from 56 to 72 years). The Wernicke's aphasic patient group was included in the present study because of our earlier work (Shapiro & Levine, 1990) that suggested that these patients might not be sensitive to the thematic properties of verbs; that is, we hoped to replicate these earlier results and extend them to include more complex sentence types.

The aphasic patients were recruited from Bethesda Memorial Hospital in Boynton Beach, Florida, Florida Atlantic University's Communications Disorders Clinic, the University of Florida Speech and Hearing Clinic, and from the Boston V. A. Medical Center. They were diagnosed on the basis of performance profiles on the BDAE, WAB, or PICA and by further clinical evaluations by speech–language pathologists and neurologists. The six Broca's aphasic patients presented with nonfluent and telegraphic verbal output and with relative sparing of auditory comprehension at the conversational level. On an independent sentence–picture matching task presented at the time of the experiment involving 10 each of reversible active, passive, cleft-object, and cleft-subject sentences, all six subjects showed above-chance performance on active and cleft-subject sentences and at-chance performance on passives and cleft-object sentences. Three of the four Wernicke's aphasic patients presented with fluent, relatively empty speech; one presented with fluent speech that appeared conversationally appropriate, although considerable word-finding problems were observed. On the sentence–picture matching task presented at the time of the experiment, two of the Wernicke's aphasic patients performed above chance on both actives and passives, although in both cases performance was worse on passives; one subject performed at chance on all sentence types; and one performed above chance on actives and at chance on passives. Thus the Wernicke's aphasic patients, unlike our Broca's aphasic patient group, performed inconsistently as a group on our screening measure.

Materials. Sentences featured verbs that varied in terms of their argument structure possibilities. We compared pure transitives, allowing a single two-place (Agent Theme) argument structure, to datives, allowing both a two-place (Agent Theme) and a three-place (Agent Theme Goal) structure. In a separate set of analyses, we compared two-complement verbs, allowing (Agent Theme) and (Agent Proposition) possibilities, to four-complement verbs, allowing (Agent Theme), (Agent Proposition), (Agent Exclamation), and (Agent Interrogative) possibilities.

For the transitive/dative comparison, there were 12 verbs in each class. Each verb was inserted in two different sentence structures (active, passive), yielding a total of 48 test sentences. For the two-complement/four-complement comparison, there were 8 verbs in each class, each inserted in an active and passive sentence, yielding a total of 32 test sentences. These 80 test sentences were included in a script of 160 sentences, half designed as foils. The appendix contains a list of the verb types, verbs, and example sentence types used in all three experiments.

Each verb was heard twice; once in an active and once in a passive sentence. Each transitive verb was paired with a dative verb resulting in sets of paired sentences that were identical except for the verb. The two- and four-complement verbs were paired as well. Table 1 shows that each passive sentence is the passivized form of its active counterpart. All sentences were of the form NP–V–NP–PP (before movement applied in the passive case). The prepositional phrases were adjuncts. Adjuncts differ from arguments in that they are not considered part of the verb phrase, do not contribute to the verb's thematic offering, and therefore do not form part of a verb's lexical entry. The adjuncts used in this experiment were locatives. The position of the locative adjunct was balanced such that in half of the passive sentences the adjunct came before the second argument; in the other half it came after the second argument.

The visual probe stimuli for the secondary CMLD were composed of 160 letter sequences—80 words and 80 nonwords. The test probes were real words that ranged from 5 to 12 letters in length, one to four syllables, and had a Francis and Kucera (1982) frequency range of 51 to 317. The real word filler probes had the same characteristics as the test probes. The nonword probes were produced from real words with the same characteristics as well; one letter was replaced, with the final result conforming to English orthographic rules.

The probes were assigned to the verbs and sentences in the following way. The test probes were designed in pairs; one of each pair was placed in an active sentence and one in a passive sentence for each verb. Additionally, the probes assigned to the transitive verbs had the same mean frequency of occurrence, length, and syllable structure as those assigned to the dative verbs. The probes assigned to the complement verb types were also balanced in the same way. Care was taken to ensure that each probe was unrelated semantically and phonologically to the sentence to which it was assigned. Two separate sets of probes with the same characteristics were produced, with roughly half of our subjects in each subject group receiving one set and the other half receiving the other set. This design feature ensured that any observed RT patterns would be attributed only to verb effects and not to any particular combination of probe and sentence. Finally, for the test sentences the probes appeared either in the immediate temporal vicinity of the verb or immediately after the direct object NP in the active sentences; in the passive sentences they appeared either immediately after the verb, or after the PP or *by*-phrase following the verb. An equal number of nonword probes also appeared at these same temporal points in the foil sentences, and the remainder of real word and nonword probes were placed at other temporal points during the unfolding of the sentence to lessen any expectations on the part of the subjects.

In summary, the overall design of this experiment involved two separate sets of analyses for each of the three subject-groups. Each set of analyses involved two probe positions (verb, downstream) and two verb types (transitive, dative in one set; two-complement, four-complement in a separate set).

Equipment. The sentences were recorded onto a Dell computer by a female speaker using normal rate and intonation and were digitized onto one channel using a SuperSound stereo card and voice editing software. On the second channel, for each sentence, a 1000-Hz tone was placed to coincide with the appropriate probe position. The digitized sentences and associated tones were then recorded onto a Sony stereo cassette recorder. Attached to the tape recorder was a Uher dia-pilot, a device that reads the tone (inaudible to the subject[2]). The tone signaled the Dell computer to present the visual probe on the computer screen and simultaneously started a hardware clock that recorded the time between onset of the visual probe and subject response. Subjects indicated their lexical decision by depressing one of two response keys set into an external response panel, using their nonpreferred hand. The visual probe remained on the screen until the subject responded. RTLAB software (ver. 9; ©Swinney & Wong, 1992) controlled the experiment, along with a clock card (Metrobyte CTM05).

Procedure. The subjects were run on the experiments in random order; they were tested individually in three sessions approximately 1 week apart. Subjects heard the sentences

---

[2] Unfortunately, some of our recordings resulted in the tones "bleeding" over to the channel in which the sentences were recorded. However, we examined the data from the subjects who were run on these tapes and found no discernible differences from those subjects who were run on tapes where the tones were inaudible.

presented over headphones and were required to show their understanding by paraphrasing randomly chosen trials (20% of the sentences). Subjects who could not appropriately verbalize either pointed to one of two pictures, one conforming to the sentence just heard, or answered questions about the sentences. The point of this query was only to ensure that the subjects were attempting to listen to the sentences for meaning. During the course of each sentence, a CMLD probe was presented visually on a computer monitor. Subjects were told to listen to the sentence for meaning and to make a lexical decision (word/nonword) on the visual probe as quickly and as accurately as possible by pressing one of two response keys; no feedback was given (before each experimental session, subjects performed a practice session consisting of 20 trials. Some feedback was given during the practice session to ensure that each subject understood the task and was responding rapidly and accurately). The taped sentence continued to unfold normally without any interruption.

Results

Transitive/dative analyses. We analyzed the RT data for each subject group separately. As a first step, we eliminated RTs to the CMLD test probes that were responded to incorrectly. For the normal control subjects, 7% of the test sentences resulted in errors on the CMLD task; for the Broca's aphasic subjects, 6.5% of the test sentences resulted in errors; and for the Wernicke's aphasic subjects, 11% of the test sentences resulted in errors. The errors were approximately evenly distributed across transitive and dative verb types, verb and downstream probe positions, and active and passive sentence types. Next, we searched and replaced outlier RT's for each subject. Outliers were defined as those RT's that were over two standard deviations above the subject's overall mean; these were replaced by the overall mean for the subject. For the normal control subjects, 2.5% of the RT's to the test probes were identified by this data comb and replaced; for the Broca's aphasic subjects, 2%; and for the Wernicke's aphasic subjects, 4.6%. Again, these outliers were approximately evenly distributed across the cells.

With the RT data in the form described above, for each subject group we performed a three-way repeated measures analysis of variance (ANOVA), with verb type (transitive, dative), probe position (verb, downstream), and sentence type (active, passive) as within-subject factors. Table 1 contains the data used in the analyses.

We present first our analyses on the normal subject data. A main effect of verb type was observed. Transitive verbs (997.45 msec) resulted in significantly faster RT's on the CMLD task than dative verbs (1036.78 msec), $F(1, 9) = 5.25$, $p = .04$. A significant interaction between verb type and probe position was observed, $F(1, 9) = 11.79$, $p < .01$. A test of simple effects of verb type at each probe position revealed a significant effect of verb type only in the immediate vicinity of the verb: Transitives (985) yielded significantly faster RT's on the CMLD task than datives (1069 msec), $F(1, 9) = 15.73$, $p < .01$. An examination of individual subject means revealed that 8 of the 10 normal control subjects showed

TABLE 1
Experiment 1: Mean Reaction Times (in msec) to CMLD for Subject Groups, Probe
Position, Verb (Transitive, Dative), and Sentence (Active, Passive)

Subject	Probe	Sentence type			
		Active		Passive	
		Transitive	Dative	Transitive	Dative
Normal	Verb	977	1062	994	1076
	Downstream	1034	1001	985	1008
Broca	Verb	1196	1303	1122	1245
	Downstream	1144	1141	1197	1172
Wernicke	Verb	1050	984	929	985
	Downstream	1029	1023	950	917

the expected transitive/dative difference in actives, and 9 of the 10 in passives. No effects or interactions involving the sentence type variable were observed.

We now present the analyses on the data from the agrammatic Broca's aphasic group. The repeated measures ANOVA revealed a main effect of verb type. Transitive verbs (1165 msec) yielded significantly faster RT's on the CMLD task than dative verbs (1215 msec), $F(1, 5) = 20.26$, $p < .001$. A significant interaction between verb type and probe position was observed, $F(1, 5) = 20.20$, $p < .01$. A test of simple effects of verb type at each probe position revealed a significant effect of verb type only when the CMLD probes were presented in the immediate vicinity of the verb: Transitives (1159 msec) yielded significantly faster RT's than datives (1274 msec), $F(1, 5) = 61.40$, $p < .001$. An examination of individual subject means revealed that all six Broca's aphasic subjects showed the expected transitive/dative difference in active sentences and five of the six in passive sentences. No effects or interactions involving the sentence type variable were observed.

The repeated measures ANOVA for the Wernicke's aphasic patient group revealed no significant effects or interactions. An examination of the individual subject means revealed no distinct group patterns. For example, one of the four subjects showed the expected transitive/dative distinction in active sentences and two in passives.

Two-complement/four-complement analyses. For the normal control subjects, 5% of the test sentences resulted in errors on the CMLD task; for the Broca's aphasic subjects, 4%; and for the Wernicke's aphasic subjects, 14%. The same search-and-replace procedure instituted for the transitive/dative comparison was performed with the complement verbs. For the normal control subjects, 3% of the RT's to the test probes were identified by the data comb and replaced; for the Broca's aphasic sub-

TABLE 2

Experiment 1: Mean Reaction Times (in msec) to CMLD for Subject Groups, Probe
Position, Verb (Two-Comp., Four-Comp.), and Sentence (Active, Passive)

| | | Sentence type | | | |
| | | Active | | Passive | |
Subject	Probe	Two-comp.	Four-comp.	Two-comp.	Four-comp.
Normal	Verb	968	1107	974	1093
	Downstream	1084	1085	1002	1031
Broca	Verb	1127	1256	1127	1223
	Downstream	1234	1197	1117	1136
Wernicke	Verb	1049	1033	1004	1021
	Downstream	949	1020	967	1074

jects, 2%; and for the Wernicke's aphasic subjects, 2.3%. Again, both
the errors and the outliers were approximately evenly distributed across
the cells.

With the RT data in the form described above, for each subject group
we performed a three-way repeated measures ANOVA with verb type
(two-complement, four-complement), probe position (verb, downstream),
and sentence type (active, passive) as the within-subject factors. Table 2
contains the data used in the analyses.

We present first our analyses on the normal subject data. A main effect
of verb type was observed. Two-complement verbs (1007 msec) yielded
significantly faster RT's on the CMLD than four-complement verbs (1079
msec), $F(1, 9) = 9.70$, $p = .01$. A significant interaction between verb
type and probe position was observed, $F(1, 9) = 8.29$, $p = .02$. A test
of simple effects of verb type at each probe position revealed a significant
effect of verb type only in the immediate vicinity of the verb: Two-
complements (971 msec) yielded significantly faster RT's than four-
complements (1100 msec), $F(1, 9) = 16.41$, $p < .01$. Eight of the 10
subjects showed this expected pattern in active sentences and 9 of 10
showed this pattern in passives. No effects or interactions involving sentence type were observed.

We now present our analyses for the Broca's aphasic group. Although
two-complement verbs (1151 msec) yielded faster RT's than four-
complement verbs (1203 msec), this difference was not significant, $F(1,
5) = 4.30$, $p = 0.09$. The verb type by probe position was not significant,
although four of the six subjects showed the normal two-complement/
four-complement distinction in active sentences and five of the six
showed the normal pattern in passives. No significant effects involving
sentence type were observed.

The repeated measures ANOVA for the Wernicke's aphasic group re-

vealed no significant effects or interactions. One of the four subjects
showed the normal two-complement/four-complement distinction in active sentences and one showed the distinction in passives.

EXPERIMENT 2

Method

The sentence types used in this experiment were cleft-subjects (e.g.,
"It was the valet who located the sports car on the lot yesterday") and
cleft-objects (e.g., "It was the sports car that the valet had located on
the lot yesterday"); all other aspects of the method were the same as
those in Experiment 1. Like Experiment 1, two separate sets of analyses
were performed, one comparing transitive to dative verbs and the other
comparing two-complement to four-complement verbs.

Results

Transitive/dative analyses. For the normal control group, 4.2% of the
test sentences resulted in errors on the CMLD task; for the Broca's
aphasic group, 5.5%; and for the Wernicke's aphasic group, 15%. The
same search-and-replace instituted in Experiment 1 was used here. For
the normal control group, 4.2% of the RT's to the test probes were identified by the data comb and replaced; for the Broca's aphasic group, 5.5%;
and for the Wernicke's aphasic group, 3%. The errors and outliers were,
again, evenly distributed across all cells.

With the data in the form described above, for each subject group
we performed a three-way repeated measures ANOVA with verb type
(transitive, dative), probe position (verb, downstream), and sentence type
(cleft-subject, cleft-object) as the within-subject factors. Table 3 contains
the data used in the analyses.

TABLE 3
Experiment 2: Mean Reaction Times (in msec) to CMLD for Subject Groups, Probe
Position, Verb (Trans., Dative), and Sentence (Cleft-Subj., Cleft-Obj.)

| Subject | Probe | Sentence type | | | |
| | | Cleft-subject | | Cleft-object | |
		Transitive	Dative	Transitive	Dative
Normal	Verb	899	984	907	1005
	Preposition	958	987	972	1000
Broca	Verb	1072	1190	1053	1149
	Preposition	1087	1110	1079	1102
Wernicke	Verb	967	971	1081	975
	Preposition	966	998	1014	1039

For the normal control group, a main effect of probe position was observed. Probes presented in the immediate vicinity of the verb (948 msec) yielded significantly faster RT's than probes presented downstream (979 msec), $F(1, 9) = 7.92$, $p < .05$. A main effect of verb type was observed. Transitive verbs (934 msec) yielded significantly faster RT's to the CMLD than dative verbs (994 msec), $F(1, 9) = 15.58$, $p < .01$. A significant probe position by verb type interaction was observed, $F(1, 9) = 5.67$, $p < .05$. A test of simple effects of verb type at each probe position revealed a significant verb effect only in the immediate vicinity of the verb: Transitives (903 msec) yielded significantly faster RT's to the CMLD than datives (994 msec), $F(1, 9) = 18.10$, $p < .01$. Eight of the 10 subjects showed this pattern with cleft-subjects and 9 showed this pattern with cleft-objects. No significant effect or interactions involving sentence type were observed.

For the Broca's aphasic group, a main effect of verb type was observed. Transitives (1072 msec) yielded significantly faster RT's on the CMLD than datives (1138 msec), $F(1, 5) = 6.33$, $p = .05$. A significant probe position by verb type interaction was observed, $F(1, 5) = 9.13$, $p < .05$. A test of simple effects of verb type at each probe position revealed a significant verb effect only in the immediate vicinity of the verb: Transitives (1062 msec) yielded significantly faster RT's than datives (1169 msec), $F(1, 5) = 45.90$, $p = .001$. All six subjects showed this pattern with both cleft-subjects and cleft-objects. No significant effect or interactions involving sentence type were observed.

For the Wernicke's aphasic group, no significant effects or interactions were observed, although cleft-subject sentences (975 msec) yielded faster RT's on the CMLD than cleft-object sentences (1027 msec), $F(1, 3) = 7.86$, $p = .07$. Two of the four subjects showed the transitive/dative distinction with cleft-subjects and two showed this pattern with cleft-objects. No significant effect or interations involving sentence type were observed.

Two-complement/four-complement analyses. For the normal control group, 4.3% of the test sentences resulted in errors on the CMLD task and 3.4% of the responses were identified as outliers; for the Broca's aphasic group, 7.8% resulted in errors and 2.6% were identified as outliers; and for the Wernicke's aphasic group, 12.8% resulted in errors and 2.7% were identified as outliers. The errors and outliers were approximately evenly distributed across all cells.

With the data in the form described above, for each subject group we performed a three-way repeated measures ANOVA with verb type (two-complement, four-complement), probe position (verb, downstream), and sentence type (cleft-subject, cleft-object) as the within-subject factors. Table 4 contains the data used in the analyses.

TABLE 4
Experiment 2: Mean Reaction Times (in msec) to CMLD for Subject Groups, Probe
Position, Verb (Two-Comp., Four-Comp.), and Sentence (Cleft-Subj., Cleft-Obj.)

Subject	Probe	Sentence type			
		Cleft-subject		Cleft-object	
		Two-comp.	Four-comp.	Two-comp.	Four-comp.
Normal	Verb	973	1087	923	1014
	Preposition	934	999	993	961
Broca	Verb	1116	1209	1108	1234
	Preposition	1217	1220	1170	1164
Wernicke	Verb	970	1047	1074	899
	Preposition	978	1026	994	989

For the normal control group, a main effect of verb type was observed. Two-complement verbs (956 msec) yielded significantly faster RT's on the CMLD than four-complement verbs (1015 msec), $F(1, 9) = 30.03$, $p < .01$. A significant sentence type by verb type interaction was observed, $F(1, 9) = 8.00$, $p = .02$. A test of simple effects of verb type within each sentence type revealed that verb effects were observed within both sentence types: Two-complement verbs (954 msec) yielded faster RT's than four-complement verbs (1043 msec) in cleft-subject sentences, $F(1, 9) = 29.43$, $p < .01$. The same pattern held in cleft-object sentences, where two-complement verbs (957 msec) also yielded significantly faster RT's than four-complement verbs (988 msec), $F(1, 9) = 4.81$, $p = .05$. A significant verb type by probe position interaction was observed, $F(1, 9) = 9.05$, $p = .01$. A test of simple effects of verb type at each probe position revealed a significant effect of verb type only in the immediate vicinity of the verb: Two-complement verbs (948 msec) yielded significantly faster RT's than four-complement verbs (1051 msec), $F(1, 9) = 40.30$, $p < .001$. Nine of the 10 subjects showed this pattern with cleft-subjects and 8 showed this pattern with cleft-objects.

For the Broca's aphasic group, a significant verb type by probe position interaction was observed, $F(1, 5) = 10.39$, $p = .02$. A test of simple effects of verb type at each probe position revealed a significant effect of verb type only in the immediate vicinity of the verb: Two-complement verbs (1112 msec) yielded significantly faster RT's than four-complement verbs (1221 msec), $F(1, 5) = 7.28$, $p < .05$. All six subjects showed this pattern with cleft-subjects and five with cleft-objects.

For the Wernicke's aphasic group, no effects or interactions were observed.

EXPERIMENT 3

Method

The sentence types used in this experiment were padded cleft-subjects (e.g., "It was the girl on the bike who hit the boy yesterday") and padded cleft-objects (e.g., "It was the boy on the bike that the girl hit yesterday"); all other aspects of the method were the same as those in Experiments 1 and 2.

Results

Transitive/dative analyses. For the normal subject group, 4.6% of the test sentences resulted in errors on the CMLD task and 2% of the responses to the test probes were identified as outliers and were replaced by the appropriate mean for each subject; for the Broca's aphasic group, 6.6% resulted in errors and 3.5% were identified as outliers and were replaced; and for the Wernicke's aphasic group, 13% resulted in errors and 2% were identified as outliers and were replaced. The errors and outliers were approximately evenly distributed across all cells.

For each subject group we again performed a repeated measures ANOVA with verb type (transitive, dative), probe position (verb, downstream), and sentence type (padded cleft-subject, padded cleft-object) as the within-subject factors. Table 5 contains the data used in the analyses.

For the normal control group, a main effect of verb type was observed. Transitives (892 msec) yielded significantly faster RT's on the CMLD than datives (985 msec), $F(1, 9) = 14.11$, $p < .01$. A significant probe position by verb type interaction was observed, $F(1, 9) = 23.00$, $p = .001$. A test of simple effects at each probe position revealed a significant verb effect only when in the immediate vicinity of the verb: Transitives (887 msec) yielded significantly faster RT's than datives (970 msec), $F(1, 9) = 36.73$, $p < .001$. Eight of the 10 subjects showed this pattern with

TABLE 5
Experiment 3: Mean RTs (in msec) to CMLD for Subject Groups, Probe Position,
Verb (Transitive, Dative), and Sentence (Padded Cleft-Subj., Cleft-Obj.)

Subject	Probe	Sentence type			
		Padded cleft-subj.		Padded cleft-obj.	
		Transitive	Dative	Transitive	Dative
Normal	Verb	887	970	880	997
	Downstream	897	921	905	871
Broca	Verb	1180	1244	1050	1152
	Downstream	1067	1046	1026	1010
Wernicke	Verb	1026	1089	956	1035
	Downstream	963	980	960	938

padded cleft-subjects and 8 showed this pattern with cleft-objects. No significant effect or interactions involving sentence type were observed.

For the Broca's aphasic group, a main effect of probe position was observed. Probes presented downstream from the verb (1037 msec) yielded significantly faster RT's on the CMLD than probes presented in the immediate vicinity of the verb (1156 msec), $F(1, 5) = 45.39$, $p = .001$. A main effect of verb type was observed. Transitives (1081 msec) yielded significantly faster RT's than datives (1113 msec), $F(1, 5) = 9.57$, $p < .05$. A significant probe position by verb type interaction was observed, $F(1, 5) = 7.65$, $p < .05$. A test of simple effects of verb type at each probe position revealed a significant verb effect only in the immediate vicinity of the verb: Transitives (1180 msec) yielded significantly faster RT's than datives (1244 msec), $F(1, 5) = 46.52$, $p = .001$. All six subjects showed this pattern with the padded cleft-subjects; five of the six showed this pattern with padded cleft-objects.

For the Wernicke's aphasic group, no significant effects or interactions were observed, although transitive verbs (976 msec) yielded faster RT's than dative verbs (1011 msec), $F(1, 3) = 4.57$, $p = .10$. Three of the four subjects showed the transitive/dative distinction with padded cleft-subjects; three showed the distinction with the padded cleft-objects.

Two-complement/four-complement analyses. For the normal control group, 4.4% of the test sentences resulted in errors on the CMLD task and 3% of the responses to the test probes were identified as outliers and were replaced by the appropriate mean for each subject; for the Broca's aphasic group, 5.7% resulted in errors and 2.1% were identified as outliers and were replaced; and for the Wernicke's aphasic group, 8% resulted in errors and 2.7% were identified as outliers and were replaced.

With the data in the form described above, for each subject group we again performed a repeated measures ANOVA with verb type (two-complement, four-complement), probe position (verb, downstream), and sentence type (padded cleft-subject and padded cleft-object) as the within-subject factors. Table 6 contains the data used in the analyses.

For the normal control group, a significant probe position by verb type interaction was observed, $F(1, 9) = 13.28$, $p < .01$. A test of simple effects of verb type at each probe position revealed a significant effect of verb type only in the immediate vicinity of the verb: Two-complement verbs (898 msec) yielded significantly faster RT's on the CMLD than four-complement verbs (979 msec), $F(1, 9) = 10.70$, $p < .01$. Eight of the 10 subjects showed this pattern with padded cleft-subjects; 8 showed this pattern with padded cleft-objects.

For the Broca's aphasic group, a main effect of verb type was observed. Two-complement verbs (1041 msec) yielded faster RT's than four-complement verbs (1104 msec), $F = 7.27$, $p < .05$. A significant sentence type by probe position interaction was observed, $F = 6.12$, p

TABLE 6

Experiment 3: Mean RTs (in msec) to CMLD for Subject Groups, Probe Position, Verb (Two-Comp., Four-Comp.), and Sentence (Padded Cleft-Sub., Cleft-Obj.)

		Sentence type			
		Padded cleft-subj.		Padded cleft-obj.	
Subject	Probe	Two-comp.	Four-comp.	Two-comp.	Four-comp.
Normal	Verb	925	1007	871	952
	Downstream	890	871	935	894
Broca	Verb	1038	1217	940	1050
	Downstream	1106	1090	1083	1059
Wernicke	Verb	990	1020	863	996
	Downstream	980	957	1068	1037

$= .056$. A test of simple effects of sentence type at each probe position revealed a significant effect of sentence type only in the immediate vicinity of the verb: Cleft-objects (995 msec) yielded significantly faster RT's than cleft-subjects (1127 msec), $F(1, 5) = 6.66$, $p = .05$. A significant probe position by verb type interaction was observed, $F(1, 5) = 7.47$, $p < .05$. A test of simple effects of verb type at each probe position revealed a significant effect of verb type only in the immediate vicinity of the verb: Two-complement verbs (1038 msec) yielded significantly faster RT's on the CMLD than four-complement verbs (1217 msec), $F(1, 5) = 12.15$, $p < .02$. Five of the six subjects showed this pattern with the cleft-subjects; five showed this pattern with cleft-objects.

For the Wernicke's aphasic group, two-complement verbs (975 msec) yielded faster RT's than four-complement verbs (1002 msec), although this difference was not significant, $F(1, 3) = 5.50$, $p = .11$. A significant sentence type by probe position interaction was observed, $F(1, 3) = 16.09$, $p < .05$. A test of simple effects of sentence type at each probe position revealed that padded cleft-subjects (968 msec) yielded significantly faster RT's than padded cleft-objects (1053) msec), but only downstream from the verb, $F(1, 3) = 63.14$, $p < .01$. Three of the four subjects showed this pattern.

DISCUSSION

We begin our discussion with the normal subject group performance. In all three experiments transitive verbs yielded significantly faster RT's than dative verbs and two-complement verbs yielded faster RT's than four-complement verbs, but only when the sentences were probed in the verb's immediate temporal vicinity. When the sentences were tapped downstream from the verb, no differences between the verb types were noted. These results add additional empirical support to the claim that when a verb is encountered in a spoken sentence, its thematic properties are exhaustively activated. Furthermore, the exhaustive activation of thematic information was observed in all four sentence types tested: actives, passives, cleft-subjects, and cleft-objects. The lexical process of accessing a verb and its thematic properties thus appears to be independent of the type of sentence in which the verb is contained.

This same normal pattern was observed with the Broca's aphasic patients. Regardless of sentence type, these subjects showed sensitivity to the thematic properties of verbs. Indeed, the Broca's aphasic patients showed normal argument structure effects even in sentences that they do not ultimately comprehend, like passives and cleft-objects. This pattern suggests that the real-time process of accessing a verb and its thematic properties must also be independent from the difficulties these patients have with comprehending complex sentences. That is, although the time course of verb-argument structure activation may be normal, the subsequent integration of this information into the temporal unfolding of the sentence may not be. We consider the Broca's aphasic patients' normal verb-argument structure access routines a strength that can be exploited in treatment programs focusing on disorders of production and comprehension. Indeed, by considering and controlling the underlying properties of verbs and sentences, we are currently training strategies to Broca's aphasic patients who show deficits in the production of complex sentences; our initial results look promising (Thompson, Shapiro, & Roberts, 1993).

Our Wernicke's aphasic patients, for the most part, did not show sensitivity to the thematic properties of verbs; they did not show the normal distinction between verbs that varied in their thematic representations regardless of sentence type (there was a suggestion of a verb effect for the padded sentences, although this effect was not significant).[3] These data buttress our previous findings where we found that a more heterogeneous group of fluent aphasic patients did not show normal thematic effects (Shapiro & Levine, 1990). Since recent linguistic accounts of the lexicon claim that thematic information is part of lexical–conceptual structure or "conceptual semantics" (Grimshaw, 1990; Jackendoff, 1990), perhaps Wernicke's aphasic patients have a disorder in either representing or, more likely, accessing this information. In this vein consider that there have been several suggestions in the literature that Wernicke's

---

[3] Three of the four Wernicke's aphasic subjects run in the present study were the same subjects run in the Zurif et al. study (1993). The lack of significant thematic effects found with these subjects in the present study cannot be attributed to some general problem with dual tasks; both studies used dual tasks (priming in the Zurif study, interference in the present study), yet Zurif et al. found that these subjects performed normally on their task when the trace–antecedent relation was at issue.

aphasia involves some sort of "semantic deficit" in terms of conceptual features, although no consensus exists on the nature of this disorder (e.g., Baker, 1986; Goodglass & Baker, 1976; McCleary & Hirst, 1986; Zurif, Caramazza, & Meyerson, 1974). Our present data provide a grammatical angle on this semantic deficit: During on-line sentence comprehension, Wernicke's aphasic patients are not provided with the set of lexical–conceptual roles associated with a verb; normal models of sentence processing require this information for further aspects of parsing and interpretation. Whether this deficit is related to that found in the existing literature remains to be seen.

Consider now a recent investigation of syntactic processing in Broca's and Wernicke's aphasia (Zurif, Swinney, Prather, Solomon, & Bushell, 1993) and how it reflects on our present work. Zurif et al. examined whether their aphasic subjects normally reactivated the antecedent to a trace in subject-relative constructions like "The gymnast loved the professor$_i$ from the northwestern city who [*trace*]$_i$ complained about the bad coffee." In this example "the professor" would normally be reactivated when the position of the trace is encountered (see Swinney & Osterhaut, 1990); "the professor" must also be linked to the trace in the subject position to receive its thematic role. Using a cross-modal lexical priming task, Zurif et al. established that their Broca's aphasic patients did not show the normal link between the trace and the antecedent, thus the moved NP cannot receive its thematic role grammatically. Yet, importantly, these patients do ultimately comprehend such subject-relative constructions, presumably relying on nongrammatical means to do so (see, for example, Grodzinsky, 1990; Hickok, Zurif, & Canseco-Gonzalez, 1993). Different from that found for the Broca's aphasic patients, the Wernicke's aphasic patients in the Zurif et al. study showed normal reactivation of the antecedent to the trace, yet typically do not show good comprehension of such structures (Grodzinsky, 1984).

Summarizing the Zurif et al. and present studies, we find the following: (1) Broca's aphasic patients are sensitive to a verb's thematic properties; Wernicke's aphasic patients are not. (2) Wernicke's aphasic patients reactivate an antecedent to a trace; Broca's aphasic patients do not. We therefore find a double-dissociation between the lexical process of accessing a verb's thematic properties and the operation of connecting a trace to its antecedent.

There are, of course, some important details to be worked out in our analyses of Broca's and Wernicke's aphasia. For example, why is it that Broca's aphasic patients do not show normal access of a noun's multiple senses at the right time in the processing stream (Swinney et al., 1989), do not show normal reactivation of the noun phrase antecedent to a trace in subject relatives (Zurif et al., 1993), and yet show normal sensitivity to the thematic representations of verbs? And, conversely, why do Wernicke's aphasic patients show both normal access of a noun's multiple senses and normal reactivation of the antecedent to a trace, yet do not show normal activation of a verb's thematic information? One possibility that we have offered previously (Prather, Shapiro, Zurif, & Swinney, 1991) deserves repeating here: Perhaps accessing a noun's "senses" is a time-dependent process that involves mapping a phonological form onto a representation in the lexicon, which in turn activates other representations that are associatively related (hence, lexical priming is observed). The same process occurs in the reactivation of an NP in a trace position, with the added syntactic operation of connecting the trace to its antecedent. But, unlike the access (or reaccess) of a noun's interpretation, the access of thematic information does not involve activation of related representations that occur over time. Instead, it involves mapping a phonological form onto a representation in the lexicon, and that representation directly yields an initially indivisible set of argument structures; the more argument structure configurations associated with the verb, the more "effort" is required to immediately access this information (hence, processing load effects are observed).

Finally, we return to the capacity limitation hypothesis. We have suggested that our experiments could shed some light on the details of this account of Broca's aphasia, and here is what we have found: Although accessing a verb's thematic information appears costly, the cost does not exceed the capacity of Broca's aphasic patients to exhaustively access this information. Moreover, the resources necessary to process sentences that contain dense phrase structures and trace–antecedent relations do not impinge on the resources necessary to access the verb's lexical properties. Recall that even when confronted with phrase structure-dense, padded cleft-object sentences, Broca's aphasic patients activated the multiple argument structures for a verb. This resource independence occurs even though the verb and the trace–antecedent relation must be computed within the same temporal range during the unfolding of the sentence.[4]

Such a result would seem to count against Caplan and colleagues' (Caplan, 1992; Caplan, Baker, & DeHaut, 1985; Caplan & Hildebrandt, 1988) claim that the combined complexity of concurrent parsing opera-

---

[4] Although Broca's aphasic patients have no problem accessing a verb's thematic properties in sentences where they also have to compute the trace–antecedent relation, perhaps they do not normally compute the trace–antecedent relation just because of the concurrent task of accessing a verb's thematic properties. To examine this possibility we would need to use verbs that vary in their thematic properties and test for reactivation of an antecedent. The single "pool" reduced capacity hypothesis would predict that as the resources necessary to access a verb with multiple argument structures increases, the ability of a Broca's aphasic patient to reactivate an antecedent to a trace would decrease. We are currently testing for this possibility.

tions can exceed the processing capacity of aphasic patients. Likewise, Frazier and Friederici (1991) claim that processing inferential chains (e.g., trace–antecedent relations) interacts with the inability to perform simultaneous operations, reduced memory capacity, and reduced speed of activation. Finally, McNeil et al. (1990) claim that aphasia is secondary to inefficient allocation of attention, suggesting that concurrent operations will tax, and overload, what is left of this attentional resource. These capacity limitation theories, although different in many important respects, commonly imply that a single "pool" of resources is shared by various sentence processing devices.[5] We suggest that there is not a single resource, but multiple resources, each dedicated to a particular process. Of course, perhaps the process of activating thematic and other lexical properties does not fall within the domain of the capacity limitation hypothesis. But if the hypothesis allowed such a restriction on its sphere of influence, other, similar, restrictions could also apply, and the account would not be falsifiable. Another alternative is that capacity limitations are only reflected in off-line performance (as measured by, for example, object manipulation and picture-pointing) where the output of various processes converge on a final decision. Although this may turn out to be the case, the capacity limitation accounts make claims about concurrent and simultaneous processing, and speed of activation—claims that are best tested under the real-time constraints of on-line processing.

Finally, our claim of dedicated resources needs to be evaluated in terms of other aspects of sentence processing that we have not directly examined here (e.g., phrase structure computations and heuristics, lexical preference effects, adjunct versus argument processing, binding relations, etc.). Nevertheless, the notion of a single pool of resources recruited for sentence processing is at least incompatible with the double-dissociation observed in the Zurif et al. and present studies: The pattern of sparing and loss that we have found in Broca's and Wernicke's aphasia appears directly related to the independence of resources recruited during the operation of computing the trace–antecedent relation and the resources recruited during the process of accessing a verb's thematic properties.

---

[5] Note the following differences among these three accounts: Caplan et al. claim a language-specific deficit in aphasia, as do Frazier and Friederici. McNeil et al., however, claim that the language problems observed in aphasia are secondary to an attentional deficit, and thus nonlinguistic processes that require "attention" should also be disrupted. So far as we can tell, McNeil et al. offer no language performance data in support of their hypothesis except for the notion of "variability"; such variability is not surprising when a wide net is cast during subject selection and when no attempt is made to characterize the kinds of sentence constructions yielding the aphasic deficits.

APPENDIX

Verb Types Used in Experiments 1 and 2

Transitive	Dative	Two-complements	Four-complements
exhibit	restore	regret	discover
locate	deliver	claim	recognize
adopt	return	maintain	remember
secure	reserve	assume	indicate
collect	address	accept	state
make	sell	expect	detect
bake	buy	demand	notice
burn	release	require	hear
fix	dig		
catch	feed		
file	lend		
measure	donate		

Sentence Type Examples

Active: The agent discovered the burglary at the dock.

Passive: The burglary was discovered by the agent at the dock.

Cleft-subject: It was the agent who discovered the burglary at the dock on Christmas.

Cleft-object: It was the burglary that the agent discovered at the dock on Christmas.

Padded cleft-subject: It was the agent in the car who discovered the burglary at the dock on Christmas.

Padded cleft-object: It was the burglary that the agent in the car discovered at the dock on Christmas.

REFERENCES

Baker, E. 1986. *Categorization of natural objects by aphasics and non-brain-damaged adults: An experimental analysis of featural dimensions.* Unpublished doctoral dissertation. Clark University, Worcester, MA.

Berwick, R. D., & Weinberg, A. 1984. *The grammatical basis of linguistic performance: Language use and acquisition.* Cambridge, MA: MIT Press.

Boland, J. E. 1991. *The use of lexical knowledge in sentence processing.* Unpublished doctoral dissertation. University of Rochester, Rochester, NY.

Canseco-Gonzalez, E., Shapiro, L. P., Zurif, E. B., & Baker, E. 1990. Predicate-argument structure as a link between linguistic and nonlinguistic representations. *Brain and Language,* **39,** 391–404.

Caplan, D. 1992. *Language: Structure, processing, and disorders.* Cambridge, MA: MIT Press.

Caplan, D., & Hildebrandt, N. 1988. *Disorders of syntactic comprehension.* Cambridge, MA: MIT Press.

Caplan, D., Baker, C., & Dehaut, F. 1985. Syntactic determinants of sentence comprehension in aphasia. *Cognition,* **21,** 117–175.

Clifton, C., Frazier, L., & Connine, C. 1984. Lexical expectations in sentence comprehension. *Journal of Verbal Learning and Verbal Behavior,* **23,** 696–708.

Ferreira, F., & Henderson, J. 1990. The use of verb information in syntactic parsing: Evidence from eye movements and word-by-word self-paced reading. *Journal of Experimental Psychology: Learning, Memory, and Cognition,* **16,** 555–568.

Fodor, J. A., Garrett, M. F., & Bever, T. G. 1968. Some syntactic determinants of sentential complexity. II. Verb structure. *Perception and Psychophysics,* **3,** 453–461.

Francis, W. N., & Kucera, H. 1982. *Frequency analysis of English usage.* Boston: Houghton-Mifflin.

Frazier, L., & Friederici, A. 1991. On deriving the properties of agrammatic comprehension. *Brain and Language,* **40,** 51–66.

Goodglass, H., & Baker, E. H. 1976. Semantic field, naming, and auditory comprehension in aphasia. *Brain and Language,* **3,** 359–374.

Grimshaw, J. 1979. Complement selection and the lexicon. *Linguistic Inquiry,* **10,** 279–326.

Grimshaw, J. 1990. *Argument structure.* Cambridge, MA: MIT Press.

Grodzinsky, Y. 1984. *Language deficits and linguistic theory.* Unpublished doctoral dissertation. Brandeis University, Waltham, MA.

Grodzinsky, Y. 1990. *Theoretical perspective on language disorders.* Cambridge, MA: MIT Press.

Haarmann, H. J., & Kolk, H. H. J. 1991. A computer model of the temporal course of agrammatic sentence understanding: The effects of variation in severity and sentence complexity. *Cognitive Science,* **15,** 49–87.

Hickok, G., Zurif, E. B., & Canseco-Gonzalez, E. 1993. Traces in the explanation of comprehension in Broca's aphasia. *Brain and Language,* **45,** 371–395.

Jackendoff, R. 1990. *Semantic structures.* Cambridge, MA: MIT Press.

Klapp, S. T., Marshburn, E. A., & Lester, P. T. 1983. Short-term memory does not involve "working memory" of information processing: The demise of a common assumption. *Journal of Experimental Psychology: General,* **112,** 240–264.

Kolk, H. H. J., & van Grunsven, M. M. F. 1985. Agrammatism as a variable phenomenon. *Cognitive Neuropsychology,* **2,** 347–384.

MacDonald, M., Just, M. A., & Carpenter, P. A. In press. Working memory constraints on the processing of syntactic ambiguity. *Cognitive Psychology.*

McCleary, C., & Hirst, W. 1986. Semantic classification in aphasia: A study of basic, superordinate, and function relations. *Brain and Language,* **27,** 199–209.

McNeil, M. R., Odell, K., & Tseng, C-H. 1990. Toward the integration of resource allocation into a general theory of aphasia. *Clinical Aphasiology,* **20,** 21–39.

Monsell, S. 1984. Components of working memory underlying verbal skills: A "distributed capacities" view—A tutorial review. In H. Bouma & and D. G. Bouwhuis (Eds.), *Attention and performance X: Control of language processes.* London: Erlbaum.

Ni, W., Fodor, J. D., Crain, S., & Shankweiler, D. 1993. *Evidence of the autonomy of syntax and pragmatics.* Paper presented in the C.U.N.Y. Sentence Processing Conference, Amherst, MA.

Pesetsky, D. 1983. *Paths and categories.* Unpublished doctoral dissertation. MIT, Cambridge, MA.

Prather, P., Shapiro, L. P., Zurif, E. B., & Swinney, D. 1991. Real-time examination of lexical processing in aphasia. *Journal of Psycholinguistic Research,* **23,** 271–281.

Schmauder, R., Kennison, S., & Clifton, C. 1991. On the conditions necessary for observing argument structure complexity effects. *Journal of Experimental Psychology: Learning, Memory, and Cognition,* **17,** 1188–1192.

Shapiro, L. P., & Levine, B. A. 1990. Verb processing during sentence comprehension in aphasia. *Brain and Language,* **38,** 21–47.

Shapiro, L. P., Nagel, N., & Levine, B. A. 1993. Preferences for a verb's complements and their use in sentence processing. *Journal of Memory and Language,* **32,** 96–114.

Shapiro, L. P., Zurif, E., & Grimshaw, J. 1987. Sentence processing and the mental representation of verbs. *Cognition*, **27**, 219–246.

Shapiro, L. P., Zurif, E., & Grimshaw, J. 1989. Verb representation and sentence processing: contextual impenetrability. *Journal of Psycholinguistic Research*, **18**, 223–243.

Shapiro, L. P., Brookins, B., Gordon, B., & Nagel, N. 1991. Verb effects during sentence processing. *Journal of Experimental Psychology: Learning, Memory, and Cognition*, **17**, 983–996.

Swinney, D., & Osterhaut, L. 1990. Inference generation during auditory language comprehension. In A. Graesser & G. Bower (Eds.), *Inferences and text comprehension*. San Diego: Academic Press.

Swinney, D., Zurif, E. B., & Nicol, J. 1989. The effects of focal brain damage on sentence processing: An examination of the neurological organization of a mental module. *Journal of Cognitive Neuroscience*, **1**, 25–37.

Stowe, L. 1989. Thematic structures and sentence comprehension. In G. N. Carlson & M. K. Tanenhaus (Eds.), *Linguistic structure in language processing*. Dordrecht: Kluwer Academic.

Tanenhaus, M. K., Carlson, G. N., & Trueswell, J. C. 1989. The role of thematic structures in interpretation and parsing. *Language and Cognitive Processing, Special Edition, Parsing and Interpretation*, **4**, 211–234.

Thompson, C. K., Shapiro, L. P., & Roberts, M. 1993. Treatment of sentence production deficits in aphasia: a linguistic-specific approach. *Aphasiology*, **7**, 111–133.

Trueswell, J. C., Tanenhaus, M. K., & Kello, C. 1993. Verb-specific constraints in sentence processing: Separating effects of lexical preference from garden-paths. Submitted for publication.

Williams, E. 1980. Predication. *Linguistic Inquiry*, **11**, 203–238.

Zurif, E., Caramazza, A., & Meyerson, R. 1974. Semantic feature representation for normal and aphasic language. *Brain and Language*, **1**, 167–187.

Zurif, E., Swinney, D., Prather, P., Solomon, J., & Bushell, C. 1993. An on-line analysis of syntactic processing in Broca's and Wernicke's aphasia. *Brain and Language*, **45**, 447–463.

BRAIN AND LANGUAGE **45,** 448–464 (1993)

An On-Line Analysis of Syntactic Processing in Broca's and Wernicke's Aphasia

E. ZURIF,*·† D. SWINNEY,‡·§ P. PRATHER,*·†·‖ J. SOLOMON,† AND C. BUSHELL§·¶

Division of Linguistics & Cognitive Science, Brandeis University; †Aphasia Research Center, Boston University School of Medicine; ‖Boston V. A. Medical Center; ‡University of California, San Diego; §Graduate Center, CUNY; ¶Manhattan V. A. Medical Center

This paper is about syntactic processing in aphasia. Specifically, we present data concerning the ability of Broca's and Wernicke's aphasic patients to link moved constituents and empty elements in real time. We show that Wernicke's aphasic patients carry out this syntactic analysis in a normal fashion, but that Broca's aphasic patients do not. We discuss these data in the context of some current grammar-based theories of comprehension limitations in aphasia and in terms of the different functional commitments of the brain regions implicated in Broca's and Wernicke's aphasia, respectively. © 1993 Academic Press, Inc.

INTRODUCTION

Comprehension in Broca's Aphasia: Representational Considerations

Most Broca's aphasic patients show sentence-level comprehension impairments.[1] Their comprehension is particularly vulnerable when one ele-

The writing of the manuscript and the research reported in it were supported by NIH Grants DC 00081 and AG10496 and by AFOSR-91-0225. We are very grateful to Hiram Brownell, Carole Palumbo, and Catherine Stern for their help. Address reprint requests to E. Zurif, Division of Linguistics & Cognitive Science, Department of Psychology, Brandeis University, Waltham, MA 02254.

[1] A few Broca's patients do not show sentence-level comprehension problems (Kolk et al., 1985; Miceli et al., 1983; Nespoulous et al., 1988). But since those that do far outweigh those that do not, the exceptional cases must be considered as checks that cannot yet be cashed. They may be anomalous (outlier) subjects. Or they might disprove the notion that lesions that cause agrammatic output also cause problems in comprehension. And partly as a response to this last possibility—but partly also because models of syntactic production are far less detailed than those for comprehension (Bock, 1991)—very few, if any, researchers still focus on the notion of an overarching agrammatism—an agrammatism that implicates the same structures in speaking and listening. Yet, as we will try to show, even if the

77

ment in a sentence must be interpreted with respect to another element
in that sentence. So, for example, given sentences of the sort "Bill
watched John bandage him," the Broca's patients perform at chance
level, often taking "him" to refer to "John" (Caplan & Hildebrandt,
1988; Grodzinsky, 1990; Grodzinsky, Wexler, Chien, Marakovitz, & Solomon, 1992).

Another type of intrasentence dependency relation that Broca's patients are unable to deal with normally, arises as a result of constituent
movement (e.g., Ansell & Flowers, 1982; Caplan & Futter, 1986; Caramazza & Zurif, 1976; Grodzinsky, 1986; Hickok, Zurif, & Canesco-
Gonzalez, 1993; Wulfeck, 1988). The relevant hypothesis here is that
movement of a phrasal constituent leaves a trace in S(urface) structures—an abstract, phonologically unrealized placeholder—in the vacated position. Traces are held to be crucial for the assignment of thematic roles in a sentence, such roles being assigned to hierarchically
structured sentence positions regardless of the identity of the assignee.
If a thematic position is filled with a lexical noun phrase then it receives
its thematic role directly, but if a thematic position contains a trace (an
empty category), then the trace is assigned the thematic role and the
moved constituent that left the trace (e.g., the first noun phrase in a
passive) gets its role only indirectly, by being coindexed (abstractly
linked) to the trace (Chomsky, 1981).

The Broca's patients' problem with traces, or empty categories, has
been foregrounded in several recent description generalizations (Grodzinsky, 1986, 1989, 1990; Hickok, 1992; Mauner, Cornell, & Fromkin, 1990).
The general hypothesis is that although Broca's patients appreciate hierarchical syntactic organization, they cannot represent traces and therefore cannot grammatically assign thematic roles to moved constituents
for comprehension purposes. Faced with thematically unassigned noun
phrases, the patients rely on nongrammatical strategies—in Grodzinsky's
(e.g., 1986) formulation, the strategy is claimed to be that of assigning
the thematic role of agent to the first encountered noun phrase (Bever,
1970); in Hickok's (1992) version, a fill-in strategy is hypothesized.

For some constructions the strategies work, for others, they do not.
Consider, for example, Grodzinsky's (e.g., 1986, 1989) treatment of object-relative and subject-relative constructions: respectively, "The girl$_i$
whom the boy is pushing (t$_i$) is tall" and "The boy$_i$ who$_i$ (t)$_i$ pushes the
girl is tall." (In each example, the vacated position, or gap, is indicated

---

question concerning parallelism remains open, Broca's aphasia—and Wernicke's aphasia,
too—continue to serve research. They continue to be mined for answers to other aspects
of brain–language relations—including in this respect the topic we focus upon here: the
neurological organization of the comprehension system alone.

by the trace (t) and the coindexation of the moved constituent (antecedent) and trace is shown by the subscript (i).) In the object-relative construction, the antecedent ("the girl") has been moved from object position—"the girl" is the theme of the action, not its agent—and so application of the agent-first strategy leads to miscomprehension. By contrast, for subject-relative constructions, the trace appears in the subject position. Thus, the agent-first strategy works—were grammatical capacity normal, it would yield the same solution.

This illustration reflects only a few of the details of Grodzinsky's (1986, 1990) trace-deletion hypothesis and none of those present in Hickok's (1992) reworking of it. What it does serve to emphasize, however, is the general point of these two accounts: namely, that for comprehension purposes Broca's aphasic patients are unable to represent intrasentence dependency relations involving traces. Indeed, in Hickok's formulations, the Broca's problem with traces is invoked even to account for their poor performance with dependencies involving overt pronouns.

Comprehension in Broca's Aphasia: Processing Considerations

The characterizations put forth by Grodzinsky and Hickok constitute efforts to describe what can and cannot be syntactically represented by Broca's aphasic patients. They are descriptive generalizations only; they do not address the *source* of the representational limitation—whether it reflects a partial loss of syntactic competence (knowledge) or whether it is due to a disruption to the processes that implement syntactic knowledge in real time.

There are data that do bear upon these alternatives, however, and they point rather convincingly to a processing explanation of the limitation. Specifically, Linebarger, Schwartz, and Saffran (1983) have reported that agrammatic Broca's aphasics who showed noticeable syntactic limitations in comprehension were, nonetheless, able to detect a wide variety of grammatical deformations, including those that required an awareness of syntactic dependencies involving traces. What emerges from this is a picture of agrammatic Broca's aphasic patients in which they can be seen to carry out quite complex syntactic judgments, yet lack the ability to exploit this sensitivity for comprehension. In effect, the patients seem to retain knowledge of syntactic structure, and, therefore, their inability to represent traces must be due to some defect in the comprehension system, itself—in the system that converts the input stream into an interpreted structure (Sproat, 1986). So, the data gained by Linebarger et al. do, indeed, suggest the need for a processing explanation of agrammatic comprehension. But of what sort?

Linebarger et al. (1983) opt for a mapping explanation. In their words, the problem arises ". . . not from a failure to parse sentences for their grammatical functions, but rather from a difficulty in assigning those functions the appropriate thematic roles."

Several points about this hypothesis warrant consideration. First, we do not think that the grammatical judgment data compel a mapping hypothesis or, more pointedly, indicate normal parsing. Sensitivity to some grammatical deformations need not depend upon the normal construction of a coherent syntactic representation. Specifically, it is one thing to notice the absence of an empty (trace) position in a deformed "sentence," and quite another matter to fill that position in a nondeformed sentence with the correct antecedent during the strictly time constrained initial structure-building stage. Sensitivity in the first instance will yield good performance on a grammatical judgment task, but only the latter capacity will yield a normally complete syntactic representation that can support subsequent thematic mapping (Wulfeck, 1988; Zurif & Grodzinsky, 1983). Indeed, this difference quite possibly implicates a hemispheric difference; as reported by Baynes and Gazzaniga (1987; Gazzaniga, 1989), the right hemisphere of "split-brain" patients can support grammaticality judgments, but cannot process syntactic information for the purpose of comprehension.

In addition, it should be noted that if there were to be a mapping problem, it would clearly not be an undifferentiated one—one that arises for all syntactic types. Schwartz and her colleagues acknowledge this by pointing to what they term a "thematic transparency effect"—viz., that agrammatic Broca's patient's have noticeably more difficulty in mapping moved noun phrases than in mapping noun phrases directly in thematic positions (Schwartz, Linebarger, Saffran, & Pate, 1987).

However, by failing to provide any evidence for the selective disruption of processing modules in terms of their real-time operating characteristics, Linebarger et al. have no basis for distinguishing mapping failures from prior parsing failures (Zurif & Swinney, in press). In fact, as the experimental work reported below indicates, when real-time processing properties are revealed through the application of an on-line analysis, parsing is observed *not* to be intact in Broca's aphasia.

The Present Approach: Broca's and Wernicke's Aphasia Compared

The analysis we present here is based on measures of early-stage lexical activation characteristics. It widens the focus to include Wernicke's aphasic patients as well as Broca's patients and it builds upon the consistently reported observation that Wernicke's aphasics have normal automatic lexical access functions and that Broca's do not. The data come from studies of lexical access involving priming (Blumstein, Milberg, & Shrier, 1982; Katz, 1986; Milberg & Blumstein, 1981; Milberg, Blumstein,

& Dworetsky, 1987; Prather, Shapiro, Zurif, & Swinney, 1991; Prather, Zurif, Stern, & Rosen, 1992; Swinney, Zurif, & Nicol, 1989). Lexical priming—facilitation in the processing of one word caused by the prior presentation of a related word—has been taken to indicate that contacting the related prime somehow lowers the recognition threshold for all words within its semantic or associative sphere (Meyer, Schvaneveldt, & Ruddy, 1975). So, to state the matter directly in terms of the data, Wernicke's patients but not Broca's patients show the normal pattern of facilitated word recognition (lexical decision) in semantically related contexts.

We hasten to emphasize, however, that Broca's patients are not completely insensitive to prime–target relations—they are not, after all, disbarred from activating lexical meanings. Rather, for Broca's patients, priming seems to be temporally protracted; lexical activation, as revealed by priming tasks, seems to have a slower-than-normal time course (Prather et al., in press; Swinney et al., 1989).

The effects of this form of aberrant lexical access may reasonably be supposed to ramify throughout the comprehension system. And our particular concern here is how an impoverished lexical data base might impinge upon the syntactic operation of linking antecedents and traces— upon just that operation that Broca's patients seem unable to carry out.

Central to this concern is the fact that traces have real-time processing consequences. Just as the presence of a relative pronoun immediately activates its antecedent, so too, in the relevant instances, traces are immediately linked to their antecedents when the traces (gaps) are encountered. This phenomenon, referred to as gap filling, reveals that antecedents actually fill the gap left by their movement. (See Swinney and Fodor (1989) and Swinney and Osterhout (1990) for reviews of this work.) This is an operation that is implemented under strict time constraints. And this being so, the inability of Broca's aphasic patients to represent antecedent–trace relations can be viewed in real-time terms as the inability to reactivate the moved constituent at the normal time in the processing sequence—in time, that is, to fill the gap left by its movement (and indexed by the trace).

In the present experiment we have examined the possibility of this scenario—and the possibility that it holds not for all aphasic patients, but for Broca's patients only—by assessing gap filling in Broca's patients and Wernicke's patients.[2] We used subject-relative constructions of the sort, "The gymnast loved the professor$_i$ from the northwestern city who$_i$ (t)$_i$ complained about the bad coffee." As shown by this example, move-

---

[2] We also assessed gap filling in 16 neurologically intact subjects of roughly the same age as the aphasic patients. The sentences used for this assessment were the same as those for the present study; in fact, the neurologically intact subjects were used to pretest the sentences.

ment from subject position is hypothesized. Technically, it is the Wh
element ("who") that has been moved from the subject position of the
relative clause. But since "who" and "the professor" (the head of the
relative clause) corefer, "who" inherits the semantics of "the professor." In sum, as indicated by the subscript (i), "the professor" must be
indirectly linked to the trace in the subject position to receive its thematic
role.

Our hypothesis that there is movement from subject position warrants
some consideration. Such movement is referred to as string-vacuous
movement; this is because the transformation does not reorder the elements in the string. Some investigators disagree with this analysis (Chomsky, 1986). Still, it remains relatively widely accepted with rather broad
cross-linguistic empirical support (e.g., Clements, McCloskey, Maling,
& Zaenen, 1983). And so for present purposes we assume that there *is*
movement from subject position. But even were future research to reveal
this not to be the optimal analysis, the main feature of our inquiry would
still stand. Specifically, were there not to be a trace following the relative
pronoun, we would be charting the formation of antecedent-relative pronoun links—we would still be assessing aphasic comprehension in terms
of the ability to establish coindexation in real time. Moreover, under one
currently active hypothesis, even in this circumstance the antecedent
must eventually link to a trace. Namely, under the verb-phrase-internal-
subject hypothesis (Burton & Grimshaw, in press; Kitagawa, 1986; Koopman & Sportiche, 1988), the relative pronoun occupies its surface position via movement from within the verb phrase. Therefore, a syntactic
chain is formed in which the antecedent is still indirectly linked to a trace
through the relative pronoun, but now the trace is in the verb phrase.
However, having entered these possibilities to make the point that our
study is not hostage to future linguistic developments, we again emphasize the current viability of our assumption of movement from subject
position.

In any event, we chose the subject-relative construction because it
offered the possibility of revealing whether the brain areas implicated
in Broca's and Wernicke's aphasia are distinguishable in terms of their
functional commitments to sentence processing. The relevant point in
this respect is that Broca's and Wernicke's differ, not only in terms of
lexical access characteristics, but also in their ability to understand the
subject-relative construction. Broca's patients, as already indicated,
show relatively normal comprehension for this construction. But Wernicke's patients are unpredictable, more often than not showing chance
comprehension (Grodzinsky, 1984; Shankweiler, personal communication, February, 1992). Our questions, then, were these: Do Broca's patients show normal parsing, as Lineberger et al. (1983) would have it?
Or does their aberrant lexical access pattern disallow normal gap filling,

requiring, in consequence, an abnormal reliance on one or another non-grammatical heuristic for thematic assignment? And to consider a reverse scenario, do Wernicke's aphasics show normal gap filling even though they often fail ultimately to achieve a normal level of comprehension for this sentence type?

Our assessment of gap filling and the range of possibilities just outlined employed an on-line task termed cross-modal lexical priming (CMLP) (Swinney, 1979; Swinney, Onifer, Prather, & Hirshkowitz, 1979). Subjects listened to a sentence over earphones (delivered uninterruptedly and at a normal speaking rate) and at one point, while listening to the sentence, were required to make a lexical decision for a visually presented letter string flashed on a screen in front of them. What we sought to discover was whether a word probe related to the moved constituent was primed at the gap—whether, in effect, the moved constituent was reactivated at the gap to serve as the prime.

METHODS

Subjects

The subjects in this experiment were eight male outpatients at either the Boston V. A. Medical Center or the Manhattan V. A. Medical Center. They all had left CVAs. Four of the eight patients were diagnosed as Broca's aphasic patients, and four as Wernicke's aphasic patients. In each case, diagnosis was based on the convergence of clinical consensus and the results of one or another standardized aphasia examination. Although the time interval between diagnosis and our experimental analysis varied considerably across patients, they had all retained the defining features of their initial diagnosis. So when tested by us, the four Broca's patients still presented with nonfluent and telegraphic verbal output and with relative sparing of auditory comprehension at the conversational level; and the four Wernicke's patients still had fluent, relatively empty speech and three of the four also had noticeable comprehension impairments.

In what follows, we list the age and educational level of each patient, the aphasia examination on which each was initially assessed, and with one exception, each patient's score on a picture matching test of active and passive voice sentence comprehension—a test that was administered around the time of our experimental inquiry. We also note when each patient suffered his stroke, and we briefly describe the available neuroradiological findings.

Broca's aphasic patients. RD is 75 years old with 2 years of college education. The Boston Diagnostic Aphasia Examination (BDAE) (Goodglass & Kaplan, 1972) administered in 1978 conformed the clinical impression of Broca's aphasia. He also exhibited the typical Broca's pattern on our test of sentence-level comprehension, performing better with semantically reversible active sentences (100%) than with semantically reversible passive sentences (60%). RD had two left CVAs—one in 1976 and the other in 1977. A CT scan administered in 1978 indicated two lesions, one in Broca's area with deep extension to left frontal horn and involving lower motor cortex (face and lip regions), the other in the left temporal lobe which spared, however, most of Wernicke's area.

FC is 59 years old with a college education. He was diagnosed as a Broca's aphasic via the BDAE administered in 1982 (and as with all other patients in this study, also on the basis of a clinical workup). On our comprehension test, he scored—in the fashion of most Broca's aphasic patients—better on actives (95%) than on passives (70%). These patterns arose consequent to a left CVA suffered in 1973, with complete occlusion of the left central artery. There are no radiological data available for this patient.

RH is 52 years old with a high school education. The BDAE administered in 1983, in agreement with clinical findings, indicated that he was a Broca's aphasic patient. And on our comprehension test he also showed the Broca's active–passive difference, scoring 90% correct for the former and 20% for the latter. He suffered a left-sided CVA in 1983. No radiological report was available for this patient.

RR is 42 years old with a high school education. His profile on the Western Aphasia Battery (WAB) (Kertesz, 1982) administered in 1991 is consistent with the clinical diagnosis of Broca's aphasia, as are his scores on our comprehension test: 80% correct for active sentences and 40% correct for passive sentences. He suffered a left-sided CVA in 1990, and a CT scan, carried out 2 months later, revealed an ischemic infarct within the territory of supply of the left middle cerebral artery, including posterior extension into the parietal lobe.

Wernicke's aphasic patients. JC is 68 years old with a college education. His performance on the WAB administered in 1986 confirmed the clinical diagnosis of Wernicke's aphasia. Although his comprehension at the sentence level was observed to be impaired on this standardized test, we have no independent assessment available—we were unable to recall him for our active–passive sentence comprehension test. He suffered a hemorrhagic left CVA in 1986. And a recent CT scan revealed solid lesions in Wernicke's area and the left temporal isthmus.

CC is 65 years old and has a high school education. He was administered the BDAE in 1984 and in accord with clinical consensus was diagnosed as a Wernicke's patient. Still, we note that he scored highly on our sentence comprehension test: 100% on actives and 90% on passives. He suffered a left CVA in 1984 and a CT scan done approximately 1 month after the stroke revealed two lesions, one involving a portion of the posterior temporal lobe, including the posterior half of Wernicke's area, with superior extension into supramarginal and angular gyrus areas (surface and deep), and a second in the occipital lobe.

WD is 67 years old with schooling through the ninth grade. The BDAE administered in 1991 confirmed the clinical diagnosis of Wernicke's aphasia. He scored 70% correct for active constructions and 40% for passive constructions on our comprehension assessment. He suffered a left CVA in 1991 and a CT scan done a month and a half later showed a lesion in the posterior half of Wernicke's area, continuing into the supramarginal gyrus and deep to angular gyrus.

JM is 55 years old with a high school education. Clinical consensus and the BDAE carried out in 1986 converged on the diagnosis of Wernicke's aphasia. On our comprehension assessment he scored at the 100% level for active sentences and at the 80% level for passives. His left CVA occurred in 1986 and a CT scan done 2–3 weeks later revealed a vague patchy lesion involving the temporal isthmus which likely interrupted the auditory fibers from the medical geniculate nucleus before reaching Heschl's gyrus and Wernicke's area. The patchy lesion extended superiorly into the posterior supramarginal and angular gyrus areas with deep extension to the border of the left lateral ventricle, interrupting fibers of the auditory contralateral pathways.

We note, in summary, two features of these patient profiles. First, although we do not have neuroradiological findings for all patients, the data that we do have broadly confirm current views on lesion localization (Benson, 1985; Mohr, 1976; Vignolo, 1988): The two Broca's patients for whom CT scan data are available both have left-sided prerolandic lesions (although, as is common, the damage is not restricted to this region). By contrast, all four Wernicke's patients have only posterior lesions, these being located mostly within the temporal lobe and the retrorolandic region of the left hemisphere. Second, the two groups were distinguished by their performance patterns on our sentence comprehension test: whereas all four Broca's patients showed the expected active–passive difference (generally good performance on actives and bad on passives), the Wernicke's patients were inconsistent in this respect. As others have observed (Caramazza & Zurif, 1976; Grodzinsky, 1990), performance for this group cannot be predicted solely on the basis of syntactic factors.

Stimulus Materials

The experimental sentences consisted of 48 auditorily presented subject-relative constructions. To use our earlier illustration, the sentences were all of the form, "The gymnast loved the professor$_i$ from the northwestern city[1] who$_i$[2] (t_i) complained about the bad coffee." Again, by hypothesis, and as indicated by the subscript (i), the trace is assigned the thematic role (the role of "complainer" and "the professor" gets this role only indirectly—by being coindexed through the relative pronoun to the trace.

For each experimental sentence, a set of two words was created to be used as visual probes for the examination of priming. One of the words—the experimental probe—was semantically related to the moved constituent (the antecedent). The other word—the control probe—was unrelated to the antecedent. It was, however, matched to the experimental probe in frequency and length (Francis & Kucera, 1982). For the above example, the experimental probe was "teacher" (related to the antecedent, "professor") and the control probe was "address." The semantically related (experimental) probes were selected, in each instance, by combining data from published norms (Jenkins, 1970; Keppel & Strand, 1970; Postman, 1970) with data obtained by polling college-age and elderly adults for their first associates to the words that were later incorporated in the sentences as moved constituents.

As indicated by the superscripts 1 and 2 in the above example, priming was examined for each sentence at two points—at the gap indexed by the trace (superscript 2) and at a pregap position (superscript 1). We assessed priming at position 2 in order to measure whether the moved constituent was reactivated, or filled, at the gap (thus providing the prime). The pregap position (position 1) allowed us to measure any residual activation from the earlier appearance of the antecedent; that is, it enabled a baseline examination of any nonsyntactic priming effects. Of course, at each position priming was determined by comparing the lexical decision time for the experimental probe to that for the control probe.

Apparatus and Stimulus Construction

The sentences were presented auditorily on a Sharp Cassette Recorder (RD-771AV) with an internal tone decoder, the recording having been made by a female speaker, speaking at a normal rate. The letter-string probes were presented visually, appearing either on a Zenith 287 video monitor connected to a Protege 286 computer or on a Sony monitor (SSM-121) connected to a Compaq Portable II computer.

Coordination of the visual and auditory components for the experimental sentences was accomplished as follows: Each of the sentences was initially recorded on one channel only of a Teac reel-to-reel recorder. On another channel, for each sentence, a tone was placed to coincide with either the pregap position or the gap position. To place these tones, all sentences were digitized on a MAC II computer and examined visually as well as auditorily.[3] This material—the sentences and their associated tones—was then transferred to the stereo cassette. The tone for each sentence—inaudible to the subjects—served to trigger (via the tone decoder) the visual presentation of the letter-string probe so that the string appeared

---

[3] The digitizer with the MAC recorder eliminates frequencies over 17 kHz, which is well above the normal range of speech.

at the center of the monitor either at the offset of the word preceding the pregap position or at the offset of the relative pronoun ("who") preceding the gap position. The tone simultaneously initiated timing for the lexical decision. Subjects indicated their lexical decision using two response buttons which could be depressed using the index and middle fingers of their left hand. As soon as either button was depressed, the reaction time for that decision (in milliseconds) was recorded under software control, and the letter string was removed from the screen. If the subject did not respond within 2750 msec, the letter string was removed and that trial terminated.

RTLAB software (V9.0) controlled the experiment. With the aid of a software-accessible clock card (Metrobyte CIM05), RTLAB enables the synchronization of stimulus presentation with monitor raster position so that lexical decision timing is accurate beginning from stimulus onset.

Design

Two scripts were created. Each script contained one-half (i.e., 24) of the experimental subject-relative sentences and 101 filler sentences. Within each script, 12 of the 24 subject-relative constructions were presented in conjunction with visual probe words appearing at the gap, and 12 with visual probes presented at the pregap position. Six of the 12 gap probes in each script were experimental probes (letter strings forming words semantically related to the antecedent) and 6 were control probes. Likewise, 6 of the 12 pregap probes in each script were experimental and 6 control. Two versions of each script were prepared, the two differing from one another only in the matter of probe location—where one version contained a particular sentence with a gap probe, the other contained that sentence with the same probe at the pregap position.

Each subject was presented with *one* version of each of the *two* scripts. Thereby, as desired, each subject heard each of the 48 experimental subject-relative sentences *once only*. As a result, each subject contributed only one data point for any one sentence—one lexical decision time for either the experimental or the control probe in either the gap or the pregap position. Thus, across all 48 sentences, each patient contributed 12 data points per condition—12 reaction-time entries for the pregap experimental probe condition, 12 reaction-time entries for the pregap control probe condition, and the same number of entries for each of these two conditions at the gap location. Given this design, four subjects per aphasic group were necessary to satisfy both probe locations and to ensure that each experimental probe could be compared to its control. And with four subjects per group, each group generated 48 data points per condition.

As for the 101 filler sentences in each script, 38 were coupled with visually presented real words and 63 with visually presented pronounceable nonwords. These filler sentences were syntactically similar to the experimental sentences. But to diminish the possibility of a "position set," the visual probes associated with the filler sentences were placed at different positions from those associated with the experimental (subject-relative) sentences.[4]

Procedure

Subjects were tested individually in two sessions not more than 2 weeks apart, each lasting 45 min to 1 hr. They were fitted with headphones and seated at a table containing the video monitor and the lexical decision keys. They were instructed on both the auditory and the visual aspects of the task.

---

[4] Actually, 24 of the 38 filler sentences coupled with real-word probes were target sentences for another experiment. But since this other experiment is irrelevant to the analysis presented here, they can be considered, for present purposes, as fillers.

With respect to the former, they were told that they would hear a series of sentences over the headphones and that their task was to listen carefully to each sentence. To encourage attention to the sentences, for each subject, we stopped the tape 14 times over the two sessions to ask a question about the sentence that was just presented. These questions did not bear on thematic assignment; ultimate interpretation of the sentences was not at issue. What was at issue was whether parsing was normal in respect to gap filling. Accordingly, we designed our questions only to reinforce the need for the subjects to listen to the sentences—using a multiple choice format, we asked only about the setting or general topic of a sentence (e.g., "Where did the activity occur—in a saloon? a classroom? or a police station?" or "Was the sentence about sports, music, or TV?") Indeed we did not even restrict the 14 questions of this sort to the experimental sentences; we also asked them of the filler sentences.

Subjects were also told that there would be a second, simultaneous task that they would have to perform: They would see a string of letters appear on the screen in front of them at some point during the presentation of each sentence, and they would have to decide as quickly and accurately as possible whether the letter string formed a word. They were instructed on the use of the response keys to indicate their decision—on pressing the "yes" key for a word and the "no" key for a nonword.

Each session consisted of 20 practice trials followed by the run-through of one version of one script.

RESULTS

Prior to a statistical analysis of the lexical decision times for the subject-relative constructions, a data screen was applied to remove errors and outliers. Errors consisted of trials on which the patients had incorrectly identified the probe words as nonwords and trials on which they had failed to respond within the maximum allotment of 2750 msec; they also included computer errors. Outliers were defined on an individual patient basis as reaction times that were more than two standard deviations above the subject's overall mean reaction time.[5] The frequencies of errors and outliers are presented in Table 1.

We cannot explain the somewhat lower error rate for the pregap experimental probes. We note, however, that the overall level of errors and outliers is of approximately the same magnitude as that observed in other reaction time studies (e.g., Prather et al., 1992; Shapiro & Levine, 1990).

The screened data for each subject in each condition were replaced by the subject's mean reaction time in each condition. The means of these screened data are presented in Table 2.

The individual reaction times for each subject in each cell were logarithmically transformed and then separately analyzed for the Broca's patients and the Wernicke's patients. For each group we performed two planned comparisons using the error term for a one-factor ANOVA. In one we compared experimental and control probe reaction times at the

---

[5] We also screened outliers on a three standard deviation criterion. Over all data entries for all subjects, this yielded only one less outlier than was found in the two standard deviation screen.

TABLE 1
Number of Errors and Outliers
(of 48 Entries per Cell)

	Pregap experimental		Pregap control		Gap experimental		Gap control	
	Errors	Outliers	Errors	Outliers	Errors	Outliers	Errors	Outliers
Wernicke's patients	2	3	8	1	9	0	5	2
Broca's patients	3	0	8	3	7	2	10	2

pregap position, and in the other, experimental and control probe reaction times at the gap site. Our use of planned comparisons was predicated on the consistent finding that priming for neurologically intact subjects is structurally governed—that is, that it occurs at gap sites and not at other locations. Indeed, we note that the 16 elderly neurologically intact subjects who were used to pretest the experimental sentences for this study (see footnote 2) also showed the expected structurally determined priming pattern: Their mean reaction times for the experimental and control probes, respectively, were 674 and 684 msec at the pregap position and 667 and 688 msec at the gap. The former comparison is not significant ($F < 1.0$), but the latter is ($F(1,15) = 5.153$, $p = .038$).

With respect to the aphasic patients, the planned comparisons straightforwardly reveal that Wernicke's patients immediately filled gaps as they were encountered and that Broca's patients did not. To be sure, the Wernicke's patients' overall base reaction times are longer than those for the neurologically intact subjects—left-sided brain damage seems usually to lessen response speed in a nonspecific way (e.g., Swinney et al., 1989).

TABLE 2
Mean Reaction Times
(msecs)
Visual Probes

	Pregap experimental	Pregap control	Gap experimental	Gap control
Wernicke's patients	1017	1061	982*	1107*
Broca's patients	1145	1125	1126	1058

* Significant difference between reaction time for experimental probe and reaction time for control probe ($F(1,9) = 7.08$, $p = .026$).

But what is relevant to the assessment of gap filling is the priming pattern, not absolute reaction time. And in this respect, the Wernicke's patients appear normal. Specifically, the Wernicke's patient group showed significant priming for the experimental probes at the gap site ($F(1,9) = 7.08, p = .026$) but not at the pregap location ($F < 1.0$). By contrast, the Broca's patient group did not show priming for the experimental probes at either location (gap site: $F < 1.0$; pregap location: $F < 1.0$).[6]

DISCUSSION

Wernicke's aphasic patients show priming of antecedents at syntactically licensed gaps (indexed by traces). Our data, however, leave several questions unanswered concerning this phenomenon. Since all of our experimental sentences contained constituents that could plausibly fill the subject position, we cannot yet tell whether the patients must rely on such plausibility or whether, like normal subjects, they fill all potential gap sites regardless of plausibility (Swinney & Osterhout, 1990) and the site from which movement actually occurred (Hickok, Canseco-Gonzalez, Zurif, & Grimshaw, 1992). What we can conclude from the present data, however, is that Wernicke's patients show a normal sensitivity to structurally licensed gaps and that they automatically reactivate available constituents at these gaps—as sentences unfold in real time.

Does the reactivation of an antecedent at a gap indicate that the patient is assigning a thematic role to that antecedent? Or does this reactivation reflect the consequences of an earlier processing stage—a stage at which elements are coindexed and dependency relations estblished *prior* to thematic assignment? In the light of recent work by Shapiro and Levine (1990), the latter possibility appears much more likely. These investigators have shown that Wernicke's aphasic patients are insensitive in real time to the argument taking properties of verbs. Unlike neurologically intact subjects, the patients are unable to access momentarily all of the possible argument structure configurations within a verb's lexical entry (Shapiro & Levine, 1990; Shapiro, Zurif, & Grimshaw, 1987, 1989). They are unable, that is, to generate a fully elaborated thematic grid (Carlson & Tanenhaus, 1987) in the normal manner. And this being so, it seems most reasonable to interpret the Wernicke's patients' ability to reactivate antecedents at gaps as being syntactically, not thematically, driven—as being the reflection of processing that occurs at a stage prior to thematic

---

[6] We emphasize that the Broca's patients' failure to show gap filling cannot be construed as some global failure to prime. In other, nonsentence circumstances—when presented either with word pairs or word lists—the patients did show priming, even if in a temporally protracted manner.

assignment (or mapping). Indeed, the fact that they were capable of filling gaps in subject-relative sentences for which they show uncertain comprehension (e.g., Grodzinsky, 1984) further strengthens this conclusion. (See also Hickok (1991) for the same interpretation of the gap-filling phenomenon based on studies of normal sentence processing.)

The conclusions we have drawn clearly do not provide a characterization of the role actually played by the cortical tissue implicated in Wernicke's aphasia. Still, we do provide a lower boundary on its functional commitment: whatever its role, it is not crucially involved in the real-time structural analysis required for the recognition and filling of gaps left by constituent movement.

By contrast, left anterior cortex—the cortical region usually implicated in Broca's aphasia—does appear to be necessary for the operation of gap filling. Contrary to Linebarger et al.'s (1983) speculations on the matter, our data show that Broca's patients do have a parsing problem—even for subject-relative sentences which they interpret at a level significantly above chance (e.g., Grodzinsky, 1986, 1989; Hickok, 1992). Either they are abnormally slow in linking antecedents and traces or they fail entirely to link the two. Either way, the consequences of this parsing problem seem relatively straightforward: Since they do not have the processing resources to establish dependency relations normally—to fill the gap at exactly the right time in the processing sequence—they cannot provide the syntactic representation necessary for supporting subsequent thematic assignment to moved constituents. Presumably, therefore, the Broca's patients rely abnormally on some nongrammatical strategy to achieve thematic role assignment for moved constituents—on a fill-in strategy (Hickok, 1992) or an agent-first strategy (Caplan & Futter, 1986; Grodzinsky, 1986). And when such strategies do not work, or when nonstructural length and complexity factors overwhelm their diminished resources,[7] their comprehension fails.

In effect, the parsing problem described here connects directly to previous analyses of the Broca's patients structural limitations. Our data indicate that these grammatical limitations are rooted to fairly elementary processing disruptions—specifically, to disruptions of automatic lexical reactivation (access) at the gap. In this view, the brain region implicated in Broca's aphasia is *not* the locus of syntactic representations per se. Rather, we suggest that this region provides processing resources that sustain one or more of the fixed operating characteristics of the lexical processing system—characteristics that are, in turn, necessary for build-

---

[7] We note, for example, that by increasing the number of main verbs in a sentence from one (the number standardly used) to two—by increasing length, in effect—even subject-relative constructions can be made difficult for Broca's aphasic patients to understand (Caplan & Hildebrandt, 1988).

ing syntactic representations in real time. Possibly these resources sustain the normal speed of lexical processing. This would be in line with independent evidence of slowed lexical processing in Broca's aphasia (Prather et al., 1993) and it is a possibility that we are currently exploring.

REFERENCES

Ansell, B., & Flowers, C. 1982. Aphasic adults' use of heuristic and structural linguistic cues for analysis. *Brain and Language,* **26,** 62–72.

Baynes, K., & Gazzaniga, M. 1987. In Plum (Ed.), *Language communication and the brain.* New York: Raven Press.

Benson, D. F. 1985. Aphasia. In K. Heilman & E. Valenstein (Eds.), *Clinical neuropsychology.* New York: Oxford Univ. Press. Vol. 2.

Bever, T. G. 1970. The cognitive basis of linguistic structures. In J. R. Hayes (Ed.), *Cognition and the development of language.* New York: Wiley.

Blumstein, S., Milberg, W., & Shrier, R. 1982. Semantic processing in aphasia: Evidence from an auditory lexical decision task. *Brain and Language,* **17,** 301–315.

Bock, K. 1991. A sketchbook of production problems. *Journal of Psycholinguistic Research* (Special Issue on Sentence Processing), **20,** 141–160.

Burton, S., & Grimshaw, J. (in press). Active–passive coordination and the VP-internal-subject hypothesis. *Linguistic Inquiry.*

Caplan, D., & Futter, C. 1986. Assignment of thematic roles by an agrammatic aphasic patient. *Brain and Language,* **27,** 117–135.

Caplan, D., & Hildebrandt, N. 1988. *Disorders of syntactic comprehension.* Cambridge, MA: MIT Press.

Caramazza, A., & Zurif, E. B. 1976. Dissociation of algorithmic and heuristic processes in language comprehension: Evidence from aphasia. *Brain and Language,* **3,** 572–582.

Carlson, G., & Tanenhaus, M. 1987. In W. Wilkens (Ed.), *Thematic relations.* New York: Academic Press.

Chomsky, N. 1981. *Lectures on government and binding.* Dordrecht: Foris.

Chomsky, N. 1986. *Barriers.* Cambridge, MA: MIT Press.

Clements, G., McCloskey, J., Mailing, J., & Zaenen, A. 1983. String-vacuous rule application. *Linguistic Inquiry,* **14,** 1–17.

Francis, W., & Kucera, H. 1982. *Frequency analysis of English usage: Lexicon and grammar.* Boston: Houghton Mifflin.

Gazzaniga, M. 1989. Organization of the human brain. *Science,* **245,** 947–951.

Goodglass, H., & Kaplan, E. 1972. *The assessment of aphasia and related disorders.* Philadelphia: Lea & Febiger.

Grodzinsky, Y. 1984. *Language deficits and linguistic theory.* Unpublished doctoral dissertation, Brandeis University, MA.

Grodzinsky, Y. 1986. Language deficits and the theory of syntax. *Brain and Language,* **27,** 135–159.

Grodzinsky, Y. 1989. Agrammatic comprehension of relative clauses. *Brain and Language,* **31,** 480–499.

Grodzinsky, Y. 1990. *Theoretical perspectives on language deficits.* Cambridge, MA: MIT Press.

Grodzinsky, Y., Wexler, K., Chien, Y.-C., Marakovitz, S., & Solomon, J. 1992. *The breakdown of binding relations.* Manuscript, Aphasia Research Center, Boston, MA.

Hickok, G. 1991. *Gaps and Garden-Paths: Studies on the architecture and computational machinery of the human sentence processor.* Unpublished doctoral dissertation, Brandeis University, MA.

Hickok, G. 1992. *Agrammatic comprehension and the trace-deletion hypothesis.* Occasional Paper No. 45, Center for Cognitive Science, MIT.

Hickok, G., Canseco-Gonzalez, E., Zurif, E. B., & Grimshaw, J. (1992). Modularity in locating wh-gaps. *Journal of Psycholinguistic Research,* **21,** 545–561.

Hickok, G., Zurif, E. B., & Canseco-Gonzalez, E. 1993. Traces in the explanation of comprehension of Broca's aphasia. *Brain and Language,* **45,** 371–395.

Jenkins, J. J. 1970. The 1952 Minnesota word association norms. In L. Postman & G. Keppel (Eds.), *Norms of word associations.* New York: Academic Press.

Katz, W. 1986. *An investigation of lexical ambiguity in Broca's aphasics using an auditory lexical priming technique.* Manuscript, Brown University, RI.

Keppel, G., & Strand, B. Z. 1970. Free-association responses to the primary responses and other responses selected from the Palermo–Jenkins norms. In L. Postman & G. Keppel (Eds.), *Norms of word associations.* New York: Academic Press.

Kertesz, A. 1982. *The Western aphasia battery.* New York: Grune & Stratton.

Kitagawa, Y. 1986. *Subjects in Japanese and English.* Unpublished doctoral dissertation, University of Massachusetts, Amherst, MA.

Kolk, H., Van Grunsven, J., & Keyser, A. 1985. One parallelism between production and comprehension in agrammatism. In M.-L. Kean (Ed.), *Agrammatism.* New York: Academic Press.

Koopman, H., & Sportiche, D. 1988. *Subjects.* Unpublished manuscript, Univ. of California, Los Angeles.

Linebarger, M., Schwartz, M., & Saffran, E. 1983. Sensitivity to grammatical structure in so-called agrammatic aphasics. *Cognition,* **13,** 361–393.

Mauner, G., Cornell, T., & Fromkin, V. 1990. *Explanatory models of agrammatism.* Paper presented at the Academy of Aphasia.

Meyer, D., Schvaneveldt, R., & Ruddy, M. 1975. Loci of contextual effects on visual word recognition. In P. Rabbit & S. Dornic (Eds.), *Attention and performance.* New York: Academic Press. Vol. 1.

Miceli, G., Mazzucchi, A., Menn, L., & Goodglass, H. 1983. Contrasting cases of Italian agrammatic aphasia without comprehension disorder. *Brain and Language,* **19,** 65–97.

Milberg, W., & Blumstein, S. 1981. Lexical decision and aphasia: Evidence for semantic processing. *Brain and Language,* **14,** 371–385.

Milberg, W., Blumstein, S., & Dworetsky, B. 1987. Processing of lexical ambiguities in aphasia. *Brain and Language,* **31,** 138–150.

Mohr, J. 1976. Broca's area and Broca's aphasia. In H. Whitaker & H. A. Whitaker (Eds.), *Studies in neurolinguistics.* New York: Academic Press. Vol. 1.

Nespoulous, J.-L., Dordain, M., Perron, C., Ska, B., Bub, D., Caplan, D., Mehler, J., & Lecours, A.-R. 1988. Agrammatism in sentence production without comprehension deficits: Reduced availability of snytactic structures and/or of grammatical morphemes? A case study. *Brain and Language,* **33,** 273–295.

Prather, P., Shapiro, L., Zurif, E., & Swinney, D. 1991. Real-time examinations of lexical processing in aphasics. *Journal of Psycholinguistic Research* (Special Issue on Sentence Processing), **20,** 271–281.

Prather, P., Zurif, E. B., Stern, C., & Rosen, T. J. 1992. Slowed lexical access in nonfluent aphasia. *Brain and Language,* **45,** 336–348.

Postman, L. 1970. The California norms: Association as a function of word frequency. In L. Postman & G. Keppel (Eds.), *Norms of word associations.* New York: Academic Press.

Schwartz, M., Linebarger, M., Saffran, E., & Pate, D. 1987. Syntactic transparency and sentence interpretation in aphasia. *Language and Cognitive Processes,* **2,** 85–113.

Shapiro, L., & Levine, B. 1990. Verb processing during sentence comprehension in aphasia. *Brain & Language,* **38,** 21–47.

Shapiro, L., Zurif, E. B., & Grimshaw, J. 1987. Sentence processing and the mental representation of verbs. *Cognition,* **27,** 219–246.

Shapiro, L., Zurif, E. B., & Grimshaw, J. 1989. Verb processing during sentence comprehension: Contextual impenetrability. *Journal of Psycholinguistic Research,* **18,** 223–243.

Sproat, R. 1986. Competence, performance and agrammatism: A reply to Grodzinsky. *Brain and Language,* **70,** 160–167.

Swinney, D. 1979. Lexical access during sentence comprehension: (Re) consideration of context effects. *Journal of Verbal Learning and Verbal Behavior,* **18,** 645–659.

Swinney, D., & Fodor, J. D. (Eds.) 1989. *Journal of Psycholinguistic Research* (Special Issue on Sentence Processing), **18,**(1).

Swinney, D., Onifer, W., Prather, P., & Hirshkowitz, M. 1979. Semantic facilitation across sensory modalities in the processing of individual words and sentences. *Memory and Cognition,* **7,** 159–165.

Swinney, D., & Osterhout, L. 1990. Inference generation during auditory language comprehension. In A. Graesser & G. Bower (Eds.), *Inferences and text comprehension.* San Diego: Academic Press.

Swinney, D., Zurif, E. B., & Nicol, J. 1989. The effects of focal brain damage on sentence processing: An examination of the neurological organization of a mental nodule. *Journal of Cognitive Neuroscience,* **1,** 25–37.

Vignolo, L. 1988. The anatomical and pathological basis of aphasia. In F. C. Rose, R. Whurr, & M. A. Wyke (Eds.), *Aphasia.* London: Whurr.

Wulfeck, B. 1988. Grammaticality judgments and sentence comprehension in agrammatic aphasia. *Journal of Speech and Hearing Research,* **31,** 72–81.

Zurif, E. B., & Grodzinsky, Y. 1983. Sensitivity of grammatical structure in agrammatic aphasics: A reply. *Cognition* **15,** 207–213.

Zurif, E. B., Swinney, D., & Fodor, J. A. 1991. An evaluation of assumptions underlying the single-patient-only position in neuropsychological research. *Brain and Cognition,* **16,** 198–210.

Zurif, E. B., & Swinney, D. (in press). The neuropsychology of language. In M. Gernsbacher (Ed.), *Handbook of psycholinguistics.* Orlando, FL: Academic Press.

BRAIN AND LANGUAGE **46**, 21–40 (1993)

Morphological Processing in Italian Agrammatic Speakers Syntactic Implementation of Inflectional Morphology

RIA DE BLESER

Department of Neurology, Klinikum RWTH, Aachen, Germany

AND

CLAUDIO LUZZATTI

Milan University, Milan, Italy

Most current linguistic and psycholinguistic characterizations of agrammatic production start from the observation that in spontaneous speech inflectional suffixes are either dropped or substituted by default forms, depending on the morphological structure of the language. So far, little experimental evidence has entered theory construction. In this paper, elicited data of two Italian patients with agrammatic speech are presented. The tasks involved the production of a past participle suffix in different sentence contexts. In Italian, the past participle has to agree in gender and number with the grammatical features of an antecedent noun, pronoun, or empty element. It is shown that both patients mastered the general principles of the agreement rule, and that they could produce correct inflectional suffixes in several tasks. Furthermore, the point of breakdown in their performance was syntactic rather than morphological, namely, when there were no overt morphological cues for the identification of the thematic roles in the sentence. These data cannot be accounted for by theories formulated in terms of the syntactic or postsyntactic deletion of suffixes or the functional elements underlying their realization. At least for the patients in this study, morphological substitutions arose as a result of an impairment in the syntactic processing of content words rather than functors. © 1994 Academic Press, Inc.

INTRODUCTION

Agrammatic spontaneous speech has traditionally been characterized by the following symptoms: (i) lack of function words like complementiz-

This study was supported by grants from the *Deutsche Forschungsgesellschaft*, the Italian *Comitato Nazionale delle Ricerche*, and the *Alexander von Humboldt Stiftung*. We are indebted to J. Bayer and L. Lonzi for suggestions and comments to a previous draft of the manuscript. We are also very grateful for the insightful comments of three anonymous reviewers. Address correspondence and reprint requests to Dr. R. De Bleser, Neurolinguistics Laboratory, Klinikum RWTH, Pauwelsstrasse, D5100 Aachen, Germany.

94

ers, auxiliaries, determiners, and pronouns; (ii) predominant use of non-functional lexical categories such as nouns and verbs; (iii) systematic use of nonfinite constructions such as participles and infinitives; (iv) lack of inflectional morphemes for congruence, tense or case (Tissot, Mounin, & Lhermitte, 1973).

Early linguistic accounts of agrammatism (Kean, 1977; Lapointe, 1985) were based on these definitions. Meanwhile, it has been shown that at least one clinical symptom, namely, inflectional suffix dropping, is not a correct characterization, since in many languages suffixes are substituted rather than stripped (Menn and Obler, 1990a,b; Bates and Wulfeck, 1989).

It has been proposed that substitution rather than deletion occurs if dropping would result in the production of a nonword. This would violate Lasnik's filter (Baker, 1988; Pesetzky, 1989), which says that the morphological subcategorization frame of a lexical element must be filled at the level of S-structure.

Grodzinsky (1990) gives examples from Russian supporting this view. He also proposes that agrammatic speech production shows changes of S-structural representations, because nonlexical terminal elements would be deleted. This includes all grammatical suffixes as well as function words. Their grammatical features would thus no longer be available for grammatical processes. Grodzinsky's theory is basically a postsyntactic morphological account. The structural representation system itself would be unaffected. Also for Bates and Wulfeck (1989), the disorder would be morphological rather than syntactic, but they place morphology in the lexicon rather than at S-structure.

A morpholexical rather than a morphosyntactic position is also taken by Miceli and Caramazza (1988) to explain the performance pattern of their Italian agrammatic patient. Moreover, these authors propose that derivation and inflection are dissociable, because the patient showed spared derivation but impaired inflection in word repetition. On the other hand, Menn and Obler (1990a) conclude for agrammatic aphasics in 14 languages that lexical morphology, derivation as well as inflection, is relatively spared in agrammatism and that the disorder should be characterized as an impairment of the syntactic frames in which morphology must be implemented. This interpretation of a dissociation between morphology and syntax was also proposed by De Bleser and Bayer (1988) on the basis of eli :ited production data with German patients.

In this paper, we report the performance of two Italian patients with agrammatic speech, MG and DR, in a variety of morphosyntactic production tasks. The morpholexical performance of these patients has been described elsewhere (Luzzatti & De Bleser, submitted). Both patients were able to extract gender features from the inflectional suffix of simple as well as derived nouns, and they could realize number inflection at least for the regular paradigm. Essentially, the patients' morpholexicon was apparently spared with respect to rule-governed access to inflection, and DR's performance only broke down if access depended crucially on a full-listing procedure (irregular inflection). Thus, the data did not support the morpholexical explanation of agrammatic speech proposed by Bates and Wulfeck (1989) and they did not conform to the morpholexical dissociation reported by Miceli and Caramazza (1988). At least the agrammatism of MG and DR seemed to result from a nonlexical disorder.

To examine the interaction of morphology and other grammatical processes, we selected the production of inflectional suffixes of past participles in different syntactic contexts. Past participles in Italian consist of the verbal root followed by $-t$ and a further inflectional ending which may have one of four forms: $-o$ (unmarked or masc.sg.), $-i$ (masc.pl.), $-a$ (fem.sg.), $-e$ (fem.pl). The inflectional ending reflects gender and number agreement with a grammatical antecedent.

If, as Grodzinsky (1990) proposes, grammatical features of suffixes are unavailable, participle agreement should be impossible already in simple sentences. A syntactic deficit hypothesis, however, would predict performance differences reflecting syntactic complexity.

Before introducing the test material, some basic facts must be described about agreement phenomena in Italian.

PARTICIPLE AGREEMENT IN ITALIAN

In linguistic theory, Italian participle agreement can simply be captured by the general principle that the past participle will agree (in gender and number) with an element holding a binding relation with its direct object (Burzio, 1987, pp. 53–56).

The descriptive situation, however, is very heterogeneous (Schwarze, 1988): There is past participle agreement with a subject in some cases and with a direct object in others, and frequently there is no agreement with any element in the sentence. Furthermore, the rule of agreement is interrelated with the distribution of the auxiliary verbs *essere* and *avere*. In *essere* sentences (ergatives and passives), there is always gender and number agreement with a surface subject (derived from an underlying direct object), but there is never subject agreement for *avere* verbs (intransitives and active transitives). In fact, the past participle of intransitive verbs always has the masculine singular form on $-o$, the default form in case of no agreement, while active transitives have obligatory agreement with a direct object only if this is cliticized, not, however, with a noncliticized direct object. In no circumstances does agreement with the indirect object take place.

The following examples should clarify this interaction.

Examples for participle agreement

Truly intransitive:
```
perfect:    [Maria]    [ha  telefonato a  Rosa]
                 fem            ø         fem
                 sg                       sg
             Maria      has telephoned to Rosa
perfect:    [Maria]    [le_i  ha    telefonato (e_i)]
clit.indir.obj.                                ø
             Maria      her has telephoned
```

Ergative "intransitive:"
```
perfect:    [Maria_i]   [è     arrivata_i   t_i]
                 fem            fem
                 sg             sg
             Maria       is ( = has) arrived
```

Transitive verbs:
```
active perfect:    [Gli amici]    [hanno     chiamato Rosa]
                                   masc    (avere)      ø    fem
                                   pl      (3rd pl.)          sg
                   The friends    have        called    Rosa

active perfect:    [Gli amici]    [la_i hanno chiamata_i (e_i)]
clit.dir.obj.                      masc fem             fem
                                   pl   sg              sg
                   The friends    her  have  called

passive present:   [Rosa_i]    [è chiamata  t_i  dagli  amici]
                       fem         fem
                       sg          sg
                   Rosa        is called      by the friends
```

The general principles of participle agreement discussed above for simple sentences also apply for complex sentences, where the agreement rules may have to refer to coindexation across clause boundaries.

Consequently, difficulties in establishing grammatical agreement may depend on variables such as (i) the lexical category of the antecedent, (ii) the argument structure of the verb, and (iii) the availability of overt cues for parsing complex sentences.

(i) The lexical category of the antecedent for agreement may be a noun or a pronoun. In Italian the subject pronoun may generally be dropped (pro-drop). In this case, the grammatical number necessary for participle agreement can be extracted only from the inflectional ending of the verb.

Examples of coindexation of participle with

Noun
```
antecedent:    la     ragazza_i è    andata_i      al cinema
               The    girl      is   ( = has) gone  to the movies
```

Pronoun
```
antecedent:    il     ragazzo la_i   ha vista_i
               The    boy      her    has seen
```

Pro-drop antecedent:
Siamo$_j$ andati (/e)$_j$ dalla nonna ($-i$:ms; $-e$:fm)
   (aux. suffix)   We are (= have) gone to the grandma

(ii) The argument structure of the verb is crucial for the application of the agreement rule. Intransitive and transitive active verbs, where the surface and deep subject are identical, take the auxiliary verb *avere*, and agreement with the subject never occurs. Ergative and passive transitive verbs, where the surface subject is the underlying object, take the auxiliary verb *essere*, and agreement occurs with the surface subject (see examples above).

(iii) In complex sentences, coindexation between antecedent and participle may be across clause boundaries.

Example of coordination

Il ragazzo$_i$ ha salutato la vicina   #   e (PRO)$_i$ è arrossito$_i$
The boy has greeted the neighbor woman and (he) is blushed

Example of subordination: object relative clause

Il ragazzo ha salutato la vicina$_i$ # che è arrossita$_i$
The boy has greeted the neighbor woman   who is blushed

A full syntactic parse may be bypassed if there are overt cues for localizing the antecedent. For example, the number of the auxiliary verb may help to determine which of two noun phrases with differing number is the grammatical antecedent of the participle.

Example of subordination: auxiliary number cue

I quadri   [che   ha   dipinto Anna]   **sono** spariti
     masc   fm   pl   masc
     pl   sg   pl
The paintings which has painted Anna   are   disappeared
''The paintings which Anna has painted have disappeared''

EXPECTATIONS

The strongest assumption one could make would be that the patients' agrammatic speech is the result of an almost total syntactic disorder. In that case, they would not be able to access the syntactic configurations necessary for participle agreement even in simple sentences, and one could expect either that the citation form of the participle (on $-o$) would be used as a default form or that the different inflected forms of the participle ($-o$, $-a$, $-i$, $-e$) would be used randomly. Alternatively, with some minimal residual sensitivity for general Italian agreement phenomena, the patients might copy an inflectional ending of some nominal element as the participle suffix.

Assuming, on the other hand, that there are some minimal syntactic abilities left, the following expectations can be formulated. Patients may still hold a simplified rule of agreement, namely, that with *essere* there is agreement with the subject, but not with *avere*. Assuming that they would use such a rule, it would be sufficient that they would have the syntactic ability to identify the subject position for them to solve the majority of the participle agreements in simple sentences.

For agrammatic patients, one could furthermore expect an asymmetry between full noun subjects vs. pronominal subjects and—in cases of pro-drop—the inflectional number information contained in the auxiliary verb suffix.

The identification of the subject in combination with a simplified agreement rule would fail to correctly realize agreement in simple sentences with a preposed cliticized direct object. In order to correctly realize participle agreement in such cases, patients need at least the syntactic abilities required to identify the subject position and the direct object case. If, however, they fail to make the correct agreement in such cases, this is not necessarily evidence for a syntactic disorder. A disturbed lexical knowledge of the clitic and its grammatical features could also lead to incorrect agreement in such cases, even if the syntactic abilities were adequate. At any rate, the extent of the syntactic preservation would need further clarification.

For agrammatic patients, the ability to produce grammatical agreement could very well be affected by syntactic complexity. Given that their spontaneous production is restricted to simple sentences which may occasionally be coordinated, one might expect a syntactically based dissociation between agreement in coordinated vs. subordinated clauses. In both cases, correct agreement depends on coindexation across a clause boundary. Alternatively, coindexation across clause boundaries could be ignored in general and patients would then resort to nonlinguistic strategies for the realization of grammatical agreement, like a minimal distance principle.

In the first case, if performance is governed by principles of syntactic complexity, patients will overgeneralize the coordinated antecedent relations for subordination also. In the second case, if performance is governed by strategies of local processing, overgeneralization would go in the opposite direction and coordinated sentences would be treated as if they were subordinated.

SUBJECTS

For the purpose of this study, two nonfluent aphasics were selected ("Broca's") with chronic prototypical "agrammatic" speech production at the time of the study, i.e., short sentences with simplified syntactic structure expressed by the overuse of direct speech, the near absence of subordinate clauses, and the almost exclusive use of nouns and verbs without the functor vocabulary which in Italian is a major means to express grammatical relations between words.

Another feature frequently cited for agrammatic speech is the omission of inflectional endings. This would, however, result in the production of nonword stems in Italian because there are no uninflected open-class elements in this language, so that problems with respect to inflection will give rise to suffix substitution rather than omission.

A further selection criterion was the absence of marked articulatory disorders and phonemic paraphasias according to the Italian version of the Aachen Aphasia Test (AAT, Luzzatti, Willmes, & De Bleser, 1991). This would make it impossible to judge the morphological form intended by the patients. The presence or absence of a syntactic comprehension disorder was not a criterion for inclusion in this study but it was examined for each patient, as was their availability of lexical morphology.

Subject 1

DR was a male dental technician. At the time of testing, he was 27 years old. He had suffered an aneurysm rupture 3 years earlier. The computerized tomography (CT) scan showed a left-hemispheric subarachnoid hemorrhage and an intraparenchymatous satellite hematoma which was evacuated surgically.

The first aphasiological examination was performed 3 months post onset with the Italian version of the AAT. At that time, the patient had right-sided hemiplegia and a global aphasia. Spontaneous speech was initially reduced to a few automatisms (e poi e poi: and then). DR had a severe disturbance in the Token Test and a complete alexia and agraphia. Whereas reading comprehension was impossible, auditory comprehension was relatively spared, as was his performance in naming and repetition, where the patient showed severe-to-medium disorders. DR was repeatedly retested over the next 3 years and showed a progressive improvement in all AAT subtests. At the time of the morphosyntactic examinations 3 years post onset, DR was still hemiplegic. He now showed a severe-to-medium disorder in the Token Test and a medium impairment in repetition. There was a medium-to-mild impairment in naming, whereas written language (reading and writing) and comprehension (auditory and reading) were only mildly disturbed. His spontaneous speech was now clearly agrammatic, as the following example shows.

Example of spontaneous speech of DR

Examiner: Could you tell me the story of Little Red Riding Hood?

Cappuccetto Rosso (CR) . . .   lupo . . . CR   . . . CR   . . . eh . .
Little Red Riding Hood (LRRH) . . . wolf . . . LRRH . . . LRRH . . . uh . .

girava (past tense, 3rd, p.sg.) . .no. . .tutto   . . . eh . un . non cosi, ma . . .
was walking around   . .no. . .completely. . .uh . an. . not thus, but . . .

(shows with hand: not in a curve, but the direct way)

diritto. . .scorciatoia. .e . . e. . .un lupo. . lupo, eh non lo so,   (. .)
straight. .shortcut . .and. .and. . .a wolf. . wolf, uhm I don't know, . . .   (. .)

eh . ."salve!" . . (. . .) poi dopo . . eh, poi dopo . .eh . . un lupo eh . .
and: "Hello!" . . . (. .) then afterward . .uh, then afterward . . uh . . a wolf uh . .

non so perche. .
(I[1]) don't know why

Examiner: Where does the wolf go to?

Lupo . . . n-nonna   . . eh. Poi   . . la bambina . . . Eh . .
Wolf . . . g-grandmother . . uh. Then . . the girl   . . . Uh . .

spalanca (pres.tense, 3rd p.sg.) e dice (pres.tense, 3rd p.sg.) . .
(subject[1]) makes wide open   and (she[1]) says   . .

Examiner: And she says?

eh . . "gli occhi" . . poi . . "la . . la voce" . . . e   . . ah no!. .
uh . . "the eyes" . . then . . "the . . the voice" . . . and . . oh no!

pero eh mangia (pres.tense, 3rd p.sg.). .nonna . .mangia, no? Poi cappuccio
but uh (subject?[1]) eats   grandma. .(he[1]) eats, right? Then   hood

(shows with hands that the previous utterances should be inserted here)

. . . Poi . . e   poi . . "grandi (masc.pl.) occhi (masc.pl) che
. . . Then . . and then . . "large   eyes   that

hai" (pres.tense, 2nd p.sg.) . . e poi   mangia . . .
(you[1]) have"   . . and then (subject?[1]) eats   . . .

Il cacciatore . . entra (pres.tense, 3rd p.sg.) e   squarcia
The hunter . . comes in   and rips

la (fem.sg.) . . . la (fem.sg.) . libera (pres.tense, 3rd p.sg.) . . la bambina
the   . . .the   . (He[1]) frees   the girl

e la nonna.
and the grandmother.

Subject 2

MG was 18 years old at the time of morphosyntactic testing. While riding a bicycle 2 years earlier, he was run over by a truck. He underwent neurosurgical treatment, was unconscious for 15 days, and woke up with right-sided hemiplegia and a severe aphasia. The CT scan taken 1 year post onset showed a large left-hemispheric cortical–subcortical fronto–central–parietal area of softening.

The first aphasiological examination with the Italian AAT 3 months

[1] In Italian, the grammatical subject is generally dropped if it is clear from the discourse in contrast to English, but the verb ending still indicates person and number.

post onset revealed a global aphasia with severe articulatory disorders and with spontaneous speech restricted to a few syllabic fragments (e.g., ce.lo, sa.co, tolco). MG had a complete alexia and agraphia, and his performance on the Token Test, repetition, naming, and comprehension was severely disturbed. Repeated retesting revealed a progressive improvement in all subtests. Three years post onset, at the time of the morphosyntactic study, there were medium-to-mild disturbances in the Token Test and in the repetition and naming subtests, whereas written language (reading and writing) and comprehension (auditory and reading) were now only mildly disturbed. MG's spontaneous speech had greatly improved and now showed characteristic features of agrammatic speech production, as the following example shows.

Example of spontaneous speech of MG

Examiner: Could you tell me the story of Adam and Eve?

Un giorno Eva . . . sull'albero . . . sull'albero . . . il serpente
One day Eve . . . on the tree . . . on the tree . . the serpent

vede . . Eva . . Dice il serpente: "Ciao! . . prova . a mangiare . .
sees . . Eve . . Says the serpent: "Hi! . . try . to eat   . .

la mela." "No, grazie . .   perche . . Dio . . Dio . . non . .   non . .
the apple." "No, thank you . .because . . God . . God . . (do) not . . (do) not

<Non mangiare!>. Non . . grazie,   perche Dio . . . non . . .
<Don't eat!>.   No . . thank you, because God . . . not . . .

non   . .   non vuole   Dio." Il serpente: "prova,
not   . . (he[1]) doesn't want (it), God." The serpent: "try,

prova, prova . . ." A un certo punto Eva lo (masc.sg., but la mela: fem.sg.)
try,   try   . . ." At a certain point Eve it

mangio . . e . . "buono (masc.sg)!"
eats   . . and . . "good!"

E . . Adamo: "Cosa hai   . . fatto? Co-cosa   fai?"
And . . Adam: "What have (you[1]) . . done? Wh-what are (you[1]) doing?"

No, niente . . Eh Dio gridava; certo punto
No, nothing . . Uh God shouted; certain point

dice Dio: "Non. ."   Dio si   . . si infuria   e   allora . .
says God: "(Do) not . ." God becomes . . becomes furious and then . .

punizione eh   dice . . morto (part.) . . . eh lei . . lui . . punizione.
punishment uh (he[1]) says . . dead   . . . uh she . . he . . punishment.

The patients' syntactic comprehension of simple reversible active and passive sentences was examined by means of a sentence–picture match-

---

[1] In Italian, the grammatical subject is generally dropped if it is clear from the discourse in contrast to English, but the verb ending still indicates person and number.

ing task. There were 70 active and 70 passive sentences. Each sentence was presented auditorily and the patients had to point to one of four pictures (target, reversal, agent of different gender, patient of different gender). Both patients were equally impaired on active and passive sentences, but DR's disorder was more severe than MG's. DR made 61% errors on active and 59% on passive sentences, MG made 29% errors on active and 30% on passive sentences. Errors were almost exclusively reversal errors.

The morpholexical abilities of both patients were extensively examined with experimental material to investigate the processing of simple, derived, and compound nouns. It was examined among others whether they could produce the plural of simple nouns by means of the appropriate noun suffix and whether they could realize the gender of nouns by means of the definite article or the gender-specific adjectival suffix. (See Luzzatti & De Bleser, submitted, for a more complete report.) MG performed normally on these tasks (95% correct plurals, 97% correct articles, 100% correct adjectival suffixes). He thus showed complete preservation of these aspects of simple noun inflection. DR's performance was subnormal though significantly above chance (74% correct plurals, 76% correct articles, 70% correct adjectival suffixes). His error pattern revealed an impairment of the irregular inflectional paradigm but regular inflection was unaffected (irregular gender: 57.5% correct, regular gender: 97% correct). Apparently, DR had an overreliance on morphological rules which led to overgeneralizations of the regular paradigms for number as well as for gender.

Given these spared morpholexical abilities of both patients, the severe agrammatism in their spontaneous speech could obviously not be traced back to a loss of morphology per se but was more likely related to a syntactic deficit. This hypothesis was examined with the materials described below.

MATERIALS AND METHODS

Experimental task. The material consisted of sentences presented in written form, one DIN A4-page for each stimulus sentence. The examiner and patient were seated opposite each other at a table, and the stimulus sentence was turned toward the patient. The examiner read the sentence aloud together with the patient. The vowel endings of the participles were indicated by dots which were read by the examiner as a gap reinforced by an audible click. The patient was told to complete the participle by the appropriate suffix, i.e., − o in cases of nonagreement and − o, − i, − a, − e, in cases where gender and number agreement had to take place with an antecedent. In other words, after the sentence with an incomplete participle had been read by examiner and patient, the patient was to produce the appropriately inflected participial form (e.g., Giovanni ha telefonat . . . a Rosa: "telefonato"; Rosa è chiamat . . . dagli amici: "chiamata"). Practice examples were trained with the patients until it was clear that they understood the task.

Experimental material. Depending on the argument structure of the verb, the antecedent for agreement was either a subject or a direct clitic object. In all sentences, gender and/or number were different for subject and object, so that the patient's choice of participle suffix could be clearly traced to one of them. In the examples to follow, target nonagreement is indicated by $x_\emptyset$, target agreement by $_i$ and $_j$, respectively, and the relevant coindexation by $x_i \ldots y_i$, $x_j \ldots y_j$.

To examine the effect of the lexical category of the antecedent and the argument structure of the verb, a total of 132 simple sentences were used. Sixty-six sentences contained a subject–NP followed by *è* or *sono* (the third person singular/plural of *essere*), the past participle of an ergative verb without the vowel suffix, and a prepositional phrase. Another 66 sentences had a subject–NP followed by *ha* or *hanno* (the third person singular/plural of *avere*), the past participle of a transitive verb without the vowel suffix, and a direct object noun.

Example of subject agreement in ergative sentences

Rosa$_i$ è cors(a)$_i$ dal padre
Rosa is (=has) run to the father

Example of nonagreement in transitive sentences

I contadini hanno nutrit (o)$_\emptyset$ le mucche
The farmers have fed the cows

In 100 cases, a second sentence was coordinated by *e* (and), the deleted subject was that of the first sentence, and the object clitic was coreferential with the direct object or the prepositional object of the first sentence. There were 80 direct objects and 20 indirect object clitics. They were followed by a finite form of *avere* followed by a past participle of a transitive verb. In cases with an indirect object clitic, a full direct object noun followed the participle.

Example of agreement with direct object clitic

Le donne hanno lavato i panni$_i$ # e li$_i$ hanno stes(i)$_i$
The women have washed the laundry and them have hung up

I turisti sono arrivati sull'isola$_i$ # e la$_i$ hanno visitat(a)$_i$
The tourists have arrived on the island and it have visited

Example of nonagreement with indirect object clitic

Carlo ha invitato una cugina$_i$ # e le$_i$ ha fatt(o)$_\emptyset$ un regalo
Carlo has invited a female cousin and her has made a gift

To investigate the patients' ability to handle *pro-drop* sentences, 24 sentences with an auxiliary in the plural form were presented where number information had to be extracted from the verbal inflection. Eight sentences were presented with *abbiamo* (we have), 16 with *siamo* (we are) immediately followed by a participle. Again, agreement of the participle with the verbal inflection in grammatical number should only take place in the case of *siamo*.

Example of nonagreement with pro-drop

(pro) abbiamo assalit(o)$_\emptyset$ la guardia
    pl   pl
We have attacked the guard

Example of agreement with pro-drop and verbal suffix cue

(pro)$_i$ siamo$_i$ andat(i/e)$_i$ dalla nonna [−i = masc; −e = fem]
    pl   pl
We are (=have) gone to the grandmother

To examine the effect of syntactic complexity, 16 relative clauses were compared with 16 coordinated clauses. The lexical material was identical, the only difference being between the relative pronoun *che* (which/whom) and the coordinating conjunction *e* (and).

Example of agreement in coordinated and subordinated sentences

Il ragazzo$_i$ ha salutato   la vicina$_j$ # (. . .)
The boy has greeted the neighbor woman

    coordination: (. . .) **e** (PRO) è arrossit(o)$_i$
                      and is (=has) become red

    object relative: (. . .) **che** è arrossit(**a**)$_j$
                      who (=has) become red

To examine the effect of a disambiguating verbal number cue, the following structures were used: 18 coordinated sentences, 12 subordinations with subject relatives, and 8 subordinations with object relatives.

Examples of complex sentences with a verbal number cue

Le   allunne$_i$ le   ha accompagnate Franco   #   **e** (PRO)$_i$ sono$_i$ partit(e)$_i$
        pl   sg   pl pl   pl
The alumnae them Franco has accompanied   and are (=have) left

Le alunne$_i$ [**che** ha accompagnato Franco   ]   sono partit(e)$_i$
      pl   sg   pl pl
The alumnae   that Franco has accompanied   are (=have) left

(pro) abbiamo   accompagnato l'alunna$_i$ # **che**$_i$ è   partit(**a**)$_i$
    pl   pl   sg   sg   sg
We   have   accompanied   the alumna who is (=has) left

The sentences were randomized and presented in four different sessions.

RESULTS AND DISCUSSION

Lexical Category and Argument Structure

The hypothesis of a total syntactic disorder as a source of the patient's agrammatic speech would have predicted the general use of the citation form of the participle (on $-o$) as a default form or the random use of the different inflected forms of the participle ($-o$, $-a$, $-i$, $-e$). The assumption of some minimal residual sensitivity for general Italian agreement phenomena would have expected the patients to copy an inflectional ending of some nominal element as the participle suffix.

Table 1 shows the results of the task for participle agreement with the gender and number features of an antecedent noun in sentences with ergative and active transitive verbs.

On the whole, both patients only made 8% incorrect agreement, in others words, they mastered the principles of participle agreement quite well in simple sentences. When agreement with ths subject was required, a few errors occurred in which gender was incorrect but number agreement was adequate.

TABLE 1
Gender and Number Agreement of the Participle with a Full NP in Simple Sentences
with Ergative and Active Transitive Verbs

Subject features and target ending	DR Response				MG Response			
	− o	− i	− a	− e	− o	− i	− a	− e
Unaccusative verbs (essere agreement)								
masc.sg.: − o	14				14			
(n = 14)	(100%)				(100%)			
masc.pl.: − i		14				12		2
(n = 14)		(100%)				(86%)		
fem.sg.: − a	6		18		1		23	
(n = 24)			(75%)				(96%)	
fem.pl.: − e		4		10		3		11
(n = 14)				(71%)				(79%)
Total	20	18	18	10	15	15	23	13
(n = 66)								
Transitive active verbs (avere agreement: default form on − o)								
masc.sg.: − o	14				12		2	
(n = 14)								
masc.pl.: − o	14				13	1		
(n = 14)								
fem.sg.: − o	24				24			
(n = 24)								
fem.pl.: − o	13			1	12	2		
(n = 14)								
Total	65			1	61	3	2	
(n = 66)								
Grand total: hits 121/132 → 92%					hits 121/132 → 92%			

Although these remarkably good results disprove the two hypotheses mentioned above, they do not necessarily provide evidence for substantially preserved syntactic abilities. The task could already be solved if patients had a simplified rule of agreement, namely, that with *essere* there is agreement with the subject but not with *avere,* in combination with a heuristic that the subject is likely to be the first position in Italian sentences.

However, identification of the subject in combination with a simplified agreement rule would fail to correctly realize agreement in simple sentences with a preposed cliticized direct object, which requires at least the additional ability of direct object identification.

Table 2 gives the results for participle agreement with a clitic object in active transitive sentences.

On the whole, DR's responses were correct in 90% of cases, MG's in

TABLE 2
Gender and Number Agreement of the Participle with the Clitic Object

Clitic features and target ending	DR Response				MG Response			
	−o	−i	−a	−e	−o	−i	−a	−e
Second sentence (avere agreement with the clitic direct object)								
masc.sg.: −o	10				8		2	
(n = 10)	(100%)				(80%)		(20%)	
masc.pl.: −i		18		2	8	8		4
(n = 20)		(90%)		(10%)	(40%)	(40%)		(20%)
fem.sg.: −a	4		26		14	1	12	3
(n = 30)	(13%)		(87%)		(47%)	(3%)	(40%)	(10%)
fem.pl.: −e	3	1		16	5	3		12
(n = 20)	(15%)	(5%)		(80%)	(25%)	(15%)		(60%)
Total	17	19	26	18	35	12	14	19
(n = 80)								
Second sentence (clitic indirect object; avere agreement: default form on −o)								
masc.sg.: −o	10				10			
(n = 10)								
fem.sg.: −o	10				10			
(n = 10)								
Total	20				20			
(n = 20)								

Note. Correct responses are in bold face. The total amount of hits for DR is 90 (90%) and for MG is 80 (80%).

60%. Neither patient ever attempted agreement with the indirect object clitic, but they showed a different pattern for agreement with direct object clitics. In fact, DR's performance here was as good as in the cases of participle agreement with a nominal subject reported in Table 1. MG's performance for participle agreement with direct object clitics was clearly disturbed. He made 50% errors here as opposed to only 9% for the subject agreement reported above. The ending −o appears as a response in 35/80 cases. However, MG produced 33/80 correct reactions on −e, −i, or −a. These can only be interpreted as the correct solution of gender and number agreement with the object clitic, which means that MG had some sensitivity left to the grammatical features of the object clitic and the principles of agreement in such cases. Furthermore, the perfect performance on indirect object clitics indicates that MG is aware of the structural case (dative versus accusative) of the clitic. His impairment on the agreement task is thus more likely the result of a disordered lexical access for the gender and number features of clitic pronouns.

Given the characteristics of agrammatic speech, it could have been expected that the performance of our patients would show an asymmetry

TABLE 3
Sensitivity to Verb Inflection for Number Agreement in Simple Sentences
(Number of Correct Responses)

	Solution							
	DR				MG			
Target	− o	− a	− i	− e	− o	− a	− i	− e
Abbiamo... (= − o)	7	—	1	—	8	—	—	—
(n = 8)								
Siamo... (= − i/ − e)	—	1	12	3	—	1	11	4
(n = 16)								

between the recognition of grammatical features contained in inflectional suffixes of auxiliary verbs as opposed to those of full nouns or pronouns.

Table 3 shows that this is not the case, as both patients are sensitive to the number information contained in the inflectional suffix of the auxiliary verb. In simple sentences with *siamo,* where the participle should agree in number with this suffix, each patient only made 1/16 errors.

Influence of Syntactic Complexity

For agrammatic patients whose spontaneous production is restricted to simple sentences, it was plausible to expect a syntactically based dissociation between preserved agreement in coordinated sentences and disturbed agreement in subordinated clauses, so that the coordinated antecedent relations would be overgeneralized for subordinations. On the other hand, since both structure types require the recovery of antecedent relations across a clause boundary, patients might ignore coindexation in general and resort to nonlinguistic, local processing strategies such as a minimum distance principle for the realization of grammatical agreement. This would favor the subordinated sentences in our task, where the antecedent immediately preceded the boundary, and coordinated sentences would then be treated as if they were subordinate.

Table 4 shows the results on the task of participle agreement in object relative versus coordinate clauses. The antecedent immediately preceded the clause boundary for object relatives (target: "short distance") but not for coordinates (target: "long distance").

Both patients were severely disturbed in this task (56% correct for DR, 44% correct for MG) but they did not resort to a simple strategy. The results indicate that they were still trying to realize grammatical agreement: There was no substitution of the default form − o by either patient, nor was there a random use of the four suffixes (− o, − i, − a, − e). In all but one item only in the case of MG, the participle suffix al-

TABLE 4
Agreement of the Participles in Relative versus Coordinate Clauses
(Number of Correct Agreement in the Second Clause)

	Solution					
	DR			MG		
Antecedent distance	Long	Short	Other (−o copy)	Long	Short	Other (−o copy)
Long (n = 16) (e clauses)	7	9	—	8	8	—
Short (n = 16) (che clauses)	5	11	—	9	6	1
Total	12	20	—	17	14	1
Target		18/32 (56%)			14/32 (44%)	

Note. e, coordinate clauses; che, relative clauses.

ways corresponded in gender and number to one of the nouns actu-
ally occurring in the sentence (*Il ragazzo$_i$ ha salutato la vicina$_j$ ed $_{-i}$
è arrosit $-$ a$_j$ $_{instead of i}$; *. . .che$_j$ è arrosit $-$ o$_i$ $_{instead of j}$).

However, the selection of the noun antecedent for agreement is obviously arbitrary for MG, whereas DR shows only a weak tendency to
select the minimally distant noun. Two alternative linguistic explanations
can be proposed for this pattern. According to a syntactic deficit account,
neither patient seems to be able to analyze syntactic structures with respect to their coindexed elements. This is necessary to identify the main
clause object (short distance) as the only possible grammatical antecedent
for the subordinate (che:who) sentences or the main clause subject (long
distance) as the only grammatically correct antecedent for coordinate
(ed:and) sentences. An alternative nonsyntactic explanation would attribute the patients' near-random choice of antecedent as a consequence of
a lexical comprehension disorder for the function words "che" (who)
and "ed" (and). The data in Table 5 on agreement in complex sentences
with a verbal number cue show this last account to be unlikely.

It is clear from Table 5 that both patients were able to discover the
correct antecedent for participle agreement if there was a disambiguating
cue within the participle clause, namely, the number of the auxiliary verb.
DR made only 1/38 errors, MG 3/38 errors. Notice that agreement could
nevertheless not be solved purely on the basis of the verbal inflection,
since the participle had to agree in both gender and number with its
antecedent, and the auxiliary verb was only marked for number. Apparently, the auxiliary number could direct the search for a noun with the
same number feature, which was then analyzed for gender and could
percolate its gender and number features to the participle.

TABLE 5
Agreement of the Participles in Sentences with a Verb Number Cue: Coordinate Clauses and Subordinate Clauses, Subject Relative versus Object Relative

Antecedent distance	Target	Solution							
		DR				MG			
		−o	−a	−i	−e	−o	−a	−i	−e
Long									
Coordinate	−i		8	1			7	2	
(n = 18)	−e			9					9
Subordinate subject relative	−i		6				5	1	
(n = 12)	−e			6					6
Short									
Subordinate object relative (n = 8)	−a	8				8			
Target		37/3				35/38			

In summary, the patients' performance in *simple sentences* showed that they recognized the argument structure of verbs (ergatives vs. intransitives and transitives) and that they mastered the basic stipulations of the agreement rule. MG only had a lexical disorder for pronominal clitics where he could often not identify the correct grammatical features. It must be noted that a full syntactic representation for the identification of subject and direct object was not necessary in these tasks, since the simple sentences contained only one nominal element which could be a candidate for antecedent. However, if there were two nominal elements preceding the participle, as in complex sentences with coordination or object relative clauses, the selection of the correct antecedent depended on a structural representation in which subject and object were specified. Obviously, neither patient could use this structural knowledge. MG's selection of antecedent became random, DR tended slightly more toward a minimal distance solution, assigning antecedent function to the noun which was closest to the participle irrespective of its grammatical function. In cases where there was an overt cue in the grammatical number of the auxiliary inflection to identify the subject of the sentence, a full syntactic analysis could again be circumvented and the performance of the patients rose to a near-normal level.

DISCUSSION

Two Italian patients were examined for agreement between a past participle and its grammatical antecedent with respect to gender and number.

For correct morphological realization, a structural representation of the sentence must be available with the thematic roles for subject and object, the gender and number features of the antecedent must be recognized and transmitted to the participle, where they are realized as a suffix.

Overall, the results on agreement in simple sentences showed that the patients had a high sensitivity for the auxiliary verb as well as for the gender and number feature of the antecedent. Especially the results on indirect object clitics showed that both patients could well discriminate these from the direct object clitics. However, the patients' performance broke down when the function of inflectional morphology had to be mapped onto a syntactically richer context like in the complex sentences of our experimental setting. In the case of the relative clauses used, the antecedent becomes available to the relative clause only via a coindexation between an empty operator before the relative pronoun and a trace relating it to the subject position of the relative clause. In the case of the coordinations used, the parser had to detect a coordinate structure such that the participle will agree with the same NP as in the first conjunct. The performance of the patients dropped dramatically in such cases. Obviously, the strategy was to match the participle agreement with one of the two preceding NPs but the structural information for the correct choice was unavailable. The errors reflected an impairment in the selection of the syntactically appropriate NP rather than a random choice of possible inflection.

The main generalization about these sets of results is that the Italian agrammatic patients could exploit very limited syntactic contexts for the determination of inflectional morphology whereas they completely failed in more elaborate contexts.

The pattern of morphosyntactic performance of patients DR and MG cannot be reconciled with linguistic explanations of agrammatic speech which assume that syntactic representations are spared but nonterminal elements are deleted at S-structure across the board (Grodzinsky, 1990). In that case, morphological agreement should not be possible in any context. Moreover, this thesis is further contradicted by the patients's ability to use a bound category of auxiliary inflection as a cue for grammatical analysis.

For similar reasons, the disorder cannot be located at the positional level in a processing model like Garrett's (Garrett, 1980; Caramazza & Hillis, 1989), where grammatical suffixes are mapped onto functional representations. The impairment is rather at this deeper functional level, where the grammatical functions of context words are specified. This is indicated by the patients' random performance in cases with multiple antecedent candidates.

On the whole, the patterns of preservation and breakdown of our Italian patients were very similar to those of three German patients reported by De Bleser & Bayer (1988). Like the Italian subjects, the German patients also had relatively well-preserved morpholexical abilities with respect to the gender and number of nouns. The syntactic implementation of morphology was investigated by means of case assignment in various syntactic contexts, German being a case-marking language. The patients' performance was astonishingly good for genitive constructions (as in "Der Arbeiter rettet den Sohn eines treuen Kumpels:" The worker saves the son (of) a dear friend), in which the second NP is inflected in local dependence on the first, structural case assigning NP. However, they were unable to inflect an uninflected subject or object NP in simple reversible sentences (as in "ein hungriger$_{nom}$ Bettler trifft einen reichen$_{acc}$Mann," "einen reichen$_{acc}$ Mann trifft ein hungriger$_{nom}$ Bettler:" A hungry beggar meets a rich man).

This breakdown pattern of the German patients might at first give the impression that they were less able to deal with syntax-relevant morphology than our Italian subjects. The German subjects were already severely disturbed in providing case morphology in simple clauses, whereas DR and MG had little difficulty with participle agreement in simple sentences.

Upon closer linguistic scrutiny, language-specific factors can be held responsible for this difference. German is a language with free NP order and the subject or object can equally appear in pre- or postverbal position. This leads to a complexity not found in Italian, which is an SVO language. The preverbal position in Italian is thus much more likely to contain the subject, so that auxiliary and verbal agreement can rely on positional information in the case of simple sentences. However, in complex Italian sentences, this information is irrelevant for agreement and the function of the NPs has to be determined structurally. Thus, what the Italian and German patients share is the inability to link thematic roles (of subject and object) with structural positions via nonlinear, nonlocal syntactic analysis. The dysmorphology in the patients' elicited speech is thus not a sign of amorphology but of dyssyntaxia.

REFERENCES

Baker, M. C. 1988. *Incorporation. A theory of grammatical function changing.* Chicago: Univ. of Chicago Press.

Bates, E., & Wulfeck, B. 1989. Comparative aphasiology: A cross linguistic approach to language breakdown. *Aphasiology*, **3**, 111–142.

Bates, E., Friederici, A., & Wulfeck, B. 1987. Grammatical morphology in aphasia: Evidence from three languages. *Cortex*, **23**, 545–574.

Burzio, L. 1987. *Italian syntax. A government-binding approach.* Dordrecht: Reidel.

Caramazza, A., & Hillis, A. 1989. The disruption of sentence production: A case of selective deficit to positional level processing. *Brain and Language*, **36**, 635–650.

De Bleser, R., & Bayer, J. 1988. On the role of inflectional morphology in agrammatism. In M. Hammond & M. Noonan (Eds.), *Theoretical morphology.* New York: Academic Press. Pp. 45–69.

Garrett, M. 1980. Levels of processing in sentence production. In B. Butterworth (Ed.), *Language production*. London: Academic Press. Vol. 1, pp. 177–220.

Grodzinsky, Y. 1990. *Theoretical perspectives on language deficits*. Cambridge, MA: MIT Press.

Kean, M. L. 1977. The linguistic interpretation of aphasic syndromes: Agrammatism in Broca's aphasia, an example. *Cognition*, **5**, 9–46.

Lapointe, S. 1985. A theory of verb form use in the speech of agrammatic aphasics. *Brain and Language*, **24**, 100–155.

Luzzatti, C., & De Bleser, R. *Morphological processing in Italian agrammatic speakers: Lexical morphology*. Submitted for publication.

Luzzatti, C., Willmes, K., & De Bleser, R. 1991. *Aachener Aphasie Test (AAT): Versione italiana*. Firenze: Organizzazioni Speciali.

Menn, L., & Obler, L. K. 1990a. *Agrammatic aphasia: A cross-language narrative sourcebook*. Amsterdam: Benjamins. Vols. 1–3.

Menn, L., & Obler, L. K. 1990b. Cross-language data and theories of agrammatism. In L. Menn and L. K. Obler (Eds.), *Agrammatic aphasia: A cross-language sourcebook*. Amsterdam: Benjamins. Vol. 2, pp. 1368–1389.

Miceli, G., & Caramazza, A. 1988. Dissociation of inflectional and derivational morphology. *Brain and Language*, **35**, 24–65.

Pesetzky, D. M. 1989. *Language-particular processes and the earliness principle*. Unpublished manuscript, MIT.

Schwarze, Ch. 1988. *Grammatik der Italienischen Sprache*. Tübingen: Niemeyer.

Tissot, R., Mounin, F., & Lhermitte, F. 1973. *L'Agrammatisme. Étude neuropsycholinguistique*. Bruxelles: Dessart.

BRAIN AND LANGUAGE **46**, 683–694 (1994)

Processing Articles and Pronouns in Agrammatic Aphasia: Evidence from French

Gonia Jarema

*Département de linguistique, Université de Montréal, Montréal, Québec; and
Laboratoire Théophile-Alajouanine, Centre de recherche, Centre hospitalier
Côte-des-Neiges, Montréal, Québec, Canada*

AND

Angela D. Friederici

*Labor für Kognitionswissenschaften, Institut für Psychologie,
Freie Universität Berlin, Berlin, Germany*

The hypothesis that closed-class items which participate in theta-role assignment are less problematic in agrammatism than items which do not (Rizzi, 1985) is put to an empirical test. Five French-speaking agrammatic patients were tested in a sentence–picture matching paradigm to probe their comprehension of sentences containing articles, which are not involved in theta-role assignment, and of sentences containing pronouns, which in the direct object position are homophonous with articles and are theta-role assignees. Gender was used as a variable to differenciate between target and distractor. The data indicate that pronouns are significantly more difficult to process than articles. This result disconfirms the claim that the availability of grammatical information encoded in closed-class items is a function of their involvement in theta-role assignement. The present study demonstrates that the ability to process gender marked articles is generally well preserved in French-speaking agrammatic patients. © 1994 Academic Press, Inc.

INTRODUCTION

In recent years, the definition of agrammatism has undergone considerable changes. In the seventies, agrammatism was predominantly viewed

Address correspondence and reprint requests to Gonia Jarema, Centre de recherche, Centre hospitalier Côte-des-Neiges, 4565 chemin de la Reine-Marie, Montréal, Québec H3W 1W5. This research was supported by a Social Sciences and Humanities Research Council of Canada Grant to the first author. Angela Friederici was supported by the Alfried Krupp von Bohlen und Halbach Science Award. The authors are grateful to the patients of the Centre hospitalier Côte-des-Neiges who participated in the study.

114

as a syntactic deficit (e.g., Caramazza & Zurif, 1976; Heilman & Scholes, 1976). The failure to process syntactic information was attributed either to an inability to construct syntactic representations or to a loss of the closed-class vocabulary (e.g., Berndt & Caramazza, 1980; Bradley, Garrett, & Zurif, 1980). This view was seriously challenged by the work of Linebarger, Schwartz, and Saffran (1983), who showed that so-called agrammatics are able to perform grammaticality judgments. Their study clearly suggested that agrammatic aphasics are capable of carrying out grammatical analyses to a certain degree, despite an inability to use grammatical information in a similarly successful way during sentence comprehension and sentence production. Independent support for this view is provided by a number of studies in different languages. Friederici (1982), for example, reported that German-speaking agrammatic patients performed well in judging the correctness of dependencies between verbs and obligatory prepositions despite poor performance on such prepositions in a production task. A disparity between relatively good performance on grammaticality tasks and impaired comprehension has also been reported for Serbo-Croatian-speaking agrammatic patients using an on-line grammaticality judgment task (Shankweiler, Crain, Correll, & Tuller, 1989) and for German-speaking patients using an off-line grammaticality judgment task with visual presentation which allowed the on-line registration of eye movements during reading (Huber, Cholewa, Wilbertz, & Friederici, 1990; but see Wulfeck (1987) reporting no difference between an off-line grammaticality judgment task and an off-line comprehension task).

These data led to a number of different redefinitions of agrammatism, mostly stressing processing aspects (for an overview, see Linebarger, 1990). Linebarger et al. (1983) proposed that the agrammatic parser may simply be less efficient, resulting in a trade-off between syntactic processes and semantic processes which comes to bear in a comprehension task, but not in a grammaticality judgment task where mainly syntactic processes operate. Others reports have stressed the inability to map from syntactic to semantic representations (e.g., Rizzi, 1985; Schwartz Linebarger, Saffran, & Pate, 1987), while Zurif, Swinney, Prather, Solomon, and Bushell (1993) claim that parsing operations prior to these mapping procedures are impaired. Again, others proposed that agrammatism may be best explained as damage to the temporal structure of language processing, in particular to pathologically slowed down parsing operations (e.g., Friederici, 1988; Haarmann & Kolk, 1990; Hagoort, 1988).

Rosenthal and Goldblum (1989) also claimed—although on different grounds—that the agrammatic deficit in comprehension cannot be interpreted as a "loss of syntactic processes and/or closed-class morphology" (p.179). Quite correctly, they argue that morphosyntactic abilities are a prerequisite for a possible dissociation for different word classes and word categories. For example, in order to be able to ignore closed-class vocabulary during production or reading as observed in agrammatism, the system must be able to identify lexical category which in turn requires morphosyntactic knowledge. They refer to a number of studies in the literature demonstrating that agrammatic subjects process lexical items as a function of their lexical category and that they must be in control of morphosyntactic knowledge (e.g., Andreewsky & Seron, 1975; Friederici & Schönle, 1980; Grossman, Carey, Zurif, & Diller, 1986). The issue, however, of what type of morphosyntactic information is available to agrammatic patients needs further specification. The goal of the present paper is to contribute to this domain.

Studies investigating the agrammatics' ability to process closed-class words and inflectional morphology have revealed that these patients are able to monitor closed-class words in a sentence, although with some delay (e.g., Friederici, 1983; Swinney, Zurif, & Cutler, 1980), that they process inflectional morphology to some degree (Jarema & Kehayia, 1992; Lukatela, Crain, & Shankweiler, 1988), and that they are sensitive to the presence or absence of closed-class elements as a marker of lexical category in an off-line judgment task (Grossman et al., 1986), as well as in an on-line comprehension task (Friederici, Wessels, Emmorey, & Bellugi, 1992). Moreover, they recognize these elements as markers of thematic roles (e.g., Friederici & Graetz, 1987; Jarema, Kądzielawa, & Waite, 1987).

More recently, it was shown that agrammatic aphasics are sensitive to grammatical gender information encoded in pronouns (Friederici, Weissenborn, & Kail, 1991) and in articles (Rosenthal & Goldblum, 1989).

Friederici and co-workers (1991) have shown that agrammatic subjects in French, Dutch and German were sensitive to gender information encoded in pronouns. The experiment required subjects to match auditory sentences to pictures. The critical variation in the linguistic material involved semantic gender and number information. The results demonstrated a clear sensitivity to gender information encoded in pronouns. Given the language material used, the study did not allow any generalization to other closed-class elements which also carry gender information. This, however, is of particular interest to theories of agrammatism as Rizzi (1985) had argued on purely theoretical grounds that agrammatic Broca's aphasics may be differentially sensitive to closed-class elements falling under the scope of the theta role module of Government-Binding Theory[1] (Chomsky, 1981) and to those which do not. According to this

---

[1] In predicate argument structures, there are thematic role assigners (e.g., verbs and prepositions heading prepositional phrases) and thematic role assignees (nominal expressions). Some linguistic expressions (e.g., prepositions which are not heads of phrases and articles) are neither thematic role assigners nor thematic role assignees and thus do not participate in theta role assignment.

distinction, pronouns fall into the former category as they are being assigned a thematic role (e.g., Agent, Theme), whereas articles, for example, falling into the latter are not. Rizzi's (1985) position thus predicts good performance on pronouns, but deficient performance on articles in agrammatic patients.

Rosenthal and Goldblum (1989) reported results from one agrammatic French-speaking subject who did well in disambiguating homophones by means of the gender information encoded in the article (*le moule*—mold vs. *la moule*—mussel). The authors take this finding to support their view of preserved morphosyntactic abilities in agrammatics. Whether the observed capacity is a feature of French-speaking agrammatic aphasics in general, and how it compares to the capacity to process gender information encoded in pronouns, remains an empirical issue.

In the present study, we compare the ability of individual subjects to process gender information encoded in articles to their ability to process this very same information encoded in pronouns in five French-speaking agrammatic aphasics. French is interesting for the study of the above-mentioned issues because it is precisely a language in which a minimal pair relevant to theta theory partitioning of linguistic phenomena is found, i.e., in which there is homophony between two distinct types of closed-class lexical items that contrast along the dimension crucial to theta-role assignment: The direct object pronoun which, being a nominal element, receives a theta role and thus becomes a theta-role assignee, and the definite article which specifies the noun and plays no part in theta-role assignment.

If Rizzi's (1985) proposal is valid, then agrammatic subjects should perform better on pronouns than on articles. If Rosenthal and Goldblum's (1989) proposal holds, then they should perform equally well on both articles and pronouns.

METHOD

Materials

A sentence–picture matching task was used to test the subjects' ability to comprehend the article or the pronoun in simple two-argument sentences. Two arrays of sets of picture were constructed. In the first, each set of pictures (*n* = 8) contained two randomly ordered line drawings presented vertically. Pictures corresponded to sentences which contrasted only in the gender of pairs of homophonous lexical items used for nouns in object position. Nouns chosen (*n* = 16) were controlled for frequency and syllable structure. Two pairs of sentences were used with each set of pictures: a pair testing the comprehension of the masculine singular article *le* versus the accusative feminine singular article *la* specifying the gender of the object (a) and a pair testing the comprehension of the accusative masculine singular pronoun *le* versus the accusative feminine singular pronoun *la* (b). The language material for the first array of sets of pictures thus consisted of 32 sentences.

(a) *Le soldat quitte le poste.*
    "The soldier is leaving the post."

    Le soldat quitte la poste.
    "The soldier is leaving the post office."

(b) *Le soldat le quitte.*
    "The soldier is leaving it (antecedent: the post)."

    Le soldat la quitte.
    "The soldier is leaving it (antecedent: the post office)."

The distinction between grammatically (as in (a) and (b) above) and semantically (as in (c) and (d) below) determined gender was also tested yielding a second array of sets of pictures ($n = 8$) and corresponding sentences ($n = 32$). All sentences ($n = 64$) were randomly ordered. Furthermore, to document the severity of the subjects' agrammatic performance, their spontaneous speech was tested in a sentence production task on the same pictures as the ones used for comprehension, as well as on the BDAE (Goodglass & Kaplan, 1972) Cookie Theft picture.

(c) *L'infirmière sert le pensionnaire.*
    "The nurse is serving the resident (male)."

    L'infirmière sert la pensionnaire.
    "The nurse is serving the resident (female)."

(d) *L'infirmière le sert.*
    "The nurse is serving him."

    L'infirmière la sert.
    "The nurse is serving her."

Procedure

Subjects were first asked to perform a naming task to ensure that the lexical items used as targets in the experiment were correctly identified and corresponded to their spontaneous productions, with regard to both lexical choice and gender identification. Pictures from the comprehension material were presented to the subjects one by one and critical lexical items were pointed at by the examiner who would then ask *"Qu'est-ce que c'est?"* (What is this?). Subjects who did not produce the elicited target were provided with the item, however, without the article. The examiner would then prompt subjects to produce the word together with its article by saying *"C'est . . . "* (This is . . .).

In the comprehension task, sentences were read to the subjects who were required to choose one of the two pictures presented to them in each set. Responses were recorded on an answering sheet. The patients' agrammatic speech was evaluated during an independent testing session on two production tasks. In the first, they were asked to describe each picture of the comprehension experiment. In the second, their spontaneous speech was further tested on the Cookie Theft picture. Each subject's production samples were tape-recorded and transcribed.

Subjects

The subjects for this study were five male, right-handed, French-speaking, agrammatic aphasics who had suffered a left CVA. Their mean age was 40 (P1, 50; P2, 57; P3, 33; P4, 30; P5, 30). All five patients had been classified on the Montréal–Toulouse Aphasia Battery (Nespoulous, Lecours, Lafond, Lemay, Puel, Joanette, Cot, & Rascol, 1986) as agrammatic Broca's aphasics. They were matched with five normal controls of the same sex, age, handedness and educational background. All subjects were tested in Montréal and were native speakers of Québec French. An evaluation of the patients' current spontaneous speech confirmed the results previously obtained in the clinical assessment of their abilities, i.e., the samples elicited for the present study showed that utterances consisted of greatly reduced subject–verb or subject–verb–object strings characterized by pauses, hesitations, and false trials. Disturbances consisted of omissions of the auxiliary (or alternatively of the production of verbs in their citation form, i.e., the infinitive) and of other closed-class items, as well as of erroneously inflected forms. The patients' agrammatic speech is exemplified in the Cookie Theft narratives presented in the appendix.

RESULTS

While the control subjects scored 100% correct in all conditions tested, errors were found in all sentence types in the performance of the aphasic subjects. Sentences containing a pronoun yielded overall more errors than did sentences with object noun phrases featuring the article (35% vs. 13.13% mean error rate). More specifically, four of five patients showed a significantly higher percentage of errors on pronouns than on articles (P1: $\chi^2 = 4.67, p < .05$; P2: $\chi^2 = 10.86, p < .01$; P3: $\chi^2 = 5.19, p < .05$; P5: $\chi^2 = 4.67, p < .05$), while the remaining patient showed no significant difference (P4: $\chi^2 = 1.29$), although his performance with twice as many errors on pronouns compared to articles pointed in the same direction. Performance on articles was above chance for each patient (P1: $\chi^2 = 10.67, p < .001$; P2: $\chi^2 = 104.53, p < .001$; P3: $\chi^2 = 41.14, p < .001$; P4: $\chi^2 = 62.16, p < .001$; P5: $\chi^2 = 41.14, p < .001$). Performance on pronouns, however, was only significantly above chance for P2 ($\chi^2 = 5.24, p < .05$) and P4 ($\chi^2 = 20.55, p < .001$), but not for P1 who performed at chance level, P3 ($\chi^2 = 3.46$) or P5 ($\chi^2 = 1.16$). Table 1 and Fig. 1 illustrate the subjects' performance on sentences containing articles versus pronouns.

Group analysis using a Mann–Whitney U test revealed that the difference between processing articles versus pronouns is also significant ($U = 1, p < .01$) at the group level. Furthermore, sentences containing pronouns in the grammatically determined gender condition proved to be

TABLE 1
Error Performance on Pronouns and Articles (32 Trials) for Individual Patients

	Pronouns	Articles
P1	16	8
P2	10	2
P3	11	4
P4	6	3
P5	13	4

the most difficult for all agrammatic subjects tested. Inspection of the individual patient data reveals that all five patients showed a tendency to perform better on naturally versus grammatically determined gender in sentences containing pronouns (see Table 2 and Fig. 2). This difference is also significant at the group level ($U = 1$, $p < .01$). No difference between grammatical and natural gender was found for sentences in which the same elements function as articles.

DISCUSSION

The results obtained in the above experiment reveal a distinction between the aphasic subjects' ability to process gender information encoded in articles and their ability to process this same information encoded in pronouns. Contrary to the predictions of Rizzi (1985), patients performed better on articles than on pronouns. Following Rizzi (1985), agrammatic aphasics are expected to show fewer difficulties with pronouns than with articles, the former being involved in theta role assignment, while the latter are not. The present findings contradict the strong form of this view.

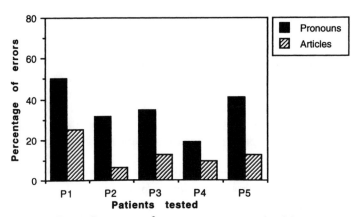

FIG. 1. Percentage of errors on pronouns and articles.

TABLE 2
Error Performance on Grammatical and Natural Gender (16 Trials) for Individual Patients

	Pronouns		Articles	
	Grammatical gender	Natural gender	Grammatical gender	Natural gender
P1	10	6	4	4
P2	8	2	1	1
P3	7	4	1	3
P4	4	2	2	1
P5	10	3	2	2

Interestingly, they further indicate that agrammatic Broca's aphasics are particularly impaired in processing pronouns when gender marking is based on grammatical gender but not when based on natural gender. While natural gender can be mapped onto a universal kind (the animate male/female contrast), grammatical gender, being arbitrary in the language, cannot. This distinction, which has been proposed to be critical in agrammatic language processing (Shapiro et al., 1989), appears to affect the processing of pronouns, but not of articles, in the agrammatic patients of this study.

Furthermore, the results reported above demonstrate that each of the five patients tested performed above chance in processing articles. This is in line with the general proposal of Rosenthal and Goldblum (1989) which predicts sensitivity to morphosyntactic information. However, the data are not entirely compatible with this proposal as only two of five patients performed significantly above chance in the pronoun condition.

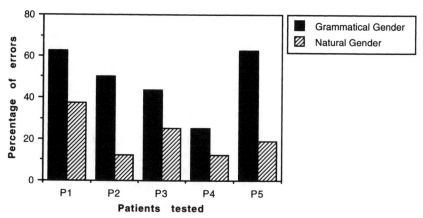

FIG. 2. Percentage of errors on grammatical and natural gender in pronouns.

Agrammatic aphasics are able to determine the lexical identity and syntactic category of words as suggested by the authors, but the processing of pronouns further requires referential operations. These additional operations may account for the problems observed in the processing of gender information encoded in pronouns by the agrammatic patients tested in the present study.

Unlike the case with articles, the interpretation of sentences containing pronouns relies on the coindexing of the pronoun with its antecedent—in our case a situational referent that can be easily inferred from the picture and which subjects had no problem identifying in the preliminary naming task. The difficulty here lies in having to assign a thematic role to a referentially dependent item which must be linked to its antecedent, an element that has to be searched for. The comprehension of sentences involving referential dependencies has been found to be problematic for aphasic patients (Caplan & Hildebrandt, 1988). The question whether the impaired performance observed in this study is due to a specific deficit at the level of pronoun coindexation remains to be addressed. Our results seem to indicate that pronoun coindexing causes more problems for agrammatic patients when they have to rely on grammatical gender information than when reliance on natural gender is possible. In the latter case, instantiation of the referential relation between closed-class element and visually presented antecedent does not require full access to the corresponding noun, but can be done on the basis of the gender information alone. The facilitatory effect observed with stimuli involving natural gender could be explained by the fact that natural gender is of a universal rather than an arbitrary kind. The finding, however, that this latter distinction only affects the processing of pronouns and not of full noun phrases suggests that the two aspects, namely gender marking and problems in coindexing, interact.

In conclusion, the present data provide evidence against the view that the availability of grammatical information encoded in closed-class elements is a function of their potential involvement in theta-role assignment, as suggested by Rizzi (1985). They rather show that the ability to process gender-marked articles is generally well preserved in French-speaking agrammatic subjects.

APPENDIX

P1 La madame . . . les les non. La madame la vaisselle. La chantepleure i'tombe . . . . Le le les . . . les enfants . . . tombent les bancs. Les enfants mang/e/ des beignes . . . . Les rideaux . . . les rideaux tombent. Les assiettes le . . . les tasses est brisée.

"The lady . . . the (pl.) the (pl.) no. The lady the dishes. The faucet it (wrong gender) falls . . . . The (sing.) the (sing.) . . . the (pl.)

children . . . fall the benches. The children eaten (past participle, or homophomous infinitive form) donuts . . . . The curtains . . . the curtains fall. The dishes, the (sing.) . . . the cups is broken.''

P2 La femme . . . tomb/e/ l'eau. Lui . . . elle et le gars s'a chaise a'tombe. La femme a'met chaussures dans l'eau. Deux chantepleures puis la pompe à eau ne fonctionne pas. Le gars prend des biscuits. Mademoiselle prend . . . des biscuits. Un deux trois quatre cinq six sept huit neuf dix. Dix armoires. La fille prend le plat. La fille essuie la vaisselle. La fille prend . . . a'regarde . . . pousser des fleurs.

"The woman . . . fallen (past participle, or homophonous infinitive form) the water. He . . . she and the boy on the chair she falls. The woman she puts shoes in the water. Two faucets then the water pump doesn't work. The boy takes cookies. Miss takes . . . cookies. One two three four five six seven eight nine ten. Ten cupboards. The girl takes the plate. The girl dries the dishes. The girl takes . . . she watches . . . flowers grow.''

P3 Le garçon . . . prend . . . les biscuits. Le garçon . . . tomb/e/ . . . le banc? La fille rit . . . rit? Non? La femme . . . essuie la vaisselle. L'eau renvers/e/ . . . . La cuisine . . . non . . . . La cuisine . . . . Dehors . . . est . . . printemps.

"The boy . . . takes . . . the cookies. The boy . . . fallen (past participle, or homophonous infinitive form) . . . the bench? The girl laughs . . . laughs? No? The woman . . . dries the dishes. The water spilled (past participle, or homophonous infinitive form) . . . . The kitchen . . . no . . . . The kitchen . . . . Outside . . . is . . . (obligatory article missing) spring.''

REFERENCES

Andreewsky, E., & Seron, X. 1975. Implicit processing of grammatical rules in a classical case of agrammatism. *Cortex*, **9**, 379–390.

Berndt, R. S., & Caramazza, A. 1980. A redefinition of the syndrome of Broca's aphasia: Implications for a neuropsychological model of language. *Applied Psycholinguistics*, **1**, 225–278.

Bradley, D. C., Garrett, M. F., & Zurif, E. B. 1980. Syntactic deficits in Broca's aphasia. In D. Caplan (Ed.), *Biological studies of mental processes*. Cambridge: MIT Press.

Caramazza, A., & Zurif, E. B. 1976. Dissociation of algorithmic and heuristic processes in language comprehension. Evidence from aphasia. *Brain and Language*, **3**, 572–582.

Caplan, D., & Hildebrandt, N. 1988. *Disorders of syntactic comprehension*. Cambridge, MA: MIT Press.

Chomsky, N. 1981. *Lectures on government and binding*. Dordrecht: Foris.

Friederici, A. D. 1982. Syntactic and semantic processes in aphasic deficits: The availability of prepositions. *Brain and Language*, **15**, 249–258.

Friederici, A. D. 1983. Aphasics' perception of words in sentential context: Some real-time processing evidence. *Neuropsychologia*, **21**, 351–358.

Friederici, A. D. 1988. Agrammatic comprehension: Picture of a computational mismatch. *Aphasiology*, **2**, 279–284.

Friederici, A. D., & Graetz, P. A. M. 1987. Processing passive sentences in aphasia: Deficits and strategies. *Brain and Language*, **30**, 93–105.

Friederici, A. D., & Schönle, P. W. 1980. Computational dissociation of two vocabulary types: Evidence from aphasia. *Neuropsychologia*, **18**, 11–20.

Friederici, A. D., Weissenborn, J., & Kail, M. 1991. Pronoun comprehension in aphasia: A comparison of three languages. *Brain and Language*, **41**, 289–310.

Friederici, A. D., Wessels, J., Emmorey, K., & Bellugi, U. 1992. Sensitivity of inflectional morphology in aphasia: A real-time processing perspective. *Brain and Language*, **43**, 774–763.

Goodglass, H., & Kaplan, E. 1972. *The assessment of aphasia and other disorders*. Philadelphia: Lea & Febiger.

Grossman, M., Carey, S., Zurif, E., & Diller, L. 1986. Proper and common nouns: From class judgments in Broca's aphasia. *Brain and Language*, **28**, 114–125.

Haarmann, H., & Kolk, H. 1990. A computer model of temporal course of agrammatic sentence understanding: The effects of variation in severity and sentence complexity. *Cognitive Science*, **15**, 49–87.

Hagoort, P. 1988. *Temporal aspects of semantic priming in aphasia*. Paper presented at the Academy of Aphasia 26th Annual Meeting, Montréal, Canada.

Heilman, K., & Scholes, R. 1976. The nature of comprehension in Broca's conduction and Wernicke's aphasics. *Cortex*, **12**, 258–265.

Huber, W., Cholewa, J., Wilbertz, A., & Friederici, A. D. 1990. *What the eyes reveal about agrammaticality judgments in aphasia*. Paper presented at the Academy of Aphasia 28th Annual Meeting, Baltimore, MD.

Jarema, G., Kądzielawa, D., & Waite, J. 1987. On comprehension of active/passive sentences and language processing in a Polish-speaking aphasic. *Brain and Language*, **32**, 215–232.

Jarema, G., & Kehayia, E. 1992. Impairment of inflectional morphology and lexical storage. *Brain and Language*, **43**, 541–564.

Linebarger, M. C. 1990. Neuropsychology of sentence parsing. In A. Caramazza (Ed.), *Advances in cognitive neuropsychology and neurolinguistics*. Hillsdale, NJ: Erlbaum.

Linebarger, M. C., Schwartz, M., & Saffran, E. M. 1983. Sensitivity to grammatical structure in so-called agrammatic aphasia. *Cognition*, **13**, 361–392.

Luketela, K., Crain, S., & Shankweiler, D. 1988. Sensitivity to inflectional morphology in agrammatism: Investigation of a highly inflected language. *Brain and Language*, **33**, 1–15.

Nespoulous, J.-L., Lecours, A. R., Lafond, D., Lemay, A., Puel, M., Joanette, Y., Cot, F., & Rascol, A. 1986. Protocole Montréal-Toulouse d'Examen Linguistique de l'Aphasie: Module Standard Initial (Version Bêta) (Laboratoire Théophile-Alajouanine, Montréal).

Rizzi, L. 1985. Two notes on the linguistic interpretation of Broca's aphasia. In M.-L. Kean (Ed.), *Agrammatism*. New York: Academic Press.

Rosenthal, V., & Goldblum, M.-C. 1989. On certain grammatical prerequisites for agrammatic behaviour in comprehension. *Journal of Neurolinguistics*, **4**, 179–211.

Schwartz, M., Linebarger, M., Saffran, E. M., & Pate, D. S. 1987. Syntactic transparency and sentence interpretation in aphasia. *Language and Cognitive Processes*, **2**, 85–113.

Shankweiler, D., Crain, S., Correll, P., & Tuller, B. 1989. Reception of language in Broca's aphasia. *Language and Cognitive Processes*, **4**, 1–33.

Shapiro, L. P., Zurif, E., Carey, S., & Grossman, M. 1989. Comprehension of lexical subcategory distinctions by aphasic patients: Proper and common, and mass and count nouns. *Journal of Speech and Hearing Research*, **32**, 481–488.

Swinney, D. A., Zurif, E., & Cutler, A. 1980. Effects of sentential stress and word class upon comprehension in Broca's aphasics. *Brain and Language,* **10,** 132–144.

Wulfeck, B. 1987. Grammatically judgments and sentence comprehension in agrammatic aphasia. *Journal of Speech and Hearing Research,* **31,** 72–81.

Zurif, E., Swinney, D., Prather, P., Solomon, J., & Bushell, C. 1993. An on-line analysis of syntactic processing in Broca's and Wernicke's aphasia. *Brain and Language,* **45,** 448–464.

BRAIN AND LANGUAGE **48,** 131–162 (1995)

Automatic Access of Lexical Information in Broca's Aphasics: Against the Automaticity Hypothesis

Lorraine K. Tyler, Ruth K. Ostrin, Mary Cooke, & Helen E. Moss

*Centre for Speech and Language, Birkbeck College, University of London,
United Kingdom*

A number of recent articles have claimed that the language comprehension
impairments of so-called agrammatic patients can be characterized as being due
to problems with the automatic access of semantic and/or syntactic information
from the lexicon. We describe three experiments, all using tasks which probe the
immediate and automatic access of lexical information and compare the performance of agrammatic patients with that of an anomic and a fluent patient. We
find no evidence in support of the automaticity hypothesis as an explanatory
account of the language deficits of agrammatic aphasics. Further, we argue that
current research does ot lend itself to a single-explanation account of agrammatic
comprehension problems, and that in-depth analyses of individual patients are
more likely to be fruitful in terms of understanding the nature of comprehension
deficits. © 1995 Academic Press, Inc.

One of the striking impressions in interacting with aphasic patients is
the difference in fluency between the most extreme non-fluent patients
on the one hand and the "press for speech" characteristic of the most
fluent patients. There is certainly the intuition that the severely non-fluent
patients are laboriously constructing their output, without the help of
the normal automatic routines that make for fluent speech in normal
speakers.

In the past decade, this clinical intuition has been turned into a theoretical account, not only of the failures in production of non-fluent patients
but also of the comprehension failures of some patients. The loss or

This research was supported by an MRC programme grant to Lorraine K. Tyler and
William D. Marslen-Wilson. We thank Greg Savage for helping with many aspects of the
research and for reading an earlier draft of this article. We also thank William Marslen-
Wilson, whose advice has been invaluable throughout all the phases of this research. Ruth
K. Ostrin is now at the Department of Psychology, Hebrew University, Jerusalem. Address
reprint requests to Professor L. K. Tyler, Centre for Speech and Language, Department
of Psychology, Birkbeck College, University of London, Malet Street, London WC1E 7HX,
UK.

slowing down of automatic access has been put forward by a number of researchers as an explanation of the comprehension difficulties of Broca's aphasics (Milberg, Blumstein, & Dworetzky, 1987; Haarmann & Kolk, 1991; Prather, Shapiro, Zurif, & Swinney, 1991; Friederici & Kilborn, 1989). Our reading of the literature, however, as well as our own research, lead us to conclude that this account does not provide a general explanation for the comprehension impairments of agrammatic patients.

First, on both empirical and theoretical grounds, we believe that there is unlikely to be any *single* account for the comprehension failures of "Broca's aphasics". The reasons for this have been argued by others in the context of the individual vs. group study debate (Bates, Applebaum, & Allard, 1991; Caramazza, 1984, 1986; Schwartz, 1984; Shallice, 1979, 1988; Zurif, Gardner & Brownell, 1989). We will simply add that, various subtests notwithstanding, clinical categories are essentially based on production and not on comprehension criteria. Even if one were to accept that the designation "Broca's aphasic" could produce a homogeneous group in terms of speech production (and we known it does not [cf. Saffran, Berndt, & Schwartz, 1989]), it is doubtful that this designation can tell us anything about language comprehension.

Nevertheless, the current suggestion that problems with the automatic access of information characterizes comprehension deficits in Broca's aphasics needs to be addressed explicitly. Over the past decade we have collected evidence directly relevant to the nature of automatic processing in aphasic patients. First, we will review the experimental evidence in the literature that has been marshalled in favor of the loss of automaticity account. We will point out what we feel are serious theoretical and methodological weaknesses and then go on to deal with two versions of the loss of automaticity hypothesis: (1) that Broca's aphasics have lost automatic access to semantic information (Milberg et al., 1987; Prather et al., 1991); (2) that Broca's aphasics are slow to activate syntactic information (Friederici & Kilborn, 1989; Haarmann & Kolk, 1991).

Our critique takes two forms. First, in our various experiments we find no evidence that impairments in the ability to automatically access either semantic or syntactic lexical information provide a general account of the comprehension deficits of Broca patients. At the most, we find that some Broca patients have problems with some aspects of syntax. This, however, could just as well be attributed to problems integrating syntactic information into an utterance as automatically accessing that information. Second, by comparing patients who are unambiguously classified on clinical tests as Broca's aphasics with those who are unambiguously classified as not being Broca's patients, we find that there is nothing homogeneous about the Broca patients as a group. Moreover, the Broca patients are not readily distinguishable from the non-Broca patients in terms of their performance on the various comprehension studies we have carried out.

BACKGROUND

In 1987, Milberg, Blumstein, and Dworetzky published a paper in which they claimed that Broca's aphasics did not exhibit the normal pattern of semantic priming in a lexical decision task, suggesting that Broca patients have a deficit either ". . . in the underlying representation of words or in accessing this information via automatic processing routines." They then went on to argue that other research suggested that the problem was one of impairment of access rather than of representation.

Although these particular results have been called into question (Hagoort, 1990), subsequent research has elaborated upon this finding in different ways, all supporting the basic point made by Milberg et al. (1987) that Broca patients have problems with the automatic access of lexical information. The specific nature of this problem is claimed to be due to the slow activation or slow rise time of lexical information (Haarmann & Kolk, 1991; Friederici & Kilborn, 1989; Prather et al., 1991; Swinney, Zurif, & Nicol, 1989). This has the effect that the relevant information for building higher-level representations is not available at the appropriate time in the processing sequence.

Experiments investigating these issues have looked at Broca's patients' ability to access either semantic (Prather et al., 1991; Swinney et al., 1989) or syntactic information (Haarmann & Kolk, 1991; Friederici & Kilborn, 1989) in the lexicon. The data, however, are used to make different kinds of generalization. Haarmann and Kolk (1991) and Friederici and Kilborn (1989) restrict the automaticity claim to syntax, whereas Swinney et al. (1989) and Prather et al. (1991) claim that this is a general problem with accessing all types of lexical information, both syntactic and semantic. In all cases, however, the interpretation is the same; that is, slow activation results in a temporal delay in the delivery of lexical information to higher-level processes. This has the consequence that information is not available at the right time in the processing sequence.

The Automatic Access of Semantic Information

The hypothesis that Broca patients are unable to automatically access information from the lexicon was originally proposed by Milberg et al. (1987). The authors used ambiguous words to find out whether aphasic patients showed priming when the ambiguous word was primed by semantically related words. Subjects heard sets of triplets which were presented auditorily and were asked to make a lexical decision to the third word of each triplet. Broca patients, unlike normal controls, showed no significant priming effects, leading the authors to conclude that the automatic processing routines involved in accessing semantic information from the lexicon may be impaired in these patients (see also: Milberg & Blumstein, 1981; Blumstein, Milberg, & Schrier, 1982).

This theme has been subsequently developed in research reported by Swinney, Zurif, and Nicol (1989) and Prather, Shapiro, Zurif, and Swinney (1991). Using a cross-modal lexical decision paradigm with ambiguous words presented in various types of sentential contexts, they found that Broca patients only showed facilitation for the most frequent meaning of an ambiguous word, irrespective of the prior context. This contrasted with the normal controls, who showed priming for both meanings of an ambiguous word. They argue that this suggests that "the lexical search module in agrammatism operates on a slower-than-normal rise time. . . ." Thus, whereas Milberg et al. (1987) claim that Brocas are unable to access lexical information automatically, Swinney et al. (1989) and Prather et al. (1991) claim that the process is intact but slowed down.

The Automatic Access of Syntactic Information

Investigations of Broca patients' ability to automatically access syntactic information have used techniques where subjects hear a sentence fragment and then make a lexical decision response to a subsequent visually presented word or non-word (Haarmann & Kolk, 1991; Baum, 1988; Friederici & Kilborn, 1989). In the Haarmann and Kolk experiment, subjects were presented with two-word sentence fragments which were followed at various ISI's (300, 700, and 1100 msec) by either a word or nonword target. The critical variable was whether the real word targets formed a grammatical or ungrammatical continuation of the fragment. They found that normal control subjects showed syntactic priming (i.e., faster lexical decision responses to the grammatical rather than the ungrammatical continuations) at all three ISIs, whereas the Broca patients only showed a significant effect at 1100 msec ISI.[1] They interpreted this pattern as showing that Broca patients take longer to activate the appropriate type of syntactic information in the lexicon.

There are two problems with this study: one concerning the data and one which is theoretical. The first issue concerns the reliability of the effect. Haarmann and Kolk, to their credit, publish the priming effects for each patient and each normal control. This enables us to see how fragile their pattern of results really is. First of all, only a small number of patients (3 out of 13) show significant priming at 1100 msec. Moreover, there is not a big difference in the number of patients showing priming at any of the 3 ISIs (1 out of 13 at 300 msec ISI, 4 out of 13 at 700 msec

---

[1] The significant effect they report for Broca patients at 1100 msec. ISI may be an outlier effect. Only 3 of 13 Broca patients show the effect on individual analyses and when the central tendency is estimated using medians instead of means, the effect disappears.

ISI, and 3 out of 13 at 1100 msec ISI). The control data are more consistent, although in the best case only 7 out of 13 subjects show significant priming.[2]

The other problem is the authors' interpretation of their data. They claim that the results support the slow-activation hypothesis. But their data are equally consistent with the claim that their patients have problems in the integration of syntactic information into the existing representation. On this account, where access and integration are separable processes (Tyler & Frauenfelder, 1987; Marslen-Wilson, 1989), access may be normal for their patients, and it may be integration which is slowed down. This is an interpretation which is more consistent with the demands of the task where priming derives from the grammatical coherence between the target and the two-word fragment which precedes it. This task does not simply tap into activation of information, it also crucially depends upon integrating the syntactic constraints derived from the sentence fragment with the syntactic properties of the target.

The same interpretation can be applied to the results of an earlier study (Baum, 1988), similar to Haarmann and Kolk's. In the Baum study, sentence fragments were presented to subjects auditorily. At a 500-msec delay after the end of the fragment, a single word was presented (also auditorily) for lexical decision. As in the Haarmann and Kolk study, the word was either a grammatical or ungrammatical continuation of the sentence fragment. Baum found that her seven agrammatic patients showed no facilitation for the grammatical target compared to the ungrammatical target. Haarmann and Kolk cite this result in support of their slow-activation hypothesis. But the Baum data can equally well be interpreted as showing that the agrammatic patients are slow to integrate syntactic information. Indeed, we would argue that this is a more plausible explanation, given the paradigm used, where the target can only be grammatical or ungrammatical to the extent that it can be integrated with the syntactic constraints generated by the prior context.

The slow-activation hypothesis is also endorsed by Friederici and Kilborn (1989), although they restrict it to elements of the closed class. They claim that agrammatic patients have lost the ". . . normal fast and automatic retrieval of structural information," which is carried by the closed class vocabulary. Lexical semantic information, in contrast, is accessed normally. This results in syntactic information becoming avail-

---

[2] To be fair, Haarmann and Kolk do not have a problem with this kind of variability. They attribute it to "within-subject fluctuation in the syntactic activation rate" of both normals and patients. However, our problem with this approach is that it makes any prediction about an individual patient difficult to refute. If the expected pattern is not found, this could be explained in terms of individual variation. However, this is not to say that variation has to be ignored.

able more slowly than lexical semantic information. As each new word is heard, the syntactic information from the previous word has not yet been assigned its structural representation and thus the immediate processing of the utterance can only be based upon lexical semantic information, which is accessed at the normal rate. This means that as agrammatic patients are listening to spoken language, they are developing an accumulating backlog of unprocessed syntactic information.

Friederici and Kilborn (1989) test this hypothesis using a cross-modal lexical decision task. The subject hears a sentence fragment (as in the previous studies) and then makes a lexical decision to a visually presented target item. The sentence fragments consist of [article + noun + auxiliary] sequences which are followed by a visual probe. The visual probe is either a grammatical or an ungrammatical continuation of the fragment. The ISI between the fragment offset and the target word was either 0 or 200 msec. This task is used in conjunction with a second task in which the same targets are presented in isolation for visual lexical decision.

There were two relevant findings in this study. The first is that their five Broca patients were slower to make a lexical decision to a visual target when the target followed a sentence fragment compared to when it was presented in isolation. The second finding was that at 0 ISI, the patients were sensitive to the grammaticality of the target, whereas at 200 msec ISI they were not. The lexical decision RTs of old-age controls were the same when targets appeared in isolation and in context, and they showed a significant grammaticality effect at both ISIs. The patient data suggest that when the visual probe is presented immediately after the sentence fragment, patients are sensitive to the grammaticality of the probe in relation to the fragment. This suggests that they are immediately sensitive to the grammatical implications of at least some closed class elements—in this case, auxiliary markers. Indeed, one could plausibly argue that these results show that their Broca patients access syntactic information normally, but that it decays more rapidly than for unimpaired listeners.

However, Friederici and Kilborn do not interpret their data in this way. They focus primarily upon the finding that the RTs of Broca patients are slower in the context condition than in the isolation condition and argue that this shows that, although the patients are sensitive to the grammaticality of the sentence, syntactic information becomes available more slowly to them than to normal listeners. However, there are other plausible interpretations of these results.

First, testing with the two ISIs was blocked and conducted on separate days so that subjects were tested on an ISI of 200 msec some (unspecified) time after being tested with an ISI of 0 msec. As Haarmann and Kolk (1991) point out, patients may have been faster at the 200 msec ISI simply due to practice effects. Second, the finding that RTs are slower in context than in isolation is entirely consistent with the view that Broca patients have problems in the integration of lexical information into sentential representations (cf. Hagoort, 1990). Third, the extra cognitive demands involved in the cross-modal lexical decision task may make it more difficult for the patients than a simple lexical decision task.

Finally, it is difficult to reconcile Friederici and Kilborn's results with their claim that the ". . . relevant syntactic information is not available when needed to do a proper parse of the incoming information." That is, that the slow activation witnessed in these patients accounts for their problems in comprehending language. If the patients are faster to respond to targets when they form a grammatical compared to an ungrammatical continuation, then they must be able to construct the appropriate kinds of syntactic representations. Without constructing these representations there would be no basis upon which a continuation (the visual probe word) could be grammatical or not. The fact that the patients are sensitive to grammatical violations—even if it takes them slightly longer than normals (for whatever reasons)—suggests that they are able to construct syntactic representations in the process of interpreting an utterance. Thus, their results do not provide an account of why these patients have problems comprehending an utterance.

Whatever the final explanation of these effects, there is still no reason to assume, as do Friederici and Kilborn, that it is syntactic context which slows down word recognition in these patients. Since subjects are presented with sentence fragments which are both grammatical and meaningful,[3] it is not possible to disentangle the contribution of semantics and syntax to their performance.

THE PRESENT RESEARCH

The claim that comprehension deficits in Broca's aphasics can be attributed to problems in the automatic access of lexical information is not supported by the data which we will report in this article. The studies which we will describe were not originally designed to address the automaticity issue, but they do so nevertheless because they test Broca patients' abilities to automatically access syntactic and semantic information. The studies all use on-line tasks, such as priming and word monitoring, where subjects produce fast, timed responses to critical aspects of the speech input.

The studies which we report here allow us to test the two versions (semantic vs. syntactic) of the automaticity claim. The first study focuses

---

[3] We are assuming that the sentences were meaningful since Friederici and Kilborn do not state otherwise.

on the ability of Broca patients to automatically access semantic information from the lexicon as rapidly as unimpaired listeners. Experiments 2 and 3 test claims about the automatic access of various types of syntactic information.

An important aspect of this research is that, in addition to testing Broca patients, we also test other aphasic patients who, on standard tests, are not classified as Broca's aphasics. This enables us to determine the range of differences and similarities within the set of Broca patients and across different kinds of patients.

Patients

In the three experiments we report in this paper, we test a variety of patients. Not all of the patients could be tested on all studies. However, in all studies we have a selection of Broca patients, one anomic and one fluent, Wernicke-type patient. These labels are based on the standard clinical classification of aphasic patients (BDAE). This combination of patients enables us to compare different patients within the Broca group, and to compare the performance of Broca patients with that of non-Broca (anomic and fluent) patients.

1. SEMANTIC INFORMATION

Experiment 1: Semantic and Associative Priming

Introduction

The original claim that Broca's aphasics are unable to automatically access semantic information from the lexicon was based on data from semantic priming experiments (Milberg & Blumstein, 1981; Blumstein, Milberg, & Shrier, 1982; Milberg et al., 1987). In this study we also use a priming task to test for the automatic activation of various kinds of semantic information in our patients.

In most semantic priming studies, the nature of the relationship between prime-target pairs is that of association. That is, the prime-target pairs are chosen from association norms. However, it has been claimed that associative and semantic priming may derive from different processes (Tanenhaus & Lucas, 1987; Moss, Ostrin, Tyler, & Marslen-Wilson, 1993). Associative relationships are based upon common co-occurrence in the language. This co-occurrence may enable activation connections among word forms to build up over time, in addition to their meaning relationships. These links would allow activation to spread between associatively related words at the level of lexical form, and result in priming effects that may not reflect the nature of semantic representations (Moss et al., 1993). Our research with unimpaired adults has shown

that pairs of words which are semantically, but not associatively, related
also prime, but to a lesser extent than pairs which are associatively related (Moss et al., 1993). We have also found pure associative priming
(*pillar–society*) and pure semantic priming (*spade–rake*) in a lexical decision task (Moss & Tyler, 1993).

If Broca's aphasics do indeed have problems with the automatic access
of semantic information from the lexicon, this may differentially affect
different types of semantic relations. They may, for example, show significant associative priming, since this can be based purely on co-
occurrence links, while at the same time not showing semantic priming
which derives solely from relationships between lexical semantic representations. Therefore, in our study, we contrast prime-target pairs which
are associatively and semantically related with those which are semantically but not associatively related.

A further consideration in our study was the nature of the semantic
relationship between prime-target pairs. There are many different types
of semantic relationships. For example, pairs of words can be near synonyms (*damp–wet*), antonyms (*hot–cold*), category co-ordinates (*cat–
dog*), functionally related (*hammer–nail*), etc. Experiments with unimpaired adults have shown that all these different varieties of semantic
relations prime each other (Colombo & Williams, 1990; Moss et al., 1992).

Given these hypothesized differences between words which are associatively or semantically related, and the fact that some patients are differentially sensitive to different types of semantic relationship (Goodglass
& Baker, 1976), we considered it to be important to test for a wide range
of semantic relationships in our patients. Thus, we modeled our experiment on the study carried out by Moss et al. (1993). In this study, the
materials consisted of pairs of words which were semantically related,
but where the degree of association varied. The study also included various types of semantic relationship between the word pairs.

We used an auditory priming task where subjects heard pairs of words
and were asked to make a lexical decision to the second member of the
pair. The target word was either preceded by a semantically related word
or by an unrelated control word. A crucial aspect of the experiment was
to ensure that we selected a task which tapped the automatic activation
of semantic representations. Thus, the timing relation between the prime
and the target was an important issue because of its implications for
controlled vs. automatic processing (Neely, 1977, 1991; Posner & Snyder,
1975). There has been considerable debate over the years about this issue,
but the emerging consensus assumes that the shorter the time between
prime and target, the greater the probability that the task reflects the
automatic processes involved in the activation of semantic information
and minimises controlled or strategic processes (de Groot, 1984; Neely,
1977). Since we were interested in the automatic activation of semantic

representations, in the present study (as in the Moss et al. study, 1993), we used an ISI of 200 msec.[4]

Method

We selected 112 target words, each of which was paired with a related prime and an unrelated control word. Half of the related primes were strongly normatively associated to their targets, and half had zero associative strength. Association was crossed with semantic type. Half of the related prime-target pairs were category coordinates (*dish–plate; dog–cat*) and half were functionally related (*theatre–play; broom–floor*).

We selected items in the associated condition from several sets of association norms (e.g., Postman & Keppel, 1970) as well as norms run in our own laboratory.[5] For the category co-ordinates, we checked ranked typicality in the Battig and Montague (1969) norms to ensure that items in the associated and non-associated sets were equally typical of their category.[6] We also ran a relatedness judgement pretest to check the degree of semantic relation between primes and targets in the functionally related conditions.[7]

Finally, the frequencies of the target words in the Associated and Nonassociated sets were matched (Median frequency of associated targets = 31; Median frequency of non-associated targets = 26).[8]

Each target was paired with an unrelated control word which acted as a baseline for lexical decision. Unrelated controls were generated by re-pairing each target with another prime in the set which was semantically and phonologically unrelated to the target. To avoid repetition within a single testing session, the materials were divided into two versions. Each target appeared only once in each version. The number of trials in each condition was fully counterbalanced across the two versions.

The same set of 224 filler pairs was added to each version. 56 of these were unrelated word/word pairs to reduce the proportion of the trials on which the target was related to

---

[4] A shorter ISI is not feasible in an auditory priming study, since the two words tend to be perceived as merging together in the speech stream.

[5] For all our association norms, we used at least 40 subjects. They heard the stimulus words over headphones, and were asked to write down the first word they thought of after hearing each word. The mean associative strength of the four categories of prime-target relations was as follows: Associated Category Coordinates = 39; Non-associated Category coordinates = 1; Associated Functionally related = 37; Non-associated Functionally related = 1. For the Non-associated condition, we used only pairs where the target was rarely (less than 2% of subjects) given as a response to the prime and the prime was rarely given as a response to the target (to avoid possible backward associative priming effects).

[6] Mean rank typicality for those items taken from the Battig and Montague norms: Associated pairs = 10; Non-associated = 6.5.

[7] We considered it to be redundant to test the coordinates in this pre-test since we had selected these pairs on the basis of their typicality ratings. Therefore, we only tested the functionally related pairs. 14 subjects were given a booklet containing all the potential functionally related test pairs as well as filler pairs of varying semantic relatedness (from highly related synonyms to unrelated rhyme pairs). Subjects were asked to indicate on a scale from 1 (very unrelated) to 9 (very related) how related in meaning they thought each pair of words were. The mean ratings for the various pairs were: synonyms = 8; rhymes = 1; functionally related pairs = 7.25. This indicates that the functionally related pairs were considered to be almost as highly related as synonyms.

[8] The median frequencies of the four conditions were: Associated/Category = 42; Non-associated category = 32; Associated functional = 34; Non-associated functional = 26.

the prime (to 33% of real word targets; 16% of all targets). It has been claimed (Neely, 1991; Tweedy, Lapinski, & Schvaneveldt, 1977) that a low proportion of related items reduces the contribution of controlled strategic effects. One hundred and sixty-eight word/ non-word trials were added so that there should be an equal number of word/non-word targets for lexical decision. All non-word targets were phonologically permissible strings in English and were matched for number of syllables to the real word targets in the list. Fillers and test items were pseudo-randomly distributed throughout the versions.

A set of 36 practice trials preceded the test list.

Procedure

The materials were recorded by a female native speaker of British English in a sound-attenuated booth. They were digitized onto computer hard disk. The experiment was controlled by the computer which played speech tokens out directly from the stored wave forms and registered the subjects' responses. Lexical decision responses were measured from the onset of the target word.

Subjects were tested individually in a quiet room and heard the materials played out over headphones. They pressed a response button labeled YES when they heard a word and another button labeled NO when they heard a non-word.

Subjects

We tested 2 non-fluent aphasic patients (DE and JG), an anomic patient (PK), and a fluent patient (FB). See Appendix for details of the patients. In addition, we tested 13 control subjects, ranging in age from 64 to 77 years (mean age = 70 years). Seven of these subjects suffered from a significant degree of hearing loss (mean: 41 db) while the other 6 did not (mean: 19 db).

Results

Controls. We cleaned each subject's data individually. Missing and extreme values (mean ± 2 *SD*) for each condition were replaced by the mean. A total of 6.2% [range: 2–10%] of the data were replaced in this way.[9] The results, collapsed across subjects, are summarized in Table 1. We have also collapsed across the functional/category variable since there was no difference between these two sets of items (see below).

We computed two ANOVAs—one with subjects and the other with items as the random factor—and calculated MinF' statistics. Each ANOVA had hearing loss as a between-subjects factor and associated/ semantic, category/functional and prime/control as within subjects factors. First of all, there was no significant effect of hearing loss (MinF' < 1.0). The mean RT of the subjects with poor hearing was 875 msec, while that of the good hearing group was 869 msec (range across subjects: 646–1108 msec), nor did this factor interact with any other variable. We will therefore ignore hearing loss in the discussion of the results.

---

[9] Eight items were removed from the analysis because subjects made a large number of errors on them. This left us with 53 non-associated items and 51 associated items.

TABLE 1
Experiment 1: Semantic Priming Study

	Prime	Control	Difference	Proportion
Controls				
+ Associated	780	902	122*	14%
− Associated	868	937	69*	7%
(Range of priming: + Associated: 7–20%; − Associated: 2–13%)				
DE				
+ Associated	776	867	91*	11%
− Associated	852	933	81*	8%
JG				
+ Associated	827	949	122*	14%
− Associated	892	997	105*	11%
PK				
+ Associated	1146	1360	214*	17%
− Associated	1192	1398	206*	16%
FB				
+ Associated	849	1032	183*	19%
− Associated	985	1155	120*	11%

Note. Mean lexical decision RTs (msec)
* Significant at the $p < .05$ level or above.

Lexical decision responses to targets preceded by a control word were significantly slower (919 msec) than to those preceded by a related prime (824 msec; MinF'[1, 26] = 77.8, $p < .01$). There was also a significant difference between the amount of priming (control-prime RTs) for associatively related pairs compared to non-associatively related pairs. For the associatively related pairs the mean difference between control and prime was 122 msec (Control = 904; Prime = 778 msec; range = 69–184 msec), whereas for the non-associates it was 70 msec (control = 899; prime = 782 msec; MinF'[1, 47] = 10.38, $p < .01$; range = 10–128 msec.). Thus, pairs of words which are semantically related get an extra priming "boost" if they are also associatively related. Finally, there was no significant interaction between the category and functionally related pairs (F^1[1, 11] = .641, $p = .44$; F^2[1, 100] = .279, $p = .598$) and both showed significant priming (category: 102 msec priming; functional: 87 msec priming).[10]

Finally, we calculated the proportion of priming for the associated and non-associated pairs for the controls. This was calculated, following Chertcow and Bub (1989), as the mean difference between prime and

[10] The mean prime/control RTs for the functional and category conditions separately were: Associated category: 778, 904 msec; Associated functional: 782, 899 msec; Non-associated category: 855, 936; Non-associated functional: 880, 937 msec.

control RTs divided by the mean control RT. The proportion of associative priming ranged from 20 to 7%, and the proportion of non-associative priming ranged from 12 to 3%.

Patients. Each patient's data was cleaned in the same way as the control subjects'. We then computed an ANOVA on each patient's data with plus/minus Association, category/functional, and prime/control as factors. The mean RTs in each condition, for each patient, are shown along with the control data in Table 1. In all respects but one the patients' data were similar to those of the control group. We will discuss the data from the two non-fluent patients first and then discuss the anomic patient (PK) and the fluent patient (FB).

Both non-fluent patients produced similar results, and their responses did not differ substantially from normal. First, their overall RTs were similar to those of the normal controls. DE's mean lexical decision latency was 857 msec, and JG's was 916 msec. These compare favorably with 872 msec for the controls (range: 645–1108 msec). Second, both showed a significant prime/control difference (DE: $F[1, 67] = 10.98$, $p < .001$;[11] JG: $F[1, 70] = 52.02$, $p < .001$)[12] with RTs to targets following control words being slower (DE, 906 msec; JG, 974 msec) than to targets following primes (DE, 830 msec; JG, 889 msec). Third, RTs to associatively related pairs were faster (DE, 839 msec; JG, 889 msec) than to non-associates (DE, 893 msec; JG, 947 msec; DE: $F[1, 75] = 3.701$, $p = .05$; JG: $F[1, 86] = 4.081$, $p < .05$). Fourth, there was no difference between category and functional in amount of priming (DE: $F[1, 75] = .504$, $p > .05$; JG: $F[1, 85] = .44$, $p > .05$).

Unlike the controls, these patients did not show a clear associative "boost." Although there was a trend toward more priming for the associatively related pairs (DE, 11%; JG, 14%) than for the non-associatively related pairs (DE, 8%; JG, 11%), this difference was not significant (DE: $F < 1.0$; JG: $F < 1.0$). However, this does not undermine our general claim since associative relationships between words may well be qualitatively different from the semantic relations which exist between lexical items. These two patients clearly show semantic priming in a task which reflects the automatic access of lexical semantic information. There is no evidence in the data that these patients, who are classically of the Broca type, are not accessing semantic information from the lexicon within the normal time-frame.[13]

The fluent patient, FB, shows a very similar pattern to the two non-

---

[11] 16% of DE's data were either extremes or errors and were replaced.

[12] 13% of JG's data were either extremes or errors and were replaced.

[13] We have also tested two other non-fluent Broca-type patients (BN and GS) on a variant of the semantic priming study. They show the same normal pattern of priming with similar RTs to those of the controls (Ostrin & Tyler, 1992).

fluent patients and the control subjects. First, he showed significantly slower RTs[14] to targets following control words rather than test words (910 vs. 1063 msec; $F[1, 81] = 20.316, p < .001$). Second, there was a significant difference between associated and non-associated pairs, with RTs being faster to associated pairs that non-associatively related pairs: 940 vs. 1044 msec ($F[1, 84] = 8.52, p < .01$). Third, there was no significant difference between functionally and categorically related pairs ($F[1, 85] = .19, p > .05$). Finally, although not significant ($F[1, 81] = .853, p = .358$), there was more priming for associated pairs (19%) than for semantically related pairs (11%).

The anomic patient, PK, produced overall latencies which were about 250–300 msec slower than the controls and the other patients. Nevertheless, he showed a significant test/control difference of 210 msec. ($F[1, 94] = 40.104, p < .001$),[15] with RTs to targets following related words being faster (1169 msec) than to those following control words (1379 msec). Unlike the normal controls, his RTs to associatively related pairs were not faster than to semantically related pairs ($F[1, 98] = 1.36, p > .05$), nor was there even a hint of additional priming for associates. This can be seen when we look at the proportion of priming in Table 1. PK shows equal proportions of priming for both sets of words.

The results of this study show, in a task which undoubtedly taps into the automatic activation of semantic information, that control subjects exhibit significant amounts of priming for a range of different types of semantic and associative relations between words (see also Moss et al., 1993). The two non-fluent patients, JG and DE, also show essentially the same pattern of results. Their performance does not differ from that of the controls, and from a fluent patient, FB. This suggests that these patients are able to access various types of semantic information from the lexicon in the same way as normals. There is no evidence here for slow activation of semantic information. If this had been the case, we would not have found significant priming that was comparable in amount and absolute latency to the results for the controls.

Hagoort (1990) reports essentially the same result. He claimed, on the basis of this, that Broca patients do not have problems with automatic processing. He claims, however, that they may have problems with controlled processing because he finds that they do not show priming at long ISIs. He argues that the locus of the impairment in lexical-semantic processing is at the level of post-lexical meaning integration and not at the level of automatic activation spreading through a semantic network. Other data we have collected on our non-fluent patients do not support this claim. We carried out a second experiment, using the materials de-

---

[14] 13% of FB's data were either extremes or errors and were replaced.
[15] 7.2% of PK's data were either extremes or errors and were replaced.

scribed above, but this time, we asked subjects to make relatedness judgements on the pair of words. It is generally agreed that this type of task taps into controlled rather than automatic processing. Our control subjects were very accurate (A' ranged from .95 to 1.0), as were the three patients we tested. Their A's were: JG, 1.0; DE, .92; PK, .94.

2. SYNTACTIC INFORMATION

In this section of the article, we will discuss the evidence against the claim that non-fluent patients have problems comprehending language because they are unable to access syntactic information from the lexicon as rapidly as normal listeners, and therefore syntactic information does not become available when the parser needs it. This claim rests on the assumption that there is a temporal discontinuity between the use of syntactic and semantic information in the process of interpreting an utterance (cf Frazier, 1987). This is a claim which is not without its opponents (Marslen-Wilson & Tyler, 1987) but it is not central to the research which we will now describe.

The claim for slow access of syntactic information has taken two forms. Haarmann and Kolk (1991) assume it applies generally to syntactic information, while Friederici and Kilborn (1989) restrict it to members of the closed class. In both cases, the claim has been translated into the following hypothesis: If patients cannot access syntactic information as rapidly as necessary to deliver it to the parser, then tests of immediate processing should reveal them to be insensitive to syntactic information. So it follows that non-fluent patients should not show sensitivity to grammatical information in an on-line task—such as word-monitoring or cross-modal lexical decision—which tests immediate processing.

Experiment 2: Argument Structure Violations

Introduction

The purpose of this study was to test for sensitivity to syntactic information in the form of subcategory restrictions on the type of arguments which a specific verb can take. We used two on-line tasks—word monitoring and cross-modal lexical decision—to test for patients' immediate sensitivity to the grammaticality of the sentence. We used these two on-line tasks because some patients perform more reliably on one than the other.

We selected verbs and constructed sentences into which they could fit such that the object noun functioned as the target word either for word monitoring or for lexical decision. For example:

(1) "The burglar was terrified. He continued to *struggle* with the DOG but he couldn't break free."

In this example, the test verb phrase is "struggle with" which is sub-categorized to take a direct object. The noun "dog" can fill this argument slot appropriately, thus subjects should have no difficulty integrating the noun into the subcategory frame specified by the verb. This condition constituted the baseline case. We compared RTs to the target word "dog" here with those to the same target word when it occurred in:

(2) "The burglar was terrified. He continued to *struggle* the DOG but he couldn't break free."

In (2), the target noun is ungrammatical because of the removal of the particle "with." The verb "struggle" alone is subcategorized as being intransitive and unable to take an object. If patients are sensitive to the syntactic restrictions on the possible arguments which the verb can take, then their RTs should be slower in condition (2) than in (1).

The syntactic violation in the contrast between conditions (1) and (2) derives from the absence of an obligatory particle in (2). Because many patients have particular problems with the closed class morphology (e.g., Goodglass & Menn, 1985), we considered it necessary to have the reverse case, where the syntactic violation was caused by the presence of a closed class word (in this case, a preposition), as in (3) and (4) where "cat" is the target word:

(3) Each person in the church had something different on his mind. The little boy *wanted* his CAT to come home.

(4) Each person in the church had something different on his mind. The litte boy *wanted* for his CAT to come home.

Materials

(a) *Word monitoring task.* We constructed sentence pairs like 1–4 above, consisting of a lead-in sentence followed by a test sentence. The structure of the test sentence was always the same. It consisted of a subject NP + verb + object NP plus a few additional words. The object NP was always the target word. In the grammatical condition (as 1 and 3 above), the object NP was syntactically appropriate in that it was consistent with the subcategory restrictions on the verb. The verb was always transitive and could take a direct object as its argument. In the ungrammatical conditions (2 and 4 above), the verb could not take an indirect object and therefore the presence of the target noun constituted a grammatical violation.

For half the sentences, the grammatical condition consisted of a verb plus a preposition, such as in 1 and the other half consisted of verbs without a subsequent closed class word (either particle or preposition), as in 3.

We created 38 sentence pairs and subjected them to a pretest to ensure (a) that subjects agreed with our intuitions about what was appropriate and what was inappropriate and (b) that subjects agreed that the violation occurred immediately prior to the target word.

For the pretest, we presented the 38 stimuli, written in a list, to subjects. We constructed two test lists so that subjects would not encounter the same sentence twice within the same session. Thirteen subjects were tested on each version. Subjects were asked to judge the grammaticality of the sentence by circling the word which they thought caused the ungrammaticality. Sentences on which subjects produced four or more errors were excluded. This left us with 30 stimuli for the experiment.

The 30 test items were pseudo-randomly interspersed with 40 filler items, half of which were grammatical and half ungrammatical. These fillers were designed to obscure the regularities of the test items in the following ways. First, half of the ungrammatical violations occurred before the target and half occurred after the target. Second, the ungrammatical fillers were ungrammatical for a variety of reasons (e.g., filled gaps, reflexive errors). Third, the position of the target word varied across the sentences.

The test and filler items were combined into two lists such that only one occurrence of each test sentence (either the grammatical or ungrammatical version) appeared in each list. Each list contained the full set of filler items. Each list was preceded by five practice items.

All the materials were recorded by a female native speaker of British English onto a CED computer. We placed a timing pulse at the onset of each target word. This served to trigger a timing device which was stopped when the subject pressed a response key to the target word.

(b) Cross-modal lexical decision task. We used the same materials as in the word monitoring task. All of the test items and five of the filler items had real word visual targets. We constructed non-words targets for each of the remaining 35 filler items. This produced a set of items which contained an equal number of real word and non-word targets. For the cross-modal experiment, after the stimuli were recorded, the target word and all subsequent words were spliced out from each sentence, leaving only the words up to the target.

Procedure

Subjects were tested individually in a quiet room. For those participating in the word monitoring task, on each trial they were presented with a target word which they read out aloud. They were told to listen to the sentences over the headphones and to press a response key as rapidly as possible when they heard the target word. Subjects who participated in the cross-modal lexical decision task were asked to listen to the sentences normally and to make a lexical decision response to each visual target which they saw on a VDU screen.

Subjects

We tested 21 control subjects ranging in age from 61 to 77 years (mean = 69 years). Half had poor hearing (mean loss: 43 db; range = 31–55 db) and half had good hearing (Mean: 19 db; range = 11–26 db). Twelve them were tested on the monitoring task and 9 on the cross-modal task.

We initially tested patients JG, GS, PK, FB, and DE on the cross-modal task. However, only DE could perform it reliably; the RTs of the other patients were long, variable, and error-prone. Therefore, they were tested on the monitoring task.

Results

Controls. (a) WORD MONITORING. Each subject's data was cleaned individually. Missing values and extremes (Mean $\pm$ 2 *SD*) were replaced. We then computed two ANOVAs, with items and subjects as the random variables and computed MinF'. Each had hearing loss and grammaticality as factors. Although the RTs of subjects with poor hearing were slower (289 msec) than those with good hearing (234 msec), this difference was not significant (MinF'' < 1.0), nor did hearing loss interact with grammaticality (F^1 < 1.0; F^2 < 1.0). For all subjects, RTs to grammatical sentences were faster (238 msec; range = 150–395 msec) than to ungrammatical sentences (285 msec; range = 170–420 msec); MinF′1, 36] = [27.18, p < .001). The size of the difference between grammatical and ungrammatical RTs varied between 24 and 80 msec, across subjects.[16]

(b) CROSS-MODAL TASK. Each subject's data was cleaned and analyzed as described above. A total of 7.5% RTs were replaced [range: 0–13%]. Just as for the monitoring study, there was a significant effect of grammaticality (MinF′[1, 26] = 8.21, p < .01), with RTs to sentences containing argument violations being significantly slower (774 msec; range = 529–1175 msec) than those to sentences which did not contain any violation (719 msec; range = 531–1069 msec.).

The results of both the word monitoring and cross-modal studies show that subjects are immediately sensitive to the subcategory constraints attached to verbs and use them as they construct a representation of an utterance. If the subcategory constraints are violated, subjects are immediately sensitive to this; they are unable to construct the appropriate syntactic representation and latencies to the following target word increase.

Patients

Each patient's data was cleaned and analyzed as described in Experiment 1. Their mean RTs are shown in Table 2.

Three out of the five patients showed the normal pattern of faster RTs to the grammatical compared to ungrammatical sentences (Word monitoring task: FB (F[1, 26] = 4.98, p < .05), GS (F[1, 26] = 5.85, p < .05); Cross-modal lexical decision task: DE (F[1, 26] = 4.4, p < .05). The other two patients (JG and PK) did not show this effect; the difference between RTs in the grammatical and ungrammatical conditions was outside the normal range (JG: (F[1, 26] = 2.32, p > .05); PK (F[1, 26] = .20, p > .05)). Moreover, just like the control subjects, the presence or absence of a preposition did not interact with the grammaticality variable for any of the patients.

These results do not support the loss of automaticity hypothesis as an explanation of the language comprehension problems of non-fluent aphasic patients. Two (DE and GS) out of the three non-fluent patients showed significant sensitivity to the presence of a grammatical violation in the sentences, as did the fluent patient. Thus, the non-fluent patients do not

---

[16] The preposition × grammaticality (good/bad) interaction was not significant [MinF′(1, 34) = 3.98, p > .05]. Sentences which were grammatical with a preposition: 245 vs. 281; Sentences which were grammatical without a preposition: 228 vs. 291 msec. Irrespective of the presence or absence of a preposition, RTs were always faster in the grammatical sentences compared to their ungrammatical counterparts.

TABLE 2
Experiment 2: Argument Structure Violations

	Grammatical	Ungrammatical	Diff	prop^n
		Word monitoring		
Controls				
Mean RT	238	285	47*	21%
Range	(140–373)	(174–390)		(5–32%)
Patients				
JG	288	267	−21	n/a
PK	325	333	8	2%
FB	354	386	32*	9%
GS	432	492	60*	14%
		Cross-modal		
Controls				
Mean RT	719	774	55*	8%
Range	(531–1069)	(579–1160)		(1–16%)
Patient				
DE	838	928	90*	11%

Note. Mean RTs in msecs and ranges (in parentheses).

* Significant at the $p < .05$ level or above.

form a consistent group in this respect, nor do they behave differently from the fluent patient, FB.

We now turn to a second experiment which looks at patients' sensitivity to a different type of syntactic information.

Experiment 3: Syntactic Violations

This study is related to the previous one in that they are both designed to investigate patients' abilities to process various kinds of syntactic information, as they listen to an utterance. The types of syntactic information we focus on differs in the two studies. In this study, we examine processing of auxilliary markers and phrase structure relations. We selected these two types of syntactic information for the following reasons. Auxiliary markers, such as the auxiliary "was" in the sentence,

(1) "It was Monday and Philip *was* making SANDWICHES for everybody's lunch,"

are members of the closed class. It has been frequently noted that Broca patients have particular problems with members of the closed class, and it was for this reason that these linguistic elements were included in the present study. We contrasted word monitoring RTs for targets occurring in sentences like (1) where the target word was "sandwiches" with those to targets occurring in sentences like (2) where the auxilliary is changed so that the sentence is ungrammatical.

(2) "It was Monday and Phillip *had* making SANDWICHES for everybody's lunch.'

The ungrammaticality in (2) can be interpreted as arising either from the wrong auxiliary or from the wrong inflection on the verb. In either case, though, the ungrammaticality involves a member of the closed class.

The second type of ungrammaticality we included in this study involved violations of phrase structure rules. These were:

(3) They went into London *to chose* CARPETS and curtains.
(4) They went into London *chose to* CARPETS and curtains.

In sentence (3) the target word CARPETS follows a verb to complete a verb phrase; the target noun is in the correct configuration with respect to the verb. In contrast, in (4) the target word follows a sequence which violates the legal configuration of grammatical categories. In all cases, the target word occurred immediately after the violation. If patients are sensitive to the syntactic coherence of the target word with respect to the prior syntactic context, then monitoring RTs should be faster when the sentence is grammatical compared to when it is ungrammatical.

These two conditions are relevant to Grodzinsky's (1989) recent claims about comprehension deficits in aphasia. He has suggested that agrammatic comprehension is best characterized as the absence of terminal nodes for closed class items. This predicts that our agrammatic patients should be sensitive to phrase structure violations but not to auxiliary violations. For auxiliary violations, the grammatical category is appropriate but the identity of the terminal node is wrong. Therefore, patients who don't "have" terminal node representations will be insensitive to incorrect auxilliaries.

Method

We constructed two types of sentences; one type consisting of sentences with the structure [NP + aux + verb + target noun], followed by additional material, as in (1) above. These sentences were then modified to produce ungrammatical versions. This was done by changing the auxilliary, as in (2). The second type of sentence was constructed such that we could introduce violations of phrase structures, as in (4), where we reordered the elements within the verb phrase to produce an illegal configuration. We constructed 10 of each type of sentence. These test items were pretested on two groups of 7 subjects; one group on version 1 and one on version 2. Subjects received written versions of the materials and were asked to indicate whether each sentence was grammatical or ungrammatical and, if ungrammatical, to indicate the point at which it became so. There were 7.8% errors, mostly on ungrammatical sentences. But no sentence was removed from the set because none was consistently misjudged as either grammatical or ungrammatical.

We also constructed 40 filler sentences. Half of the fillers contained various types of syntactic violations and half were fully grammatical. We varied the position of the target word in the fillers so that it did not always occur immediately following a grammatical violation.

We made two versions of the materials, each containing all the fillers and all the test sentences, pseudo-randomly interspersed. Half of the test sentences in each version were grammatical and half were ungrammatical. A set of eight practice items preceded each version.

The materials were recorded by a female native speaker of British English. They were then digitized on a Mac II using Audiomedia, and a timing pulse was placed exactly at the onset of each target word. These speech files were then transferred onto a DAT tape and the experiment was run on a pc using a software programme which presented the monitoring target words on a screen, controlled the delivery of the speech and collected monitoring RTs.

Subjects

We tested 10 control subjects; 5 with good hearing (mean age = 69 years; range = 61–76 years; mean hearing loss = 18 db; range = 11–26 db) and 5 with poor hearing (mean age = 70 years; range = 64–77 years; mean hearing loss = 43 db; range = 30–55 db). We also tested four aphasic patients (DE, GS, PK, and FB).

Results

Controls. We cleaned each person's data individually and replaced extreme and missing data (7%: range = 2–11%) with the mean for the appropriate condition for each subject. We then computed two ANOVAs (items and subjects) on the combined data with hearing loss, sentence type and grammaticality as factors. The main effect of hearing loss was not significant (MinF' < 1.0), nor was sentence type (MinF' < 1.0). The mean RT for the sentences containing auxilliary violations was 252 msec, and for the set containing phrase structure violations it was 267 msec. There was a significant effect of grammaticality (MinF'[1, 23] = 5.93, *p* < .05) with targets in grammatical sentences being responded to faster (242 msec; range = 160–357 msec) than in ungrammatical sentences (278 msec; range = 208–400 msec). There were no significant interactions. The mean RTs for the grammatical and ungrammatical versions of both types of sentence are shown in Table 3. The Table also shows the proportion by which RTs in the ungrammatical condition are slower than RTs in the grammatical condition. The proportion increase is very similar for the two types of sentences.

Patients. The patient data were cleaned in the same way as the control data.[17] Each patient's data were analyzed separately as described in Experiment 2.

The patient who was most similar to normal was DE. Like the control subjects, he produced slower RTs in the ungrammatical conditions compared to the grammatical conditions (*F*[1, 13] = 4.23, *p* = .054). He also showed a trend toward being more sensitive to violations involving auxilliaries than to those involving phrase structures. This can be seen by

[17] The percentage of replaced data for each patient ranged from 3 to 7%.

TABLE 3
Experiment 3: Syntactic Violations

	Auxilliary			Phrase		
	Gram	Ungram	Prop^n increase	Gram	Ungram	Prop^n increase
Controls	247	287*	16%	236	269*	14%
	(176–337)	(218–426)	(5–42%)	(222–334)	(217–385)	(0–26%)
DE	174	232*	33%	201	234*	16%
GS	496	547	10%	505	469	−7%
PK	301	392*	30%	320	327	2%
FB	307	322	5%	354	358	1%

Note. Mean monitoring RTs in msec and ranges in parentheses.
* Significant at the $p < .05$ level or above.

comparing the proportion by which RTs in the ungrammatical conditions increased compared to the grammatical conditions in Table 3. For the auxilliary violations there was an increase of 33% and for the phrase violations, the increase was only 16%. However, the interaction between the two types of violation was not significant. ($F < 1$).

PK's RTs were not, overall, faster in the grammatical sentences compared to the sentences which contained grammatical violations ($F(1, 13) = 2.084$, $p = .173$). However, he showed a substantial increase in RTs for the set of sentences involving auxilliary violations ($t[18] = 2.1$, $p < .05$) but not phrase structure violations ($t[18] < 1.0$). GS showed a similar trend (see Table 3), although the grammaticality effect was not significant (GS: $F < 1.0$). The only patient who appeared to be completely insensitive to the grammaticality of the sentences was FB. His RTs barely increased when he encountered either type of ungrammatical sentence.

Our patients, in general, show a trend toward being more sensitive to auxilliary violations than to phrase structure violations. We interpret the patients' sensitivity to auxilliary violations as indicating that they are able to immediately access and use this type of syntactic information in the on-line interpretation of an utterance. Friederici & Kilborn (1989)'s patients (in a cross-modal lexical decision task) also showed sensitivity to auxilliary markers; however, their RTs were slower than those of the normal controls. Friederici & Kilborn focussed mainly on the patients' absolute RTs and argued that because they were slow, this suggested that the syntactic information carried by Aux had become available more slowly than normal (even though they found significant grammaticality effects for Aux at a 0 ISI.)

In our study, one of our agrammatic patients, DE, produced fast RTs which were indistinguishable from normal in terms of speed. In addition, he was sensitive to the grammatical information carried by the auxilliary marker, as shown by a significantly slower RT for the ungrammatical continuation compared to the grammatical continuation. This patient, then, provides counter-evidence to the Friederici and Kilborn claim that Broca patients are characterized by their slow access of syntactic information from the lexicon, especially when it involves members of the closed class. These data also do not support Grodzinsky's (1989) claim that agrammatic patients should have particular problems with auxilliaries. We found the opposite pattern.

Finally, once again, we find that we cannot distinguish Broca patients from other "types" of patients on the basis of their RT data. Both DE, a Broca patient, and PK, an anomic, show significant effects of auxilliary violations in a task which, we claim, taps the immediate processing of these linguistic elements.

Summary

The two studies described in this section show that not all Broca patients have problems accessing syntactic information and using it to constrain the interpretation of an utterance. We saw in Experiment 2 that two of our Broca patients (DE and GS) were sensitive to argument structure violations, and in Experiment 3, all of our Broca patients showed some degree of sensitivity to the syntactic constraints on auxilliary markers. Moreover, we found no evidence in support of either the claim that Broca patients are slow to access syntactic information in general (Haarmann & Kolk, 1991), or the more specific claim that they are slow to access syntactic information carried by members of the closed class (Friederici & Kilborn, 1989), as evidenced by slower than normal RTs. When tested in two different on-line tasks, we found that some of our Broca patients showed immediate sensitivity to various types of ungrammaticality. Some patients also showed grammaticality effects involving members of the closed class (auxilliaries and prepositions), with RTs which were well within the normal range.

GENERAL DISCUSSION

In the experiments reported here, we have found no strong evidence that Broca patients cannot access lexical semantic information as rapidly as unimpaired subjects (cf Ostrin & Tyler, 1993). In an auditory semantic priming study, Broca patients showed significant priming for a range of semantic relationships, with latencies which were within the normal range.

Similarly, we found no evidence supporting either the claim that Broca patients are slow to access syntactic information in general or the more specific claim that they are slow to access members of the closed class.

In both Experiments 2 and 3, some of our violations involved members of the closed class; in Experiment 2, subcategory violations involved prepositions, and in Experiment 3 we included violations of auxilliary markers. In both studies, we found that some of our Broca patients were sensitive to these violations and, crucially for the Friederici and Kilborn (1989) claim, they produced latencies which were either within the normal range or just outside it. Thus, following Friederici and Kilborn's line of argument, our patients are accessing syntactic information within the normal time-frame.

Finally, we also found that it is difficult to characterize the comprehension deficits of Broca patients in such a way as to differentiate them from other types of patients (fluents and anomics). Our Broca patients do not all show the same pattern of results, and across the various experiments, their performance is sometimes more similar to either the anomic or fluent patient than it is to other Broca patients.

The results reported in this article differ markedly from those described by Haarmon and Kolk (1991), Prather et al. (1991), and Friederici and Kilborn (1989). The different results obtained may stem from a variety of factors; for example, both patients and tasks differ. However, the fact that we study different patients should not, in principle, have a significant impact on the results since the automaticity account is intended as an explanation of the comprehension deficit of all Broca-type patients. However, the fact that different tasks are involved may be very important.

In this article we have described two types of study: one which investigates the access of meaning from the lexicon and which uses single words as the test stimuli and the other which examines patients' abilities to process words when they occur in sentences and thus uses sentences as the test stimuli. To investigate the access of single word meanings, we used an intra-modal auditory lexical decision task. Most of our evidence concerning the processing of words in sentences used the word-monitoring paradigm. In general, we find that patients can produce enough reliable data when tested with spoken materials.

However, we found that many patients had difficulty with tasks involving both written and spoken materials, such as the cross-modal lexical decision task. Most of them produced too many errors (between 15 and 45%) and long RTs to be able to use the data. Yet these same patients can perform the word-monitoring task without any difficulty. Their RTs are usually within the normal range and they do not make many errors. The cross-modal lexical decision task requires patients to switch attention from what they hear to what they see, and this may be difficult for them. In addition, they are required to read the target word. But many nonfluent patients suffer from reading disorders and this will interfere with their ability to carry out the task. These two factors—attention-switching and reading difficulty—could well explain why their RTs are longer than normal, without the additional claim that they are slow to access lexical information.

The picture which emerges from the studies described in this paper is consistent with studies we have previously reported using the word monitoring task as a measure of immediate sentence processing (Tyler, 1985, 1988, 1992). Two word-monitoring experiments are particularly relevant. In one, we looked at patients' abilities to exploit syntactic and semantic information in the process of interpreting an utterance by having them monitor for target words in normal, anomalous and scrambled prose. For normal listeners, word monitoring RTs get progressively faster across normal and anomalous prose sentences (we refer to this as the "word-position effect") but not across scrambled lists (Marslen-Wilson & Tyler, 1975; 1980), reflecting the listener's ability to use semantic and syntactic information to immediately interpret an utterance. If Broca patients are slowed down in their ability to access semantic and/or syntactic information, then they should not show the word-position effects typical of normal listeners and their RTs should be slowed down relative to those of the controls. However, this is not what we found; four non-fluent patients (DE, JG, BN, and GS) showed the normal word-position effect in normal prose—significantly faster RTs the later the target word occurs in the sentence[18]—and monitoring RTs which were not substantially slower than the controls.[19] These results support and extend the findings from Experiment 1; both studies show that non-fluent patients not only access semantic information rapidly but they also integrate it into the developing context within the same time-frame as normal listeners. For anomalous prose we found a variable pattern for all patient groups, with some non-fluents and fluents showing a word-position effect and others not. Thus, there were no clear distinctions between the different types of patients, and therefore no support for the claim that it is only non-fluents who have problems processing syntax in real time.

A second word-monitoring study (Tyler, 1985; Marslen-Wilson, Brown, & Tyler, 1987) underscores these points. In that study, we examined listeners' immediate sensitivity to the pragmatic, semantic, and syntactic implications of verb-argument structures. We had subjects monitor for target nouns which immediately followed particular verbs. We manip-

---

[18] Moreover, the proportion of facilitation across the normal prose materials was comparable for the patients and the controls. For old controls, RTs were on average 22% faster at the late word-positions compared to the early word-positions (range for old people = 11–30%). All of the patients showed a similar amount of facilitation. Their RTs decreased by 14–33%, with the smallest decrease being attributable to the fluent patient FB.

[19] The non-fluent patients produced mean RTs ranging from 258–559 msec (mean 406 msec.) compared with the control mean of 352 msec. (range = 336–501 msec.). Thus, they are on average only 50 msec. slower than the controls, in spite of having suffered brain damage which tends to slow down psychomotor performance.

ulated the pragmatic, semantic, and subcategory relations between the verb and the target noun. We found that out of our four non-fluent patients (JG, BN, GS, and DE), only JG was not like normal controls. The three other non-fluent patients, as well as the anomic (PK) and the fluent (FB) patients, were sensitive to all aspects of verb-argument relations—as witnessed by significantly slower RTs whenever the semantic, syntactic or pragmatic constraints on verb-argument structures were violated (see Tyler, 1992). Moreover, the mean RTs of the patients were within the normal range.[20]

In conclusion, on the basis of our findings, we argue that even if it turns out to be the case that the language comprehension deficits of some Broca patients can be attributed to the abnormal activation of lexical information, this is certainly not a characterization that is appropriate for all Broca's aphasics. In general, we think that the evidence does not yet favor a single-explanation account of the comprehension difficulties which Broca patients exhibit. When a patient's language comprehension is examined in detail, we usually find that each patient suffers from a cluster of deficits, some of which are shared with other patients and some which differ (see Tyler, 1992). We believe that it is only by probing the nature of each patient's comprehension problems in detail that an explanatory account of their deficit is likely to emerge.

APPENDIX: PATIENT DETAILS[21]
Non-fluent, Broca-Type Patients

1. DE

Date of birth: 1954
Date of onset (accident): 11.6.70
Occupation: Storekeeper

General details
Hearing loss: 7.0 db
Digit span: 3 digits
Digit matching task: 6/6 correct on 4 and 5 digits; 4/6 correct on 6 digits
Simple RT: 121 msec

Standard aphasia tests
Trail Making Test: 39 sec
Token Test: 24/36 (moderate impairment)
BDAF (administered June 1983):

---

[20] Mean RTs of the patients: DE = 288 msec; GS = 556 msec; BN = 531; JG = 485 msec.; PK = 573 msec.; FB = 486 msec. Normal range = 287–531 msec.

[21] Reprinted, by permission, from L. K. Tyler, *Spoken Language Comprehension: An Experimental Approach to Disordered and Normal Processing*, MIT Press: Cambridge, MA. © 1992 by MIT Press.

(a) Auditory comprehension: $z = +.75$

(b) Repetition: Good repetition of single words, poor repetition of phrases.

(c) Spontaneous speech: His speech is slow and hesitant. He rarely produces more than two word utterances which primarily consist of content words.

Sample of Spontaneous Speech: Cookie Theft Picture (4.11.89)

E: So if you could just describe what's going on here.

DE: Right .. children first .. alright .. like chair tip over wrong ... you got cookies high up.. wrong again right.. like ask. um ... Lady right washing um ... dry up right .. washing right .. right .... Full up with water ..right ..turn it off right ..wrong.. overflowing right.. on the floor .. everywhere on the floor, and that's it.

2. GS

Date of birth: 1927
Date of onset (cva): 14.4.78
Previous occupation: Computer operator/clerk

General adults
Hearing loss: 29.6 db
Digit span: 3 digits
Digit matching task: 5/6 correct on 4 and 5 digits; 3/6 correct on 6 digits
Simple RT: 360 msec.

Standard aphasia tests
Trail Making Test: 46 sec
Token Test: 29/36 (no significant impairment)
BDAE (administered January 1983):

(a) auditory comprehension: $z = +1$

(b) repetition: only very slightly worse than normal

(c) Spontaneous speech: She produces speech slowly and carefully. Her utterances are short and relatively simple.

Sample of spontaneous speech: Cookie theft picture (9.11.89)

E: Could you describe whats happening in this picture?

GS: The pictures of a kitchenette... erm.. er.. mother and two children a boy ... and a girl.. erm.. she's got the tap running and the water running over the floor. She's.. erm.. she's washing, driving, dry up. The boy's on the stool to get the cookies and he goin to fall erm an anylarhute The girl the girls wants. erm.. a cookie.. erm.. the window's open an you see the garden an the path and.. er another window there an trees an grass and bushes er....

3. BN

Date of birth: 1944
Date of onset (cva): 25.4.84
Previous occupation: Chemical engineer

General details

Hearing Loss: 5.5 dB
Digit span: 4 digits
Digit matching task: 6/6 correct on 4 digits; 5/6 correct on 5 and 6 digits
Simple RT: 143 msec

Standard aphasia tests

Trail Making Test: 53 sec
Token Test: 11/36 (severe impairment)
BDAE (administered January 1985):

(a) Auditory comprehension: $z = +.5$

(b) Repetition: Normal repetition of single words, poor repetition of phrases.

(c) Spontaneous speech: BN's speech is very limited. He has problems with articulation which makes it hard for him to produce even the limited amount of speech he does produce. The fragments below are very typical, with long pauses between words (usually nouns) and no grammatical structure. His speech lacks intonational contour, it is effortful and he typically produces single word utterances.

Sample of spontaneous speech: Cookie theft picture (3.11.89)

BN: ER ... man ... no ... no ... nay man cookies right, fall over um fall over .. stool ummmm water er water .. er ... over rightn and greemin reamin umm ...

E: What else is she doing?

BN: Dreamin say .. look no water umm ...

E: Is she?

BN: Ohh .... oh god ....woman no .....woman ....woman ordin .. ordin tachin.

4. JG

Date of birth: 1929
Date of onset (cva): 22.11.80
Previous occupation: Groundsman

General details

Hearing loss: 22.1 db
Digit span: 3 digits

Digit matching task: 5/6 on 4 digits; 6/6 correct on 5 digits; 3.6 correct on 6 digits

Simple RT: 185 msec

Standard aphasia tests

Trail Making Test: 67 sec

Token Test: 10/36 (severe impairment)

BDAE (administered October 1981):

(a) Auditory comprehension: $z = -.75$

(b) Repetition: Normal repetition of single words, poor repetition of phrases.

(c) Spontaneous speech: He produces short utterances, consisting of one or two words. His speech is hesitant and effortful.

Sample of spontaneous speech: Cookie theft picture (23.11.89)

E: Could you just describe for me what's happening in this picture?

JC: Yeh. The boy is fallin down because the chocolate in.. in.. then the stool is woompy and the water is a... taps is on and drippin down. And a.. and the boy girl.. and the father.. er.. father.. no.. the yeh far.. father... ha ha ha. And ......a.. an boy and.. and still its carryin on.. an and an.. an the y'know. There is water an there is runnin' an that boy and y'know ....this ole boy.

Anomic:

5. PK

Date of birth: 1945

Date of onset (cva): 16.4.84

Previous occupation: Architect

General details

Hearing loss: 12.9 db

Digit span: 4 digits

Digit matching task: 5/6 correct on 4 digits; 3/6 correct on 5 and 6 digits

Simple RT: 242 msec

Standard aphasia tests

Trail Making Test: 72 sec

Token Test: 9/36 (severe impairment)

BDAE (administered October 1984):

(a) Auditory comprehension: $z = +.5$

(b) Repetition: normal

(c) Spontaneous speech: His output is fluent, well-intoned and grammatically correct. He does, however, show a severe word finding problem. In addition, he tends to produce verbal (semantic) paraphasias.

Samples of spontaneous speech: Cookie theft picture (3.11.89)

PK: Right you have a mother, daughter and a son. The son and daughter are in the process of picking out coconut coco jam umm ... high level and to get up there he has gone on a er ... one two three pinned sort of ... it's a kind of very tall um ... what do they call it a tall table not table er chair. And he has climbed up to get the um .. the er .. urm ......anyhow gone up to get two, one for his one one for his er daughter no his um son no no his er younger son keep on and the chair has slipped. Sorry that is all that was in that one. Um .. the wife is busy washing up and she seems to have forgotten the er sink and whereas one would normally pull out the plug she has left it in and it's all poured down the front and on the floor um ... That's it.

Fluent:

5. FB

Date of birth: 1921
Date of onset (cva): 25.9.79
Previous occupation: Solicitor

General details

Hearing loss: 37.9 db
Digit span: 4 digits
Digit matching task: 6/6 correct on 4 and 5 digits; 5/6 correct on 6 digits
Simple RT: 221 msec

Standard aphasia tests

Trail Making Test: 65 seconds
Token Test: 11/36 (severe impairment)
BDAE (administered November 1980):

(a) Auditory comprehension: $z = +.5$

(b) Repetition: Moderate repetition of single words, poor repetition of phrases.

(c) Spontaneous speech: His speech is fluent, with normal intonational contour. His speech is fairly typical of a fluent patient in that it is semantically "empty" and contains paragrammatisms.

Sample of spontaneous speech: Cookie theft picture (9.11.89)

E: Describe for me whats going on in that picture.

FB: Oh yes it obviously the first thing that you see here is is is of course the the the wife if you like or or the mother of the two children erm is er all all the waters is gone over over her sink erm and she still showin that them an she hasn't even bothered about that obviously with that because she's she's still sort of em erm erm cleanin cleanin washin washin...the the the plate erm but I would've thought sh what she what she what she should've done should er put put the plate allon some some there took took and took and took the erm got away with the got away with the er away from from the water but there you are.Ha ha ha. Now you wan't eh....

REFERENCES

Battig, W. F., & Montague, W. E. 1969. Category norms for verbal items in 56 categories: A replication and extension of the Connecticut category norms. *Journal of Experimental Psychology Monograph*, **80**, No. 3, Part 2.

Baum, S. 1988. Syntactic processing in agrammatism: evidence from lexical decision and grammaticality judgement tasks. *Aphasiology*, **2**, 117–135.

Blumstein, S. E., Milberg, W., & Schrier, R. 1982. Semantic processing in aphasia: Evidence from an auditory lexical decision task. *Brain and Language*, **17**, 301–315.

Caramazza, A. 1984. The logic of neuropsychological research and the problem of patient classification. *Brain and Language*, **21**, 9–20.

Caramazza, A. 1986. On drawing inferences about the structure of normal cognitive systems from the analysis of patterns of impaired performance: The case for single-patient studies. *Brain and Cognition*, **5**, 41–66.

Chertcow, H., Bub, D., & Seidenberg, M. 1989. Priming and semantic memory loss in Alzheimer's disease. *Brain and Language*, **36**, 420–446.

Colombo, L., & Williams, J. N. 1990. Effects of word and sentence-level contexts upon word recognition. *Memory and Cognition*, **18**, 153–163.

de Groot, A. 1984. Primed lexical decision: Combined effects of the proportion of related prime-target pairs and the stimulus onset asynchrony of prime and target. *Quarterly Journal of Experimental Psychology*, **36**, 253–280.

Frazier, L. 1987. Sentence processing: A tutorial review. In M. Coltheart (Ed.), *The psychology of reading*. London: LEA.

Friederici, A. 1988. Agrammatic comprehension: Picture of a computational mismatch. *Aphasiology*, **2**(4/4), 279–284.

Friederici, A., & Kilborn, K. 1989. Temporal constraints on language processing: Syntactic priming in Broca's aphasia. *Journal of Cognitive Neuroscience*, **1**(3), 262–272.

Goodglass, H., & Baker, E. 1976. Semantic field, naming and auditory comprehension. *Brain and Language*, **3**, 359–374.

Goodglass, H., & Kaplan, E. 1983. *The assessment of aphasia and related disorders*. Philadelphia, PA: Lea & Febiger.

Goodglass, H., & Menn, L. 1985. Is agrammatism a unitary phenomenon? In M-L. Kean (Ed.), *Agrammatism*. New York: Academic Press.

Grodzinsky, Y. 1989. Agrammatic comprehension of relative clauses. *Brain and Language*, **37**, 480–499.

Haarmon, H., & Kolk, H. 1991. Syntactic priming in Broca's aphasics: Evidence for slow activation. *Aphasiology*, **5**, 247–263.

Hagoort, P. 1990. *Tracking the time course of language understanding in aphasia*. Doctoral Dissertation, Nijmegen.

Marslen-Wilson, W. D. (Ed.) 1989. Access and integration: Projecting sound onto meaning. In W. D. Marslen-Wilson (Ed.), *Lexical representation and process*. Cambridge, MA: MIT Press.

Marslen-Wilson, W. D., & Tyler, L. K. 1975. Processing structure of sentence perception. *Nature*, **257**, 784–786.

Marslen-Wilson, W. D., Brown, C., & Tyler, L. K. 1988. Lexical representations and language comprehension. *Language and Cognitive Processes*, **3**, 1–17.

Marslen-Wilson, W. D., & Tyler, L. K. 1980. The temporal structure of spoken language. *Cognition*, **8**, 1–71.

Marslen-Wilson, W. D., & Tyler, L. K. 1987. Against modularity. In J. L. Garfield (Ed.), *Modularity in knowledge representation and natural language understanding*. Cambridge, MA: MIT Press.

Milberg, W., & Blumstein, S. E. 1981. Lexical decision and aphasia: Evidence for semantic processing. *Brain and Language*, **14**, 371–385.

Milberg, W., Blumstein, S., & Dworetzky, B. 1987. Processing of lexical ambiguities in aphasia. *Brain and Language*, **31**, 138–150.

Moss, H., Ostrin, R. K., Tyler, L. K., & Marslen-Wilson, W. D. *Accessing different types of lexical semantic information: Evidence from priming*. Submitted for publication.

Moss, H., & Tyler, L. K. 1993. *Semantic priming without an associative boost in aphasia*. Paper presented at the American Academy of Aphasia, Tucson, AZ.

Neely, J. H. 1977. Semantic priming and retrieval from lexical memory: Roles of inhibitionless spreading activation and limited-capacity attention. *Journal of Experimental Psychology: General*, **106**, 226–254.

Neely, J. H. 1991. Semantic priming in visual word recognition: a selective review of current theories and findings. In D. Besner & C. Humphries (Eds.), *Basic processes in reading: Visual word recognition*. Hillsdale, NJ: Erlbaum.

Ostrin, R. K., & Tyler, L. K. 1993. Automatic access to lexical semantics in aphasia: Evidence from semantic and associative priming. *Brain and Language*, **45**, 147–159.

Posner, M. I., & Snyder, C. R. R. 1975. Attention and cognitive control. In R. L. Solso (Ed.), *Information processing and cognition: The Loyola Symposium*. Hillsdale, NJ: Erlbaum.

Postman, L., & Kepple, G. 1970. *Norms of word association*. New York: Academic Press.

Prather, P., Shapiro, L., Zurif, E., & Swinney, D. 1991. Real-time examinations of lexical processing in aphasics. *Journal of Psycholinguistic Research*, **20**(3), 271–281.

Saffran, E. M., Berndt, R. S., & Schwartz, M. F. 1989. The quantitative analysis of agrammatic production: Procedure and data. *Brain and Language*, **37**, 440–479.

Schwartz, M. F. 1984. What the classical aphasia categories don't do for us and why. *Brain and Language*, **21**, 3–8.

Shallice, T. 1979. Case-study approach in neuropsychological research. *Journal of Clinical Neuropsychology*, **1**, 183–211.

Shallice, T. 1988. *From neuropsychology to mental structure*. Cambridge University Press: Cambridge.

Swinney, D., Zurif, E., & Nicol, J. 1989. The effects of focal brain damage on sentence processing: an examination of the neurological organisation of a mental module. *Journal of Cognitive Neuroscience*, **1**(1), 25–37.

Tanenhaus, M., & Lucas, M. 1987. Context effects in lexical processing. In U. Frauenfelder & L. K. Tyler (Eds.), *Spoken word recognition*. Cambridge, MA: Bradford Books.

Tweedy, J., Lapinsky, R., & Schvaneveldt, R. 1977. Semantic context effects on word recognition. *Cognition*, **25**, 213–234.

Tyler, L. K. 1985. Real-time comprehension processes in agrammatism: a case study. *Brain and Language*, **26**, 259–275.

Tyler, L. K. 1988. Spoken language comprehension in a fluent aphasic patient. *Cognitive Neuropsychology*, **5**, 375–400.

Tyler, L. K. 1992. *Spoken language comprehension: An experimental approach to disordered and normal processing*. MIT Press: Cambridge, MA.

Tyler, L. K., & Frauenfelder, U. 1987. The process of spoken word recognition: An introduction. In: U. Frauenfelder & L. K. Tyler (Eds.), *Spoken word recognition*. MIT Press: Cambridge, MA.

Tyler, L. K., & Warren, P. 1987. Local and global structure in spoken language comprehension. *Journal of Memory and Language*, **26**, 638–657.

Zurif, E., Gardner, H., & Brownell, H. 1989. The case against group studies. *Brain and Cognition*, **10**, 237–255.

BRAIN AND LANGUAGE **49**, 50–76 (1995)

Syntactic Processing in Agrammatic Aphasia by Speakers of a Slavic Language

KATARINA LUKATELA, DONALD SHANKWEILER, AND STEPHEN CRAIN

Haskins Laboratories and University of Connecticut

It is widely believed that agrammatic aphasics have lost the ability to assign complete syntactic representations. This view stems from indications that agrammatics often fail to comprehend complex syntactic structures, as for example, some types of relative clauses. The present study presents an alternative account. Comprehension by Serbo-Croatian-speaking agrammatic aphasics was tested on four types of relative clause structures and on conjoined clauses. The relative clauses varied in type of embedding (embedded vs. nonembedded) and in the location of the gap (subject position vs. object position). There were two control groups: Wernicke-type aphasics and normal subjects. The findings from a sentence–picture matching task indicated that agrammatic aphasics were able to process complex syntactic structures, as evidenced by their well-above chance performances. The success rate varied across different types of relative clauses, with object-gap relatives yielding more errors than subject-gap relatives in all groups. Each group showed the same pattern of errors: agrammatic subjects were distinguished from Wernicke subjects and normal subjects only in quantity of errors. These findings are incompatible with the view that the agrammatics are missing portions of the syntax. Instead, their comprehension deficits reflect varying degrees of processing impairment in the context of spared syntactic knowledge. © 1995 Academic Press, Inc.

EXPLAINING COMPREHENSION DIFFICULTIES IN AGRAMMATISM

The view that the "agrammatism" of Broca's aphasia represents a disorder involving loss of some structural component of the language apparatus has enjoyed considerable influence in the last two decades (Berndt & Caramazza, 1980; Schwartz, Saffran, & Marin, 1980; Zurif, 1984). The appeal to missing structural knowledge rested in part on the promise it seemed to hold for explaining parallel deficits in language pro-

Address correspondence and reprint requests to Katarina Lukatela, Haskins Laboratories, 270 Crown Street, New Haven, CT 06511.

158

duction and comprehension. Just as agrammatic aphasics produce syntactically deficient speech largely as a result of a tendency to omit function words and to distort inflections, so, too, it might be supposed that they understand sentences by inferring meaning without recourse to normal syntactic operations, using non-syntactic, lexically based strategies instead. Several specific proposals have been offered, each seeking to ground the difficulties involving the closed-class vocabulary and the inflectional system on one or another level of linguistic representation: phonological (Kean, 1977), lexical (Bradley, Garrett, & Zurif, 1980), morphological (Lapointe, 1983), or syntactic (Caramazza & Zurif, 1976; Caplan & Futter, 1986; Grodzinsky, 1986, 1990; Hickok, Zurif, & Canseco-Gonzales, 1993; Mauner, Fromkin, & Cornell, 1993). Collectively, we call these proposals the Structural Deficit Hypothesis.

Whatever the plausibility of these proposals, there is mounting evidence that calls into question any form of the Structural Deficit Hypothesis. First, several case studies have reported patients who fail to show parallel deficits in production and perception. Some patients present agrammatic symptoms in production, but not in comprehension (Miceli, Mazzucchi, Mann, & Goodglass, 1983). Additionally, there are reports of patients who show agrammatic symptoms in comprehension despite fluent production of well-formed sentences (Caramazza, Basili, Koller, & Berndt, 1981; Smith & Bates, 1987). These findings suggest that expressive and receptive agrammatism may represent different deficits, though they often occur together.

The finding that agrammatic aphasics retain the ability to make metalinguistic judgments of grammatical acceptability presents a further challenge to the Structural Deficit Hypothesis. Retained ability to detect syntactic violations has been demonstrated even in patients who were severely agrammatic in both production and comprehension (Linebarger, Schwartz, & Saffran, 1983). Preserved sensitivity to syntactic structure in doubly agrammatic patients cannot readily be explained by a syntactic account of agrammatism. Spared ability to judge the grammaticality of complex syntactic structures has been confirmed in additional studies of English-speaking agrammatics (Shankweiler, Crain, Gorrell, & Tuller, 1989; Wulfeck, 1988). Sensitivity to violations of the inflectional morphology has also been demonstrated in Italian, German, and Serbo-Croatian agrammatics (Lukatela, Crain, & Shankweiler, 1988; Kolk & van Grunsven, 1985; Bates, Friederici, & Wulfeck, 1987, Friederici, Wessels, Emmorey, & Bellugi, 1992).

Central to the Structural Deficit Hypothesis is the assumption that the comprehension deficit in agrammatism is syndrome-specific. This assumption, too, is challenged by findings with other language impaired populations and with normal subjects. For example, sentence comprehension in children with reading problems shows the same ordering of

difficulty across syntactic structures as is displayed by agrammatic aphasics (Smith, Macaruso, Shankweiler, & Crain, 1989). Moreover, normal
adults working under time pressure have been found to conform to the
same pattern (Milekic, 1993; Ni, 1988). Such consistencies that cut across
diagnostic groups and normal subjects point to a common source of variation that would implicate a processing explanation, not a structural explanation.

Spurred by findings that are unfavorable to the Structural Deficit Hypothesis, an alternative has begun to crystallize. We call it the Processing
Limitation Hypothesis.[1] This hypothesis appeals to the distinction between structural and processing components of the language apparatus.
The structural components include the lexicon and the different levels of
linguistic representation: phonology, syntax, and semantics. According
to the Processing Limitation Hypothesis, impaired comprehension need
not reflect loss of critical linguistic structures. Language processing involves not only the assignment of structural representations, it also requires a series of operations for storing and retrieving linguistic information and for coordinating the transfer of information between levels of
linguistic representation. The Processing Limitation Hypothesis directs
us to consider linguistic *processing* as a possible source of the comprehension deficits that are characteristic of aphasia.

In addition to giving direction to the quest for the source of sentence
comprehension difficulties in agrammatism, the Structural Deficit Hypothesis and the Processing Limitation Hypothesis have implications for
accounts of normal sentence processing. If an obtained pattern of preserved and impaired comprehension can be accounted for on the basis
of the disruption of a particular component of syntactic representation
postulated in one theory but not in others, then the data would provide
support for that theory. However, if the pattern of performance can be
accounted for on the basis of a limitation in processing capacity, then the
data could not decide among linguistic theories, but would require a
model of sentence processing that incorporates the appropriate processing components.

The intent of the present study was to compare a structural deficit
versus a processing limitation account of syntactic comprehension difficulties in agrammatic aphasia. We proceed by examining a structure often
implicated in agrammatism, *the relative clause*. We then present the rationale for a study of comprehension of relative clauses in agrammatic subjects who are speakers of the Slavic language, Serbo-Croatian. The highly

---

[1] The term "processing impairment" has been used differently by different authors.
Tzeng, Chen, and Hung (1991) use the term much as we do to refer to an account of
language breakdown based on deficits in the processes by which a preserved knowledge
base is accessed and deployed.

inflected morphology of the Serbo-Croatian language is exploited to provide the appropriate experimental conditions for distinguishing between the two accounts and for testing specific proposals regarding difficulties in processing relative clauses.

Some initial comments about Serbo-Croatian are in order. The closed-class morphology, consisting of grammatical words and inflections, plays a somewhat different role in syntactic operations in a free word-order language, like Serbo-Croatian, than in a fixed word-order language, like English. In order to construct a grammatically correct sentence in Serbo-Croatian, words must match in gender, number, person, and noun case. This is accomplished by an appropriate suffix (an inflectional morpheme) added to the word root. In English, word order is used to indicate, for example, agent/object relations, both semantically and syntactically (e.g., "The girl pushed the boy"). Case is generally conveyed either by word order or by free-standing prepositions or pronouns in English. Case is conveyed by noun-inflections in Serbo-Croatian, however. In the absence of a consistent word order pattern, a Serbo-Croatian listener must rely on case markers and other agreement markers (subject–verb agreement, modifier–noun agreement, agreement between pronouns and their referents, etc.). Consequently, the English sentence from the example above can be translated into two Serbo-Croatian sentences having the same meaning but different word orders (e.g., "Devojčica$_{(nom)}$ je gurnula dečka$_{(accus)}$" and "Dečka$_{(nom)}$ je gurnula devojčica$_{(accus)}$"). The present study was designed to exploit this cross-language difference in the use of inflectional morphology to evaluate difficulties agrammatics experience in comprehending relative clauses. We proceed by examining relevant findings that have been reported in the literature.

Evidence from Studies with Relative Clauses

Among the earliest evidence of a specific sentence processing deficit in agrammatism is the finding by Caramazza and Zurif (1976) of difficulties in comprehension of semantically reversible relative clause sentences. It is presently well established that agrammatic aphasics often fail to understand correctly certain sentences with relative clauses if they are presented without the support of semantic content and/or pragmatic context. All types of relative clauses have not proven equally difficult, however. There appear to be selective difficulties on sentences with object-gap relatives, as compared to subject-gap relatives. For example, Caplan and Futter (1986) report such a pattern, based on a study of an agrammatic subject using an object manipulation test. Object-gap relatives contain a superficially empty noun phrase in object position (e.g., "The monkey that the rabbit grabbed _ shook the goat"). Caplan and Futter's subject performed more accurately with subject-gap relative clauses, i.e., where the empty noun phrase is in subject position, (e.g., "The sheep that _ pushed the cat jumped over the cow") . The authors suggest that the subject had lost the ability to interpret sentences using the rules of normal English syntax. On their view, the subject attempted to map thematic roles (agent, patient, theme, etc.) directly to linear sequences of words. This strategy could sometimes result in the correct linguistic interpretation even for subjects who lacked the relevant grammatical knowledge. This would happen with structures that conform to the canonical word order of the language in question. Canonical word order provides the right results in sentences of English that contain subject-gap relative clauses. This strategy would lead to consistent misinterpretation of sentences that depart from canonical S-V-O form of English sentences, however. One example is object-gap relatives.

The distinction between object-gap and subject-gap relatives has received a specific structural interpretation by Grodzinsky (1986, 1989). Grodzinsky explains agrammatics' comprehension difficulties within the framework of Chomsky's theory of Generative Grammar known as Government and Binding theory. One aspect of this theory is the postulation of a 'trace" whenever a constituent is moved by a transformational rule from one level of representation, D-structure, to another level, S-structure. What is missing in the representations of agrammatics, according to this view, is the trace left behind by the transformation. Therefore the affected individuals are unable to maintain the crucial grammatical link between the "trace" and the moved constituent. Although Grodzinsky discussed several structures that involve constituent movement, we are concerned here specifically with his discussion of relative clauses. One of the assumptions of Government and Binding theory is that traces are the bearers and transmitters of thematic roles. From this assumption it follows that the thematic role of a moved NP inside a relative clause will be unspecified in the absence of the trace. Accordingly, Grodzinsky proposes that agrammatics must resort to a default strategy for heuristically assigning thematic roles to disenfranchised NPs in relative clauses. In an SVO word-order language like English, the heuristic strategy assigns roles according to word order conventions: the initial NP would receive the role of agent. This strategy gives the right interpretation for sentences with subject-gap relatives such as, "The boy that kissed the girl is tall." In such a sentence, the transformation preserves the original NP order; therefore, comprehension is preserved in spite of loss of traces in the S-structure representations. However, in object-gap relatives, as a result of trace deletion, the S-structure representation has two NPs preceding the verb (e.g., "The boy that the girl kissed was tall"). Because there are two possible agent candidates, the assignment of thematic roles cannot be determined. Therefore, agrammatic patients should perform at chance in responding to object-gap relatives. According to Grodzinsky's theory, then, agrammatics generate complete syntactic representations except in the case of constructions that involve movement transformations, such as relative clauses and verbal passives.

A test of this conceptualization of the comprehension deficit in agrammatism is presented by Grodzinsky (1989). In this study, agrammatic subjects were tested using a sentence–picture matching task for comprehension of four types of relative clauses (embedding vs. nonembedding and subject- vs. object-gap). The results are interpreted in favor of the trace deletion account. We question whether the results do constitute unequivocal support for this hypothesis, however. For one thing, Grodzinsky's analysis is based on averaging across sentence types. Each sentence type should be considered separately, in our view. By pooling the results of two types of subject-gap relatives and comparing them with two types of object-gap relatives, and by comparing two types of embedded structures with two types of nonembedded structures, one is liable to lose sight of relevant variability. In addition, there were marked individual differences among the subjects. For example, the performance of the four subjects varied from 20 to 80% error in response to nonembedded object relatives. These differences cannot be explained on Grodzinsky's account.

We have presented two structurally based accounts of agrammatic comprehension difficulties, indicating how each applies to sentences containing relative clauses. The accounts differ in their diagnosis of where within the structural apparatus the problem lies, but each assumes that critical syntactic information for the assignment of thematic roles is not available to agrammatics. We now consider how the two accounts might be differentiated empirically—Grodzinsky's specific trace deletion hypothesis and Caplan and Futter's more general syntactic simplification account—and how each, in turn, may be distinguished from the Processing Limitation Hypothesis.

Testing between the Two Hypotheses

Though differing in their assignment of the specific source of comprehension difficulty, each version of the Structural Deficit Hypothesis leads to specific predictions concerning the comprehension performance of an agrammatic subject. It is important to spell out the expectations in detail. (1) The affected individual would perform poorly on all sentences in which the correct interpretation depends on a full syntactic analysis that would bring into play the damaged component. Thus, if there is loss of syntactic knowledge there should be no significant variation across any sentence type that conforms to a specific syntactic pattern (this prediction would apply only if the putative syntactic loss was complete). If agrammatics construct incomplete syntactic representations, as on Grodzinsky's theory, they lack the means to determine the thematic role played by the moved NP. Therefore, they must apply a guessing strategy which should be reflected in chance performance on sentences with object-gap relatives. On the other hand, if agrammatics fail to construct hierarchical syntactic representations, but rely on simplified structures that are governed by word order, as Caplan and Futter supposed, then, similarly, they should consistently err in responding to object-gap relatives. (2) There should be no significant variability in performance level across patients on a given sentence type. If in order to understand a particular construction, it is necessary to apply the syntactic rule that is assumed to be missing (for example, a rule for assigning thematic roles in relative clauses), all agrammatic subjects would be expected to perform deficiently (i.e., at chance, if syntactic roles are randomly assigned, or below chance, if some specific non-syntactic strategy is used). (3) If the syntactic deficit is structural, one could expect it to be syndrome-specific. Thus, a given pattern of results would characterize agrammatism but not other syndromes which differ in the underlying deficit. Agrammatic patients would be forced to rely on non-syntactic comprehension strategies and to assign a syntactic structure that deviates from that assigned by the normal population, or by another aphasic group whose syntactic problems, if any, are not identified with those of Broca-type aphasics (for example, Wernicke-type aphasics). In consequence, the pattern of performance on any structures that tax the damaged component (for example, relative clauses) should be qualitatively different in agrammatic subjects than in other aphasics, or in normal subjects. (4) If a missing structure is part of Universal Grammar, agrammatics in any language would be expected to erroneously process the critical structures. Thus, if one tests the critical syntactic structure across different languages, agrammatics from a non-English-speaking population would be expected to fail in processing the missing structure just as their English-speaking counterparts.

The Processing Limitation Hypothesis makes different predictions about the comprehension difficulties associated with agrammatism. On this view, particular sentences place greater processing demands upon the language apparatus, and particular tasks further augment the difficulties imposed by these sentences. The processing limitations account makes specific predictions about the performance of agrammatic subjects. (1) Variability in performance levels across different sentence types is expected because processing difficulties are on a continuum. Agrammatic subjects are predicted to demonstrate more difficulty with syntactic structures that impose heavy demands on the processing system (e.g., object-gap relatives) as compared with structures that do not (e.g., subject-gap relatives). (2) Variability in performance levels across individuals on a given sentence type is expected, but each agrammatic subject should display the same rank order of sentence difficulty. The level of performance should vary according to the severity of each individual's processing impairment. Thus, we would expect a continuous distribution of scores across subjects, but with a consistent ordering of sentence types. (3) The relative difficulty of each syntactic structure should be the same in both aphasic subjects and normal subjects; the sentences that are most difficult for normal subjects should also be most difficult for agrammatic aphasics. Although, the pattern of performance across different syntactic structures should be the same for agrammatic aphasics and normals, the level of performance may well differ. If difficulties in comprehension are caused by a processing limitation, then we would expect that when normal subjects are pressed (e.g., by artificially speeded speech or text) they would show the same pattern of performance as agrammatic aphasics. (4) Variability in performance across languages is expected because languages use different means to accomplish the same syntactic ends. These may vary in their costs to the processing system.

The present study was designed to take advantage of the manner in which inflectional morphology is used syntactically in a free word-order language, Serbo-Croatian. Four types of relative clauses varied in their place of attachment (embedded vs. nonembedded), and in the grammatical role of the missing NP inside the relative clause (subject- vs. object-gap). These sentence types are abbreviated as SS, SO, OO, and OS. The abbreviations use the first letter (S or O) to indicate the place of attachment (S = embedded, O = nonembedded). The second letter indicates the role of the missing NP (S = subject, O = object). In some relative clauses in Serbo-Croatian, as in subject-gap relatives (SS, OS) and nonembedded object-gap relatives (OO), the thematic role of an NP is determined by a noun-inflection marking the moved NP. Examples with underlined case-inflections are given in 1–3:

(1) SS: Žena$_{(nom)}$ koja$_{(nom)}$ ljubi čoveka$_{(accus)}$ drži kišobran _ (nom, accus).
The lady who is kissing the man is holding an umbrella.

(2) OS: Žena$_{(nom)}$ ljubi čoveka$_{(accus)}$ koji$_{(nom)}$ drži kišobran _ (nom, accus)·
The lady is kissing the man who is holding an umbrella.

(3) OO: Žena$_{(nom)}$ ljubi čoveka$_{(accus)}$ koga$_{(accus)}$ štiti kišobran _ (nom, accus)·
The man is kissing the lady that the umbrella is covering.

Thus, in these sentence types the inflectional morphology aids in coindexation of the moved constituent and trace. However, in embedded object-gap relatives, as in (4), both NPs have the same nominative-case inflection and, therefore, thematic roles cannot be assigned by processing the noun-case inflection only.

(4) SO: Čovek_ (nom) koga (accus) žena$_{(nom)}$ ljubi drži kišobran_(nom, accus)·
The man that the lady is kissing is holding an umbrella.

The relative pronoun of the relative clause is invariably marked by the thematically appropriate case inflection. Thus, although in SO sentences, the NPs cannot be thematically differentiated by processing only NP inflections, the thematic roles can nonetheless be differentiated by processing the relative pronoun-case inflection.

The fact that moved constituents are marked not only by traces but also by case inflections provides an additional cue for Serbo-Croatian users (which is unavailable to English users) when assessing thematic roles. It is this feature that enables us to test Grodzinsky's trace-deletion hypothesis. The trace-deletion account predicts that agrammatics will perform successfully on subject-gap relative clause sentences (OS, SS), but will be at chance on object-gap sentences (SO, OO). However, if, agrammatics have retained the inflectional morphology and are missing only traces of movement in their syntactic representations, as this hypothesis proposes, then Serbo-Croatian agrammatics are expected to have an advantage over English-speaking agrammatics because their preserved inflectional morphology would be sufficient for determining the thematic role. According to this account, therefore, Serbo-Croatian agrammatics are expected to perform at chance only on SO sentences but equally well on the other three types of relative clauses. Alternatively, if Serbo-Croatian agrammatics have intact inflectional morphology, their performance can be expected to be equally successful on all four types of relative clauses, since the relative pronoun in the SO sentences is marked by the thematically appropriate case inflection.

On the other hand, if Serbo-Croatian agrammatics are unable to make syntactic use of inflections, as an account of parsing deficiency resulting in incomplete, simplified syntactic representations would state, then noun and pronoun case inflections could not aid their comprehension of relative clauses. On this account Serbo-Croatian agrammatics are expected to err on all sentences that depart from canonical word order (SO, OO), systematically choosing the conjoined-clause interpretation instead. In consequence, Serbo-Croatian agrammatics should demonstrate a similar degree of difficulty as their English-speaking counterparts in comprehension of object-gap relatives.

In addition to testing agrammatics' ability to assign thematic roles in relative clauses we also asked whether they tend to simplify the syntactic structure of a relative clause. One possibility is that object-gap relative clauses might be treated as though they consisted of two conjoined clauses. This would be expected on the suggestion that agrammatics lose the ability to construct complete syntactic representations, regressing by default to simpler structures (e.g., Caplan & Futter, 1986). Thus, conjoined-clause sentences can be used to test the proposal that agrammatics fail in comprehension of relative clauses because they tend to simplify complex syntactic structures and employ heuristic, non-syntactic strategies (e.g., a canonical word-order strategy) when interpreting some relative clauses. Studies previously cited have focused on testing for ability to assign correct agent/patient (thematic) relations. The present study offers the first test of the possibility that agrammatics tend to simplify the complex syntax of relative clauses in certain sentences by construing them as though they contained two conjoined clauses (CC). A conjoined clause simplification of, for example, an SO sentence (4) would be:

(5) CC: Čovek ljubi ženu i drži kišobran.
The man is kissing the woman and holding an umbrella.

A test of this possibility was made by requiring subjects to choose between two pictures, one of which depicted the conjoined-clause analysis and the other the relative clause analysis. This technique was used successfully in previous research examining comprehension of relative clauses by agrammatic aphasics (Zurif & Caramazza, 1976, Wulfeck, 1988; Grodzinsky, 1989).

The present study makes use of the forgoing features of the Serbo-Croatian language to investigate comprehension of relative clauses by Serbo-Croatian speaking agrammatics. The fact that inflectional morphology plays such an important role in Serbo-Croatian syntax makes it an ideal language to contrast with English for testing theoretical claims about the basis of comprehension deficiencies in agrammatism. The experiment was designed to distinguish between versions of the Structural Deficit Hypothesis as well as between either version and the Processing Limitation Hypothesis. The study therefore addressed the following questions:

1. Are there systematic variations in performance among agrammatic subjects across different types of reversible relative clauses and conjoined clauses. Do these variations form a graded continuum or are they all-or-none?

2. Are there cross-language differences in comprehension of relative clause sentences between agrammatic speakers of a highly inflected language (Serbo-Croatian) and a fixed word-order language (English)?

3. Are there systematic differences between subject groups? Will Broca-type aphasics, Wernicke-type aphasics, and normal subjects each show a distinctive pattern of errors? If a hierarchy of difficulty of sentence types is found, will it differ for the three subject groups, or will it be the same.

METHOD

Subjects

The aphasic subjects were seven non-fluent Broca-type aphasics (three females and four males) and five fluent Wernicke-type aphasics (one female and four males). All were outpatients of the Neurological Clinic or the Institute for Psychophysiology and Speech Pathol-

TABLE 1
Aphasic Subjects: Background Data

Aphasic subjects	Sex	Age	Educ.	Etiology	Lesion
Broca subjects					
S.P.	M	53	16	CVA (1981)	L inf. frontal at the depth of the ventricle
D.R.	M	62	16	CVA (1983)	Large subcortical Broca's area, L motor strip, parietal area, patchy Wernicke's area
V.P.	M	46	12	CVA (1986)	Cortical and subcortical Broca's area
D.T.	F	52	16	CVA (1984)	L basal ganglia and int. capsule
A.T.	M	46	10	CVA (1985)	L frontal, lower motor cortex
V.M.	F	44	14	CVA (1986)	L inf. fronto-temporal cortex
M.J.	F	47	10	CVA (1985)	L inf. frontal
Wernicke subjects					
M.C.	M	57	14	CVA (1983)	L subcortical tempo-parietal, supramarginal and angular gyri
A.B.	M	59	14	CVA (1985)	L fronto-parietal cortex and basal ganglia
V.V.	M	48	16	CVA (1987)	L fronto-parietal cortex
M.B.	M	59	16	CVA (1981)	L temporo-parietal cortex
D.D.	F	60	12	CVA (1980)	L temporo-parietal cortex

ogy, in Belgrade, Yugoslavia. All were native speakers of Serbo-Croatian. The age range was 44–62 for Broca-type aphasics and 48–60 for Wernicke-type aphasics. All subjects had at least a secondary education and all were right-handed. Further details are given in Table 1.

The control group comprised seven neurologically normal subjects (four females and three males), roughly matched to the aphasic group in age and years of education.

All patients were categorized according to a neurological examination, the results of a CT-scan, and the results of tests of language function based on the Serbo-Croatian version of the Boston Diagnostic Aphasia Examination (BDAE, Goodglass and Kaplan, 1972). The etiology in all cases was a single cerebrovascular accident confined to the left cerebral hemisphere. Time since onset of the symptoms varied from 6 months to 7 years. There was no history of drug abuse and no significant disabilities in vision or hearing among either the patients or the control subjects.

All Broca-type patients showed the characteristic nonfluent speech and all displayed some degree of agrammatism (see Table 2). Their sentences were short with impoverished syntactic structure, consisting mainly of nouns and verbs with frequent omission of free-standing functors and occasional substitution of bound morphemes. A common error was to use the nominative case, in place of the appropriate noun case. All Broca-type subjects had measurable losses in language comprehension when tested with the BDAE (results by individual subjects on the comprehension subtests of the BDAE are given in Appendix A).

The Wernicke-type aphasics had fluent speech with an apparently normal melodic line. Their sentences were rife with semantic and phonetic paraphasias and paragrammatically inappropriate grammatical forms. Their comprehension was markedly impaired as measured with the BDAE (results by individual subjects on the comprehension subtests of the BDAE are given in Appendix A).

Materials

In designing semantically reversible sentences containing relative clause, steps were taken to minimize possible difficulties in pragmatic interpretation that these sentences might induce: (a) to this end only two animate noun phrases were allowed in each sentence (in contrast, for example to Caplan & Futter, 1986); (b) semantic relations among noun phrases were always plausible; (c) the third noun phrase in each test sentence was inanimate and conveyed descriptive information. The last restriction was imposed because findings with young children have shown that performance on an act-out task improved when the number of animate noun phrases in relative clause sentences was reduced from three to two (Goodluck & Tavakolian, 1982).

Experimental sentences. Four types of semantically reversible relative clause sentences were created and recorded on audiotape. The relative clauses varied in their place of attachment (embedded vs. nonembedded), and in the role of the missing noun phrase inside the relative clause (subject- vs. object-gap). See 1–4 above.

Control sentences. In addition to relative clause sentences, conjoined-clause (CC) sentences were included in the test materials. As noted, CC sentences have structures that are hypothesized to be syntactically less complex than relative clause sentences and are considered to be mastered earlier in development (Tavakolian, 1981). The CC sentences were derived from OS sentences. Each contained one empty noun phrase in the second clause, which is coreferential with the subject of the first clause, as illustrated below.

(6) CC: Žena drži kišobran i ljubi čoveka.
      The lady is holding the umbrella and kissing the man.

Additional sentences were added as controls to ascertain that the subjects were attending to the entire sentence. These control sentences were of the same form as three of the sentence types (SS, OS, CC), but their respective foils differed. The picture foils for all sentence types are described later.

Picture materials. Given that the task is a forced choice among alternative pictures, the design and choice of picture materials is critical. Steps were taken to create pictures depicting possible nonreversible situations. The so-called "felicity conditions" (Hamburger & Crain, 1982) were met by providing a natural context for the relative clause. This was accomplished by depicting more than one character corresponding to the head NP. These felicity conditions were not met in the sentences used to test comprehension in previous studies of aphasia.

A two-choice picture task was adapted from materials constructed by Smith et al. (1989). Both picture choices depicted plausible events. Since a relation between two animate noun phrases was depicted in each picture, the location of agents (left or right side of the picture) was randomized within sentence sets. In half of the arrays, the correct picture was in the top position, and in the other half the correct picture was in the bottom position (sample test materials for an experimental sentence are displayed in Appendix B).

Picture foils. The conjoined-clause analysis was used as the picture-foil, that is, the correct interpretation of SO, OS, and OO sentences was contrasted with foils depicting the conjoined-clause analysis interpretation. This misanalysis was chosen for the reasons indicated above.

The following examples are descriptions of correct target pictures and the incorrect foils that were used for stimulus sentences.

(7) SO:[2]   The man that the lady is kissing is holding an umbrella.
    Target picture: a man holding an umbrella while a lady is kissing him.
    Foil picture: a man holding an umbrella and kissing a lady.

(8) OS: The lady is kissing the man who is holding an umbrella.
    Target picture: a lady kissing a man while this man is holding an umbrella.
    Foil picture: a lady kissing a man and holding the umbrella.

(9) OO:[3]   The man is kissing the lady that the umbrella is covering.
    Target picture: a man is kissing a lady while she is protected by an umbrella.
    Foil picture: a man is kissing a lady and he is protected by an umbrella.

For the SS sentences a conjoined-clause analysis would yield the same result as interpretation of the relative clause. Therefore, a foil depicting a main clause only interpretation was used for the SS sentences (10).

(10) SS: The lady who is kissing the man is holding an umbrella.
     Target picture: a lady while holding an umbrella is kissing a man.
     Foil picture: a lady is holding an umbrella.

For the CC sentences, however, the foil depicted an erroneous minimum-distance principle interpretation (11).

(11) Stimulus sentence (CC): The man is kissing the lady and holding an umbrella.
     Target picture: a man kissing a lady and holding the umbrella.
     Foil picture: a man kissing a lady and the lady holding an umbrella.

For the control SS and OS sentences a relative-clause only interpretation was depicted in the foil. Finally, a first-clause-only interpretation was used for the control CC sentences.

Test Design

The test contained 65 sentences: 10 sentences in each set (OO, SO, SS, OS, CC), plus 5 sentences in each set of foil-control sentences (SS, OS, CC). Two test orders were prepared, with the control sentences interspersed randomly. Practice trials consisting of four sentences and their picture sets were used to familiarize subjects with the procedure.

Procedure

When performing a sentence–picture matching task, the subject is asked to listen to each sentence and then to decide which picture, among simultaneously present alternatives, depicts the meaning of the sentence correctly. The dependent variable is error rate since performance on this task is not timed. Subjects were tested individually in a single, 1-hr session. Before each sentence was presented, the picture array was exposed. A practice session was administered to familiarize subjects with the materials and the procedure. Subjects were instructed to listen carefully to the entire sentence, to look carefully at both

[2] For the SO sentences there are two possible erroneous conjoined-clause analyses. One of these was the most commonly observed conjoined-clause response in studies with children (Tavakolian, 1981). Therefore this response type was selected to be the foil for this sentence type.

[3] The OO sentences, like the SO, offer two conjoined-clause analyses. Again, young children choose one conjoined clause response more often than the other (Tavakolian, 1981) and that is why it was used as a foil.

pictures in the array, and then to point to the picture that matched the meaning of the sentence.

RESULTS

There is clear separation between the subject groups on overall accuracy. The Broca subjects averaged 22% errors, (range 10–34%), Wernicke subjects averaged 37% errors, (range 28–54%), and normal control subjects averaged 6% errors (range 2–10%). Thus the Wernicke subjects were more impaired in sentence-picture matching of relative clause sentences than Broca subjects or normals.

Since the task consisted of two-picture choices, chance performance would be 50%. We define chance performance conservatively: as an error rate between 40 and 60%. Error rates less than 40% were considered to be above chance, whereas error rates above 60% were considered to reflect systematic application of a nonlinguistic strategy.

Table 2 displays the mean number of errors by individual subjects. Although all subjects demonstrated better comprehension of subject-gap sentences than of object-gap sentences, there is much individual variability in error rates, with Wernicke subjects performing overall worse than Broca subjects. All Broca subjects exhibited overall above-chance ability to match the correct picture to the experimental sentence. On the SO sentences the Broca subjects manifested performance that ranged from

TABLE 2
Percentage of Errors on Each Sentence Type for Broca and Wernicke Subjects

	Sentence type					
Individual subjects	OO	OS	SO	SS	CC	Mean
Broca aphasics						
S.P.	40*	10	30	10	30	24
D.R.	30	30	60*	20	30	34
V.P	10	10	30	20	20	18
D.T.	60*	40*	60*	0	0	32
A.T.	30	20	40*	10	10	22
V.M.	20	10	20	0	0	10
M.J.	10	20	30	0	10	15
Mean	29	20	40*	9	14	
Wernicke's aphasics						
M.D.	70	40*	60*	50*	50*	54*
A.B.	50*	50*	50*	10	50*	42*
V.V.	40*	30	60*	20	30	33
M.Dj.	50*	20	80	0	0	30
D.D.	40*	20	60*	10	10	28
Mean	50*	32	62*	18	28	

* Chance performance.

highly above chance (20% error) to chance (60% error). Four of the seven Broca subjects performed with an above chance success rate of this sentence type. However, subject D.T. performed at chance on all object-gap relatives (OO, SO), and, in addition, on some of the subject-gap sentences (OS). All five Wernicke aphasics performed at chance level on the SO sentences. Moreover, one subject (M.Dj.) chose the conjoined clause option very frequently (80% error). Another Wernicke subject (M.D.) performed at chance on all sentence types, and a third (A.B.) performed at chance on all sentence types except the SS sentences. The task was evidently too difficult for these latter subjects, so that they judged sentences in a random manner. For the OO sentences the mean error rate was smaller but there was high variability. The range of errors for Broca patients was 10–60% and for the Wernicke patients 40–70%. Only two Broca patients performed at chance, whereas all of the Wernicke patients did so. The pattern of performance within each aphasic group (with exception of two Wernicke patients who performed equally poorly on all sentence types) shows the same hierarchy of sentence difficulty.

Factorial analyses of variance were performed separately on the experimental and conjoined-clause control sentences, and on the foil-control sentences. Since there was no effect of test order on the accuracy score, the data from both orders were combined for analysis. The error scores were analyzed by an ANOVA which compared the factors of Group (Broca, Wernicke, Control) and Sentence type (OO, OS, SO, SS, CC). Both main effects were significant. The main effect of Group ($F(2, 16) = 26.35$, $p < .001$) indicates that there were differences between types of aphasia and the normal control group. The significant effect of Sentence type ($F(4, 64) = 21.83$, $p < .001$) indicates that all sentence types were not equally difficult. The interaction between Group and Sentence type was also significant ($F(8, 64) = 2.39$, $p < .02$). Its interpretation will be considered presently.

A post hoc Tukey test ($p = .01$) indicated that each subject group was significantly different from the others with the normal control group exhibiting the fewest errors and the Wernicke group exhibiting the most.

The rank order of difficulty for the sentence types was similar in both aphasic groups: The SO sentences were the most difficult. Three of the seven agrammatic subjects performed at chance level on these sentences, and four performed with above-chance success. The SO sentences were the most difficult for all the subjects including the control subjects, although the Sentence-type effect did not reach significance in this group because performance was at the ceiling level. A Post hoc Tukey test ($p = .01$) indicated that there were significantly more errors on SO sentences than on all others, with the exception of the OO type, from which they differed only at the $p = .05$ level. More errors occurred on the OO type than on either SS or CC sentences. The latter were not significantly

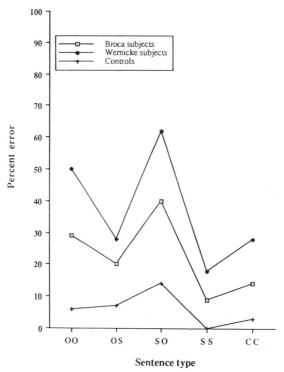

FIG. 1. Percentage of errors by sentence type.

different from each other. OS sentences gave rise to more errors than SS sentences but did not differ from OO or CC types. As was expected, the control CC sentences and the SS sentences were the easiest for all three groups of subjects.

The mean percent error per sentence type for the three groups of subjects is displayed in Fig. 1. The figure shows the same pattern of performance across sentence types in all three subject groups. When the Broca group and the Wernicke group were compared, there was a significant effect of aphasia type $(F(1, 11) = 9.19, p < .01)$, but no aphasia-type by sentence-type interaction. The most difficult sentence type, the SO sentences, produced the only significant difference between aphasic groups $(p < .02)$. Group differences on OO and OS sentence types were in the same direction, but failed to reach significance (each with $p < .09$). There was no significant difference between the two patient groups in the number of errors on control CC sentences and SS sentences.

Given the absence of interaction of type of aphasia and sentence type, we should ask why an interaction with subject group was obtained in the analysis that included all subjects. Figure 1 shows that few errors were made by control subjects; for them, the plot of errors against sentence type is relatively flat. Thus, the presence of an interaction in the composite analysis is clearly attributable to the ceiling level performance of the control group.

Foil-control Sentences

On the foil-control sentences both aphasic groups performed at a high level of accuracy. Broca's aphasics averaged 4% errors (range 0–13%); Wernicke's aphasics averaged 7% errors (range 0–20%). The difference was not significant ($F(1, 10) = .46$, $p < .51$). The control group performed with 100% accuracy on these sentences.

DISCUSSION

Our purpose was to obtain evidence that could distinguish between the explanatory adequacy of two accounts of comprehension impairment in agrammatism. One explanation, the Structural Deficit Hypotheses, states that syntactic structures critical for sentence interpretation are lost or are unavailable. The other explanation appeals to a processing deficiency. To distinguish the two hypotheses we have studied one complex structure intensively, the relative clause. This structure is well suited also to our additional goal of bringing data from different languages bear on the problem.

This study is the first to present data from an inflected language on comprehension of a complete set of relative clause structures by Broca's and Wernicke's aphasics. The Structural Deficit Hypothesis predicts that agrammatics would fail to assign correct syntactic representations to relative clauses. If the requisite structures are lost, agrammatics would have no recourse but to apply nonsyntactic strategies. In the case of object-gap relatives, they might be expected, to assign thematic roles randomly (Grodzinsky, 1989) or to apply a canonical word-order strategy indiscriminately (Caplan & Futter, 1986). We therefore asked whether agrammatics do, in fact, lack the necessary syntactic structures to analyze object-gap relative clauses and, if so, whether they tend to simplify these structures by treating them as conjoined clauses. The first question was addressed by comparing the comprehension of relative clauses that differed in place of attachment (i.e., embedded and nonembedded relatives) and in the location of the gap (i.e., subject- and object-gap relatives). This was accomplished by exploiting particular features of the grammar of Serbo-Croatian, taking advantage of the fact that Serbo-Croatian marks thematic roles in relative clauses by case inflections. This characteristic enabled us to tease apart two possible sources of syntactic deficiency: syntactic simplification amounting to loss of hierarchic structure and deletion of the traces of movement. The second question was addressed by using conjoined-clause sentences as controls, a syntactic structure that could plausibly result from simplification of a relative clause. Accordingly, four types of reversible relative clauses and conjoined clauses provided the critical materials for testing between the two hypotheses.

Notably, the agrammatic aphasics found the different relative clause structures to be unequal in difficulty. Object-gap relatives yielded the highest error rates, in keeping with the earlier findings with English-speaking agrammatics (Caramazza & Zurif, 1976; Grodzinsky, 1989; Caplan & Futter, 1986) and in agreement with both Grodzinsky's and Caplan and Futter's predictions concerning the expected order of difficulty. If one were to draw conclusions about agrammatic subjects' competence only by taking average performance into account, one might be led to conclude that the subjects of the present study had lost a portion of their agrammatical knowledge and, consequently, were forced to rely on nonlinguistic strategies. However, the prediction of the Structural Deficit Hypothesis that agrammatics would perform at chance on object-gap sentences was not met, at least for a majority of subjects. Four out of seven of the agrammatic subjects performed well above chance on these structures. Thus, this result offers, at best, only partial support for the theoretical conceptions of Caplan and Futter and Grodzinsky.

It could be expected that trace deletion in object-gap relatives should impair Serbo-Croatian speaking subjects less than English-speaking subjects, since critical information about the subject/object distinction can be extracted from noun case inflections regardless of word order. But these subjects, like their English-speaking counterparts would be expected to be at chance on SO sentences if they lacked traces, even if they were able to rely on noun-phrase inflectional morphology. That is because, as we explained, these sentences have ambiguous inflectional markings because both noun phrases are marked for the nominative case. On the other hand, performance on OO sentences should not differ from subject-gap relatives because on these sentences the inflections indicate thematic roles unambiguously.[4]

However, although in all subjects object-gap relatives gave rise to significantly more errors than subject-gap relatives neither of these expectations based on Grodzinsky's hypothesis (1989) finds support in the data. Concerning the first prediction, although SO sentences were more diffi-

---

[4] Grodzinsky's description of agrammatic *production* proposes a more inclusive deficit at the level of S-structure than the putative deficit underlying comprehension disorder (Grodzinsky, 1990). On this account nonlexical terminals are deleted, including case markers and other aspects of inflectional morphology as well as traces of movement. If this description of the agrammatic deficit were extended to comprehension, additional difficulties in interpretation of the inflectional morphology would be anticipated.

cult than OO sentences, performance was at chance only for three of the
seven agrammatic subjects. One of those (D.T.) who performed at chance
on SO sentences also performed at chance on OO and OS sentences,
which indicates that this subject was not taking advantage of the inflectional morphology. Concerning the second prediction, the OO sentences
were comprehended with more errors than the subject-gap sentences.
Additionally, the comprehension difficulties in these agrammatics cannot
be explained on the trace deletion account, since difficulties in comprehension were also present to a lesser degree on other structures (subject-
gap relatives) which would be expected on the trace deletion account to
be analyzed normally.[5] On the other hand, diffuse difficulties are expected when there is a special limitation in processing. Only on the processing limitation account is it expected that the comprehension difficulties in agrammatics would be most severe on specific syntactic structures,
but also present to a lesser degree with other structures.

The results of the present study lend no support to Caplan and Futter's
(1986) conjecture that the syntactic apparatus of agrammatics has undergone simplification that would necessitate use of word-order strategy in
the absence of syntactic parsing. On this proposal, agrammatics should
choose the erroneous conjoined-clause interpretation on all relative
clauses that fail to preserve canonical word order (OO, SO). That clearly
did not happen. The possibilities for varying word order that are permitted by the grammar of Serbo-Croatian enabled us to hold word-order
constant and to construct OS and OO sentences with the same sequencing
of NPs and VPs. Keeping the same word order in OO and OS sentences
would induce agrammatics to be incorrect on the OO sentences as often
as they are correct on the OS sentences if they relied solely on a word-
order strategy. Although, in fact, the agrammatics produced more errors
on OO sentences than on OS sentences, their performance on OO sentences was above chance. They were successful in distinguishing different syntactic structures even though these structures had the same noun–
verb sequences. Above-chance interpretation of the OO sentences is
incompatible with the hypothesis that these agrammatics were using a
linear word-order strategy.

A further test between the differing accounts of comprehension disorder in agrammatic aphasia was made by comparing the performances
of agrammatic subjects with those of Wernicke's aphasics and with the
neurologically-normal control group. The Processing-Limitation Hypoth-

---

[5] A recent paper by Hickok, Zurif, and Canseco-Gonzales (1993) also reports that agrammatics can experience difficulties with subject relatives. In addition to their failure on
object-gap relatives, Hickok et al.'s subjects showed a deficit in comprehension of matrix
sentences in subject relatives. The latter finding, the authors note, is incompatible with the
trace-deletion hypothesis as framed by Grodzinsky (1990).

esis predicts that the pattern of performance across sentence types should be consistent across subject groups. The present results showed that, in fact, both agrammatic Broca and Wernicke subjects experienced difficulties with interpretation of semantically reversible relative clauses. The significant group differences were differences of degree, not qualitative differences in pattern. Both types of aphasic subjects were similarly affected by the variations in syntactic structure that were introduced by inclusion of different types of relative clauses; the same rank order of difficulty among sentence types was found for each group with the object-relatives (SO, OO) being the more difficult structures. This order of difficulty was also observed in the normal control group. The agrammatic group performed better overall than the Wernicke group, creating the significant between-group interactions. Finally, a consistent pattern of performance across sentence types was observed in the individual subject data.

In this connection it is relevant to note that the ordering of difficulty on the four relative clause structures obtained in this study is consistent with that which has been found in several research studies that explored acquisition of relative clauses in young children (deVilliers et al. 1979; Tavakolian, 1981). In addition, this pattern has also been demonstrated in dyslexic children (Smith et al., 1989; Crain et al., 1990). These similarities are unlikely to be mere coincidences. The existence of parallel findings across such diverse groups fits with the failure of the present study to find evidence for a syndrome-specific comprehension deficit in agrammatism.[6]

Taken together, these findings give us reason to prefer an account on agrammatism that appeals to damaged processors in favor of an account that evokes loss of grammatical structures. The processing limitation account is to be preferred because it shows itself capable of tying together

---

[6] The processing account gains further support from the finding that the performance gap between agrammatics and normal subjects can be eliminated when normal speakers are tested in a way that places them under a heavy processing load. Word-by-word reading, in which previous words disappear as new ones come into view, is a technique that was employed by Ni (1988) in studies of sentence processing in normal adult subjects. The task was to detect an anomalous word which occurred at the beginning, middle, or end of the test sentence. Comparing the results of Ni's study with the results obtained by Shankweiler et al. (1989) with agrammatic aphasics who were tested (in a listening test) with the same set of sentences, we find a similar pattern of latencies and errors across structures. The strong similarities between the normal subjects under pressure and the aphasics led Ni to infer that each group used syntactic mechanisms in the same way. The same conclusion was reached by Milekic (1993) in a comparison between performance patterns of Serbo-Croatian-speaking agrammatics and normals in a word-by-word reading test. Milekic's findings yield further evidence that sentence processing in normal subjects can be profoundly affected by variation in processing demands, and that the relative difficulty of different structures mirrors the pattern exhibited by agrammatic aphasics.

a wider variety of findings. An adequate theory of "agrammatic" comprehension would account for syntax-related variations in performance among agrammatics and for parallels across different populations.

It remains to give positive underpinnings to the proposal that the source of the comprehension deficit in aphasia is in processing limitations. The question becomes: What is the origin of the difficulties in sentence processing that cause comprehension failures? Elsewhere, we have developed a proposal that appeals to an extended version of Fodor's (1983) modularity hypothesis (Crain & Shankweiler, 1990). On this view, language processing is carried out in discrete stages, organized in a hierarchical, bottom-up fashion (Forster, 1979). Language comprehension involves a series of translations between levels of representation: phonological, syntactic and semantic. A processing limitation view of aphasics' comprehension difficulties assumes at least two distinct ways in which syntactic processing could be impaired. On one possibility, although syntactic knowledge is preserved, its access and utilization are restricted during the process of parsing in which syntactic structures are assigned to the incoming string of lexical categories. One consequence of impaired parsing capacity may be that agrammatics, contrary to normals, do not access syntactic information in an automatic fashion but via a slow and controlled process (Kolk & vanGrunsven, 1985; Friederici et al., 1992; Zurif et al., 1993). Under this assumption, although the input to the syntactic parser is normal, processing at the syntactic level is disrupted.[7] On the other possibility (which we have discussed at length elsewhere, Crain et al., 1990), difficulties in processing syntax ultimately derive from deficient phonological input and memory processes. The phonology is especially vulnerable because it is the first level at which the input engages the language apparatus. Under this assumption, although syntactic processing per se is intact, the input to the parser is deficient, thus resulting in comprehension failure.

This notion is consistent with our findings concerning sentence comprehension in young children, normal adults, and the reading impaired, and we suggest a possible source of comprehension deficits in agrammatism that could also account for parallel findings in other populations. One resource limitation that young children, dyslexics, and aphasics may have in common concerns the processing of phonological input. The pro-

---

[7] Recently, we have begun to use other paradigms to assess specific syntactic abilities in agrammatic subjects (Lukatela, Ocic, & Shankweiler, 1991). In an on-line study that used the syntactic priming paradigm, the same agrammatic subjects that participated in the present study demonstrated sensitivity to syntactic priming when case was primed by a preposition. These results, however, do not necessarily indicate intact on-line sentence processing ability given that priming was demonstrated within a "minimal" syntactic context; a test trial consisted of a sentence fragment.

cessing account can provide a basis for the observed parallels in syntactic comprehension performance. If the hypothesis is correct, then any group that suffers from a bottleneck in phonological processing, for any reason, should display limitations at sentence level.

In a subsequent study we obtained confirmation of phonological deficiencies in some of our agrammatic subjects. The capacity of phonological short-term memory was tested in the same Broca-type aphasics that participated in the present study (Lukatela & Shankweiler, 1990). The aphasic and control subjects were compared on verbal and nonverbal retention of rhyming and nonrhyming word strings, and nonsense drawings, testing in each case memory for serial order. The results indicated that these subjects had a material-specific deficit in short-term retention. They differed from the control group on word strings but not on nonsense drawings. The deficit was exacerbated when all the words were phonologically similar (rhyming). Arguably, a phonological processing deficiency of this nature could impair the working memory sufficiently to impede comprehension, at least for sentences that are likely to require reanalysis (McCarthy & Warrington, 1987). These findings, therefore, lend further substance to the speculations that our agrammatic subjects' comprehension difficulties may stem at least in part from deficiencies in phonological processing that curtail the efficient use of working memory in comprehension tasks.[8]

In sum, the comprehension difficulties encountered by the agrammatic aphasics are more consistent on several counts with a Processing Limitation Hypothesis than with a Syntactic Deficit Hypothesis involving trace deletion or failure to interpret grammatical inflections: (1) Comprehension accuracy for agrammatic speakers of Serbo-Croatian was overall above chance for all types of relative clauses. (2) Agrammatics' difficulties in comprehending these structures proved remarkably similar to those displayed by Wernicke's aphasics: the pattern of performance did not distinguish syndromes. (3) Comparisons from the literature based on dyslexic

---

[8] The research literature presents a confusing picture of the relationship between sentence comprehension and working memory. Researchers have often noted that some aphasic patients with a severely restricted phonological short-term store are sometimes capable of sentence comprehension at a level far exceeding what would be expected on the basis of their span limitations (Martin & Feher, 1990; Caplan & Waters, 1990; McCarthy & Warrington, 1987). However, it is important to note that memory in these studies was assessed by measuring patients' span for unorganized material. In our theoretical model of working memory we have assumed that there are two components: a storage buffer and a mechanism whose primary task is to relay the results of lower-level analyses of linguistic input upward through the language apparatus (Shankweiler & Crain, 1986; Crain et al., 1990). In the studies cited above the patients may have suffered impairment of only one of the proposed memory components, the storage buffer, and have preserved a relay mechanism which maintained the ability to synchronize information flow.

children and normals tested under stressful conditions reveals an order of difficulty of relative clause structures consistent with that displayed by the aphasics. (4) Agrammatics can succeed in detecting syntactic violations of these and other sentence types with a high degree of accuracy,[9] and they are sensitive to syntactic priming. (5) There is independent evidence of phonological impairments in the agrammatic subjects of this study.

[9] The subjects of the present study were tested on another occasion for detection of syntactic violations in relative clause sentences that were structurally identical to those of the sentence picture matching study (Lukatela, Shankweiler, & Crain, 1988). Although the results of the grammaticality judgment test cannot be compared directly with those of the sentence picture matching test, it is instructive to note that performance on judgments was appreciably more accurate averaging 90.6% correct for subject-gap relatives and 85.5% for object-gap sentences.

APPENDIX A

Aphasic Subjects: Comprehension Data

Subjects	BDAE comprehension			Speech production: Description of "cookie theft" picture
	A (15)	B (12)	C (10)	
Broca				
S.P.	14	6	7	Kujna. Mama pere...ovaj tanjir. A ovaj decak i devojcica. Ova je voda pri..pri..E, voda je pr-li-la. Kitchen. Mama is washing...this plate. Boy and girl. This water..is li..li..Water is li-king.
D.R.	6	3	2	Seka...kolač...Majka...Čaše...Vodu Girl...cookie...Mother...Glasses..Water
V.P.	10	9	6	Mama...pe-re. Sestra i brat. Ne mogu da kazem. Vidi ovde... Mama...wa-shing. Sister and brother. I can not say. Look here....
D.T.	11	9	7	Uzimaju kolače. Bo..bori se da ne..Tu..mama..pere. Taking the cookies. Is try-trying not to... Here..mama..washing.
A.T.	10	11	9	Ovde žena pere sudove a klin-ci se igraju. Jedan pao sa sto-lice. To..pere sudove. Here a woman washing dishes, kids are playing. One is fallen from the chair. This.. washing dishes..
V.M.	15	10	10	Deca uzimaju kolače. Devojčica gleda. Dečak je pao. Majka pere a voda curi. Children are taking cookies. The girl is watching. The boy is fallen. Mother is washing and water is liking.

APPENDIX A—*Continued*

M.J.	13	10	9	Majka pere sudje. Deca se igraju. Uzi-maju keks. Stol-ica..stolica..seka i braca..Pašće sa stolice. Mother is washing dishes. Children are playing. They are taking cookies. The chair..chair..brother and sister..they are going to fall from the chair.
Wernicke				
M.C.	8	3	3	Majka radi, je bila je radila jedva za hranu, sa jedne strane to su radnici. A deca su uzela da jedu čokoladu. The mother is working, she was, she was working barely to support them, from one point this are workers. And children are eating the chocolate.
A.B.	2	0	0	Ovaj...dete je ustalo da pojede pekmez a ova žena je pro-sula vodu što je htela da pere pa je sve oprala. Well..the child stood up to eat the jelly and this woman has spilled the water, because she want to wash, she washed everything.
V.V.	6	1	1	Devojčica...ova stolica se valjda slomila. Ukrali su..ne mogu da se setim. Drugarica je donela kolače i sada deca kradu kolače. The girl...this chair, looks like it has broken. They are stealing..I can't say. The woman brought the cookies and the children are stealing cookies.
M.B.	4	0	0	Vidite ovde decu, devojcica, vidite ovaj stolnjak. Stolnjak nije u redu, a majka to ne vidi. U..kako se to zove. You see, here are children, the girl, you see this table-cloth. The tablecloth is not OK., and mother doesn't see that. Well, what's the name for this.
D.D.	5	3	4	Šta je ovo? Neka deca ovde su se popela,hoće da uzmu ko-lače. Žena pere..šta je ovo..tanjir. Ona stalno gleda kroz prozor. What's this? Some children have climbed here, they wont to take cookies. The woman is washing..what is this..the plate. She is looking through the window.

Note. A, Commands (max. score 15); B, Complex ideational materials (max. score 12); C, Reading sentences and paragraph (max score 10).

REFERENCES

Bates, E., Friederici, A., & Wulfeck, B. 1987. Comprehension in aphasia: A cross-linguistic study. *Brain and Language*, **32**, 19–67.

Berndt, R. S., & Caramazza, A. 1980. A redefinition of Broca's aphasia: Implications for a neuropsychological model of language. *Applied Psycholinguistics*, **1**, 225–278.

Bradley, D., Garrett, M., & Zurif, E. 1980. Syntactic deficits in Broca's aphasia. In D. Caplan (Ed.), *Biological studies of mental processes*. Cambridge, MA: MIT Press.

Caplan, D., & Futter, C. 1986. Assignment of thematic roles to nouns in sentence comprehension by an agrammatic patient. *Brain and Language*, **27**, 117–134.

Caplan, D., & Waters, G. 1990. Short-term memory and language comprehension: A critical review of neuropsychological literature. In G. Vallar & T. Shallice (Eds.), *Neuropsy-*

APPENDIX B

Sample Picture Array for the Sentence–Picture Task

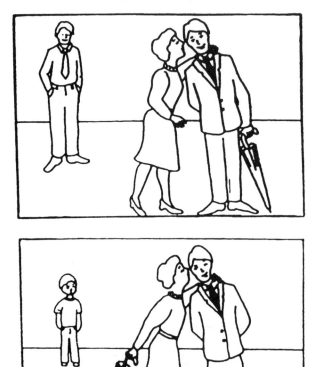

OS: The lady is kissing the man who is holding an umbrella.

chological impairments of short-term memory. Cambridge: Cambridge Univ. Press. Pp. 337–389.

Caramazza, A., & Zurif, E. 1976. Dissociation of algorithmic and heuristic processes in language comprehension: Evidence from aphasia. *Brain and Language*, **3,** 572–582.

Caramazza, A., Basili, A. G., Koller, J., & Berndt, R. S. 1981. An investigation of repetition and language processing in a case of conduction aphasia. *Brain and Language*, **14,** 235–271.

Crain, S., Shankweiler, D., Macaruso, P., & Bar-Shalom, E. 1990. Working memory and sentence comprehension: Investigations of children with reading disorder. In G. Vallar, & T. Shallice (Eds.), *Impairments of short-term memory.* Cambridge: Cambridge Univ. Press.

Crain, S., & Shankweiler, D. 1990. Explaining failures in spoken language comprehension by children with reading disabilities. In D. Balota, F. d'Arcais, & K. Rayner (Eds.), *Comprehension processes in reading*. Hillsdale, NJ: Erlbaum.

de Villiers, J. G., Tager-Flusberg, H. B., Hakuta, K., & Cohen, M. 1979. Children's comprehension of relative clauses. *J Psycholinguistic Research*, **8**, 499–518.

Fodor, J. A. 1983. *The Modularity of Mind*. Cambridge, MA: MIT Press.

Friederici, D. A., Wessels, M. J., Emmorey, K., & Bellugi, U. 1992. Sensitivity to inflectional morphology in aphasia: A real-time processing perspective. *Brain and Language*, **43**, 747–763.

Forster, K. I. 1979. Levels of processing and the structure of the language processor. In W. E. Cooper & E. C. T. Walker (Eds.), *Sentence processing: Psycholinguistic studies presented to Merrill Garrett*. Hillsdale, NJ: Erlbaum.

Goodglass, H., & Kaplan, E. 1972. *The assessment of aphasia and related disorders*. Philadelphia: Lea & Febiger.

Goodluck, H., & Tavakolian, S. 1982. Competence and processing in children's grammar of relative clauses. *Cognition*, **11**, 1–27.

Grodzinsky, Y. 1986. Language deficits and the theory of syntax. *Brain and Language*, **27**, 135–159.

Grodzinsky, Y. 1990. *Theoretical perspectives on language deficits*. Cambridge, MA: MIT Press.

Grodzinsky, Y. 1989. Agrammatic comprehension of relative clauses. *Brain and Language*, **37**, 480–499.

Hamburger, H., & Crain, S. 1982. Relative acquisition. In S. Kuczaj, II (Ed.), *Language development, Volume 1: Syntax and semantics*. Hillsdale, NJ: Erlbaum.

Hickok, G., Zurif, E., & Canseco-Gonzales, E. 1993. Structural description of agrammatic comprehension. *Brain and Language*, **45**, 371–395.

Kean, M. L. 1977. The linguistic interpretation of aphasic syndromes. *Cognition*, **5**, 9–46.

Kolk, H. H. J., & vanGrunsven, M. M. F. 1985. Agrammatism as a variable phenomenon. *Cognitive Neuropsychology*, **2**, 347–384.

Lapointe, S. G. 1983. Some issues in the description of aggrammatism. *Cognition*, **14**, 1–39.

Linebarger, M., Schwartz, M., & Saffran, E. 1983. Sensitivity to grammatical structures in so-called agrammatic aphasics. *Cognition*, **13**, 361–392.

Lukatela, K., Crain, S., & Shankweiler, D. 1988. Sensitivity to inflectional morphology in agrammatism: Investigation of highly inflected language. *Brain and Language*, **33**, 1–15.

Lukatela, K., & Shankweiler, D. 1990. *Working memory, phonological decoding and agrammatic aphasia*. Paper presented at the Academy of Aphasia, Baltimore.

Lukatela, K., Ocic, G., & Shankweiler, D. 1991. *Syntactic priming of inflected nouns in agrammatic aphasia*. Poster presented at the Academy of Aphasia, Rome.

Lukatela, K., Shankweiler, D., & Crain, S. 1988. *Sentence comprehension in fluent and non-fluent aphasia*. Paper presented at the Academy of Aphasia, Montreal.

Martin, C. R., & Feher, E. 1990. The consequences of reduced memory span for the comprehension of semantic versus syntactic information. *Brain and Language*, **38**, 1–20.

Mauner, G., Fromkin, A. V., & Cornell, T. L. 1993. Comprehension and acceptability judgments in agrammatism: Disruptions in the syntax of referential dependency. *Brain and Language*, **45**, 340–370.

McCarthy, R. A., & Warrington, E. K. 1987. Understanding: A function of short-term memory? *Brain*, **110**, 1565–1578.

Miceli, G., Mazzucchi, A., Menn, L., & Goodglass, H. 1983. Contrasting cases of Italian agrammatic aphasia without comprehension disorder. *Brain and Language*, **19**, 65–97.

Milekic, S. 1993. *Distance and position effects in sentence processing by agrammatic aphasics*. Unpublished Ph.D. thesis, University of Connecticut, Storrs.

Ni, W. 1988. *An investigation of grammatical knowledge and processing mechanisms using RSVP*. University of Connecticut Working Papers in Linguistics, pp. 69–81.

Schwartz, M. F., Saffran, E. M., & Marin, O. S. M. 1980. The word order problem in agrammatism. I. Comprehension. *Brain and Language*, **10**, 249–262.

Shankweiler, D., & Crain, S. 1986. Language mechanisms and reading disorders: A modular approach. *Cognition*, **24**, 139–168.

Shankweiler, D., Crain, S., Gorell, P., & Tuller, B. 1989. Reception of language in Broca's aphasia. *Language and Cognitive Processes*, **4**, 1–33.

Smith, S., & Bates, E. 1987. Accessibility of case and gender contrasts for assignment of agent-object relations in Broca's aphasics and fluent anomics. *Brain and Language*, **30**, 49–60.

Smith, S., Macaruso, P., Shankweiler, D., & Crain, D. 1989. Syntactic comprehension in young poor readers. *Applied Psycholinguistics*, **10**, 429–454.

Tavakolian, S. L. 1981. The conjoined-clause analysis of relative clauses. In S. L. Tavakolian (Ed.), *Language acquisition and linguistic theory*. Cambridge, MA: MIT Press.

Tzeng, O., Chen, S., & Hung, D. 1991. The classifier problem in Chinese aphasia. *Brain and Language*, **41**, 187–202.

Wulfeck, B. B. 1988. Grammaticality judgments and sentence comprehension in agrammatic aphasia. *Journal of Speech and Hearing Research*, **31**, 72–81.

Zurif, E. 1984. Psycholinguistic interpretation of the aphasias. In D. Caplan, A. R. Lecours, & A. Smith (Eds.), *Biological perspectives on language*. Cambridge, MA: MIT Press.

Zurif, E., Swinney, D., Prather, P., Solomon, J., & Bushell, C. 1993. An on-line analysis of syntactic processing in Broca's and Wernicke's aphasia. *Brain and Language*, **45**, 448–464.

BRAIN AND LANGUAGE **50,** 10–26 (1993)

Representation, Referentiality, and Processing in Agrammatic Comprehension: Two Case Studies

Gregory Hickok

The Salk Institute for Biological Studies

AND

Sergey Avrutin

University of Pennsylvania

A number of investigators have argued that agrammatic comprehension, the pattern of sentence comprehension often associated with Broca's aphasia, can be characterized in terms of a representational disruption in one or another module of the normal grammar. In this study, these proposals are reviewed and their adequacy is examined in light of two case studies of agrammatic comprehension. In particular, we present data from sentences that have composed the core of the agrammatic comprehension pattern, as well as data from three different classes of sentences including comprehension of the matrix clause of center-embedded relative constructions, pronoun and anaphor dependencies, and Wh-questions. Our conclusion is that none of the existing representational models provides a fully adequate account of the data, and we propose some alternative approaches that distinguish between referential and nonreferential elements and potential processing differences between the two. © 1995 Academic Press, Inc.

This study explores questions surrounding representational generalizations relevant to agrammatic comprehension. A number of recent proposals hold that the pattern of sentence comprehension typical of many Broca's aphasia patients can be characterized in terms of a representational limitation in one or another module of the normal grammar (Grodzinsky, 1986, 1990; Hickok, 1992; Hickok & Avrutin, 1995; Hickok, Zurif, & Canseco-Gonzalez, 1993; Mauner, Fromkin, & Cornell, 1993). We examine the adequacy of these proposals in light of two case studies of agrammatic comprehension.

Address correspondence and reprint requests to Gregory Hickok, Laboratory for Cognitive Neuroscience, The Salk Institute for Biological Studies, 10010 North Torrey Pines Road, La Jolla, CA 92037. E-mail: hickok@crl.ucsd.edu. Sergey Avrutin is now at Yale University.

PRELIMINARIES

Two related points are worth making here. The first concerns the issue of patient classification; that is, over what population the generalizations we discuss are supposed to hold. The proposals put forth in this paper are intended to account for the pattern of comprehension documented in the two case studies presented here. We hypothesize, however, that the comprehension deficit found in our two patients is a fairly reliable feature of agrammatic aphasia, and thus we will draw on data from studies of clinically similar patients where these data provide new insights. This hypothesis will, of course, require empirical verification and these data should be viewed accordingly. The second point concerns whether the data set generally presumed to hold for agrammatic comprehenders as a group (see below) *actually* holds for any given patient or whether a data set has been abstracted from a number of studies of disparate groups of agrammatics, each study testing performance on a different sentence type. The entire set of data motivating our discussion of representational generalizations in agrammatic comprehension—and much of the work of those authors cited above—has been demonstrated in the two patients discussed below. (See Caramazza & Badecker (1989) for related discussion.)

This work will assume a basic familiarity with the proposals of Grodzinsky (1990), Hickok (1992; see also Hickok et al., 1993), and Mauner et al. (1993) and their underlying linguistic assumptions. We begin by presenting what has formed the core of the data defining agrammatic comprehension and provide a cursory review of the major representational accounts of this pattern of performance with emphasis on the differences. We then discuss recent comprehension data from three different classes of sentences and consider how the descriptive accounts fare in light of these data. Our conclusion is that none of the existing proposals, including our own (Hickok & Avrutin, 1995), provides a fully satisfactory account. Finally, drawing on processing data from normal subjects, we suggest an alternative approach that may prove more satisfactory. As noted, two agrammatic patients will serve as the source of data for our discussion. These data are presented in the Appendix. Patient descriptions are presented below.

THE PATIENTS

RD is a 75-year-old right-handed man with 2 years of college education. He had two left-hemisphere strokes, one in July 1976 and the other in November 1977. In 1978 he was diagnosed with Broca's aphasia on the basis of the BDAE (Goodglass & Kaplan, 1976) and clinical workup. Currently, he still presents with features of Broca's aphasia. His verbal output is nonfluent, effortful, and telegraphic; his comprehension is good at the conversational level. A CT scan administered in 1978 revealed two left-hemisphere lesions, one in Broca's area with deep extension to the left frontal horn and involving lower motor cortex and the other in the temporal lobe which, however, spared most of Wernicke's area. This patient has served as a subject in a number of studies (Grodzinsky, 1989; Grodzinsky, Wexler, Chien, Marakovitz, & Solomon, 1993; Hickok & Avrutin, 1995; Hickok et al., 1993; Sherman & Schweickert, 1989; Zurif, Swinney, Prather, Solomon, & Bushell, 1993).

FC is a 59-year-old college-educated man who suffered a left-hemisphere stroke in 1973. He was diagnosed with Broca's aphasia on the basis of clinical workup and the BDAE administered in 1982. A CT scan revealed a large infarction in the distribution of the left middle cerebral artery. FC still presents with the features of Broca's aphasia. This patient has also served as a subject in a number of studies (Grodzinsky, 1989; Grodzinsky et al., 1993; Hickok & Avrutin, 1995; Sherman & Schweickert, 1989; Zurif et al., 1993).

AGRAMMATIC COMPREHENSION: THE CORE DATA

The core set of data defining agrammatic comprehension is given below in (1) and (2). Comprehension is typically tested using sentence-to-picture matching with semantically reversible sentences (Caplan & Futter, 1986; Caramazza & Zurif, 1976; Grodzinsky, 1986, 1989; Hickok et al., 1993; Schwartz, Saffran, & Marin, 1980; Sherman & Schweickert, 1989), although similar results have been obtained using less demanding tasks (Hickok et al., 1993).

(1) Relatively Good Performance
    (a) Actives: *The psychologist attacked the linguist*
    (b) Subject-Gap Relative Clauses: *It was the psychologist that attacked the linguist*

(2) Relatively Poor Performance
    (a) Passives: *The psychologist was attacked by the linguist*
    (b) Object-Gap Relative Clauses: *It was the psychologist that the linguist attacked*

RD and FC's performance on these structures can be found in the Appendix. Their performance is consistent with the pattern above.

All three representational models cited above account for the pattern of performance in (1) and (2) in terms of a disruption in assigning thematic roles to moved elements. These models differ in a number of respects. One difference concerns which syntactic component is presumed to be disrupted in the process of linking a moved element to its thematic role (e.g., trace, chain, index). For Grodzinsky (1990) and for Hickok (1992) the choice of a particular syntactic entity as the source of the disruption is noncritical: both of these authors have chosen to discuss the notion of "trace-deletion" in the agrammatic representation, but this choice was merely intended to provide one possible formalization of the hypothesis that thematic roles are not being assigned to moved elements. Mauner et al. (1993), however, have a more specified model in that their implication of a particular syntactic limitation—a failure to mark referential dependencies with appropriate referential indices—is crucial to account for both the comprehension data in (1) and (2) and data from acceptability judgments in agrammatism (Linebarger, Schwartz, & Saffran, 1983; Shankweiler, Crain, Gorrell, & Tuller, 1989; Wulfeck, Bates, & Capasso, 1991). For our purposes, in which only comprehension data are considered, we will adopt a relatively agnostic position on the issue of which particular syntactic component (of those involved in theta role transmission) might be implicated. We will use the term "chain-disruption" generically to refer to a failure in thematic role assignment to moved elements.

Another difference concerns the underlying syntactic representation. Hickok and Mauner et al. assume the VP-Internal Subjects Hypothesis (Kitagawa, 1986; Koopman & Sportiche, 1988, among others), which states that grammatical subjects are base generated inside the verb phrase and move out to a case-assigning position, thus necessitating a chain for thematic role assignment to all subjects in English. In contrast, Grodzinsky (1986, 1990), who developed his model in the context of an older version of Government and Binding Theory, does not make this assumption. Both Hickok and Mauner et al. have argued that adopting VP-Internal Subjects improves upon Grodzinsky's (1990) account. Without VP-internal subjects, a chain-disruption hypothesis does not differentiate subject-gap sentences from object-gap sentences; both contain one chain, the only difference being the position from which an element was moved. In order to capture the difference between movement of a subject versus an object, Grodzinsky proposed the Default Principle, which assigns the role "agent" to a noun phrase that does not receive a role grammatically. Assuming VP-internal subjects, however, subject- and object-gap constructions differ in the number of chains they contain with the former containing only one chain and the latter two chains. Relatively preserved comprehension of subject-gap sentences can thus be accounted for on the basis of knowledge derived from the grammatically assigned role, and poor performance on object-gap sentences results from a failure to assign *any* thematic roles in the sentence. For example, in (1b) an agrammatic comprehender would know, on the basis of lexical knowledge and the grammatically assigned roles, that there was an attack and that the linguist was the object of this attack. This information alone is enough to produce a correct response in a typical comprehension paradigm. (Presumably the patient would also know that a psychologist was somehow involved and by inference could determine that this person was the agent of the attack.) The same would hold for the simple active case (1a). In (2b), on the other hand, all NPs require thematic role assignment via a chain, and thus no roles will be assigned. The patient would know only that there was an attack and that a psychologist and a linguist were involved but not who is attacking whom; poor performance is predicted, as desired. The Default Principle can thus be eliminated completely.[1] We note also that a purely structural difference in terms of the number of chains involved in sentence types like (1) versus (2) is consistent with working memory limitation accounts of agrammatic comprehension (Miyake, Carpenter, & Just, 1993; Shankweiler et al., 1989) and indeed may provide a principled explanation for such effects in the normal case.

There are also differences in the treatment of the passive. Grodzinsky assumes that in the agrammatic representation the agent role is assigned to the NP in the *by*-phrase grammatically. The default assignment of the agent role to the subject thus yields a representation with two agents, and poor performance results. Hickok assumes that in the passive, the external (agent) argument is suppressed and the *by*-phrase is simply a kind of adjunct that does not receive a thematic role at all (Grimshaw, 1990).[2] Because of the disrupted chain, the representation contains one unassigned role and two NPs in the input string. This situation is ambiguous and the patient guesses. Mauner et al. adopt yet another analysis of the passive in which the agent role is normally assigned to the NP in the *by*-phrase, although it is assigned indirectly with mediation by referential indices (Baker, Johnson, & Roberts, 1989). Passives, then, in Mauner et al.'s account contain two referential dependencies just like object-gap sentences and poor performance results. Part of the reason for these disparate accounts of the passive in agrammatic comprehension is that Passivization is poorly understood in the normal case (Goodall, 1993). Nonetheless, all authors provide a reasonable explanation for poor performance on these constructions given the current state of knowledge. Additional basic linguistic research on Passivization is needed before the question of agrammatic comprehension of passives can be settled.

In sum, all three models provide a reasonable account of the core data. Hickok and Mauner et al.'s accounts are preferable, in our view, because the additional assumption of a default strategy is unnecessary. We now turn to some recent findings from agrammatic comprehension of three

---

[1] In fact, the Default Principle seems to become problematic under the VP-Internal Subjects Hypothesis. An object-gap sentence will contain two NPs that do not receive a theta role. In order to maintain the application of the Default Principle and still derive the comprehension data, one would have to assume that *both* NPs in a sentence like (2b) are assigned the agent role by default. This seems untenable.

[2] Adjunct status is consistent with the optionality of *by*-phrases; arguments by definition are obligatory.

different types of sentences and consider how these models fare in light of these data.

MATRIX CLAUSE OF CENTER-EMBEDDED RELATIVES

Hickok et al. (1993) report a case study of an agrammatic patient (RD) who performed well on subject cleft constructions (e.g., (1b)), yet performed significantly worse on sentences like (3) (below) when knowledge of the information in the *matrix clause* was probed (i.e., who is tall), rather than information in the relative clause. In an unpublished study (G. Hickok, 1992) FC performed equally poorly on these stimuli (see Appendix).

(3) *The psychologist that attacked the linguist is tall*

These data pose a serious challenge to Grodzinsky's (1990) account. Because Grodzinsky's work did not incorporate VP-internal subjects and hence no trace mediates the relation between the subject and the predicate adjective, comprehension of the matrix clause should be intact, yet clearly in our patients it is not. Hickok however, suggests that if one assumes VP-internal subjects along with chain-disruption, this finding can be accounted for. The relativized subject, like all subjects in English, receives its theta role via a chain; if this chain is disrupted, then the role normally assigned to the NP *the psychologist* by the predicate *is tall* will not be assigned. The grammar thus fails to yield a viable structure and normal grammatically driven interpretation procedures fail. Given that there are two NPs in the input, the choice of the correct response is not sufficiently constrained, and poor performance results (Hickok, 1992; Hickok et al., 1993).

Some have argued that in sentences like (3) the correct choice *is* sufficiently constrained by linguistic information, such as the fact that the embedded NP receives a grammatically assigned role whereas the matrix NP does not, suggesting that agrammatics should be able to deduce that the unassigned role goes with the one NP that has not yet received a role (e.g., Linebarger, this issue). Before proceeding it is important to be very clear about what is at stake here. The question is *not* whether there is a disruption in the chain between matrix subject and predicate—this is predicted by the theory. The question is, assuming that there is such a disruption, is there reason to believe that the agrammatic will have enough information to deduce the correct answer anyway in a nongrammatical problem-solving fashion.

That said, let us return to the above suggestion. Consider the sentence in (4) where in the agrammatic representation *the psychologist* has not received a role, *the linguist* has, and the subject role associated with *is tall* has not been assigned.

(4) *The psychologist attacked the linguist that is tall*

Here if we apply the algorithm suggested above, the subject role of *is tall* would be incorrectly assigned to *the psychologist*. The correct assignment is to a NP that already has a role in the representation,[3] an assignment that differs from that needed to arrive at the correct response in (3). It would seem then, that a simple act of reasoning will not deterministically derive the correct answer for sentences like (3). However, perhaps a more linguistically sophisticated piece of information might be argued to be available to the patient. For example, it is a fact of syntax that embedded NPs cannot serve as the subject of a matrix clause. Yet this is apparently the interpretation given to structures like (3) by our patients on some portion of the trials. This observation can be interpreted in at least two ways: (i) the agrammatic linguistic system is incapable of computing the appropriate structural relations, and thus potentially constraining structural information is unavailable. This would imply a much more severe deficit than is being proposed here, and to the extent that acceptability judgment performance elicited from other agrammatics can be generalized to our patients, this seems an unlikely possibility (Linebarger et al., 1983; Shankweiler et al., 1989; Wulfeck et al., 1991); (ii) the patients can, in principle, compute such structural relations but for some reason are unable to use this information in practice. Two possible scenarios come to mind in this respect: One is that information of this type is simply not used by the cognitive system of a nonlinguist in a problem-solving situation, and the other is that the incomplete thematic structure in the agrammatic representation of these sentences leads to an increase in processing load (Gibson, 1991; Gibson & Hickok, 1993), which in turn impacts the ability to use structural information in a problem-solving situation.

While we must leave as unresolved the question of how much information can be brought to bear on the comprehension task in lieu of intact grammatical representations, it is clear that comprehension of the matrix clause in sentences like (3) is poor in our two patients, and these data must be accounted for in any theory of agrammatic comprehension. This pattern is inconsistent with Grodzinsky's (1990) hypothesis, but is consistent with Hickok's and with Mauner et al.'s proposals in that the latter two predict a disrupted chain in these constructions.

PRONOUNS AND REFLEXIVES

Grodzinsky et al. (1993) recently published a study that examined agrammatic comprehension of binding relations. They tested a group

---

[3] Of course the role assignment is not literally to the head of the relative because it would violate the Theta Criterion, but rather to the relative pronoun which in turn bears some syntactic relation to the head supporting thematic interpretation.

of agrammatics (including RD and FC) for comprehension of sentences like (5) and (6) using a Yes/No judgment paradigm.

(5) Is Mama Bear touching her?

(6) Is Mama Bear touching herself?

As a group, the agrammatic patients performed more poorly on the pronoun sentences (5) than on the reflexive sentences (6). RD and FC's performance was true to this pattern (pronouns: RD, 58% correct, FC, 42% correct; reflexives: RD, 100% correct, FC, 83% correct), suggesting that they interpret sentences like (5) reflexively on some portion of the trials. Grodzinsky's (1990) Trace-Deletion Hypothesis does not predict poor performance on either of these sentences since no traces are involved on his assumptions. In fact Grodzinsky et al. (1993) interpret their results as indicative of a processing deficit independent of the limitation with traces.

Hickok (1992), however, has argued that these data can be explained straightforwardly on the joint assumptions of VP-Internal Subjects and chain disruption. Recall that co-reference between *her* and *Mama Bear* is ruled out in the normal case under Principle B of the Binding Theory, which states that a pronoun must be free (i.e., not co-indexed) in its binding category. In the framework of the VP-Internal Subjects Hypothesis, Kitagawa (1986) argues that the binding catagory for the pronoun in (5) is VP.[4] The relevant normal structure for (5) is given below in (7). Since in the normal representation the trace of the subject is inside VP (and therefore by virtue of its link with the trace, the subject is also) co-reference is impossible in (7). However, in the agrammatic representation (8), the subject *Mama Bear* is not linked to a position internal to the VP, and hence is outside of the binding category of the pronoun, and co-reference is possible without a violation of Principle B.

(7) Is $[_{IP}$ Mama Bear$_i$ $[_{VP}$ t$_i$ touching her]]? ("i" = chain relation)

(8) Is $[_{IP}$ Mama Bear$_{\#}$ $[_{VP}$ t$_{\#}$ touching her]]? ("#" = disrupted chain)

The sentence in (6), for which performance is relatively good in the two patients, seems at first glance to be problematic. Like the case of pronouns, the subject NP would seem to be outside the binding category of the reflexive in the agrammatic representation of (6), given below in (9). Since Principle A of the Binding Theory states that a reflexive must be bound in its binding category, these sentences should be uninterpretable for the agrammatic because there is no allowable antecedent for the

---

[4] In particular, Kitagawa argues that "The binding category for β is the maximal projection of β's lexical case marker, where β = an anaphor or a pronominal" (p. 307). In (5), *her* is case-marked by the verb *touch;* the maximal projection of that verb is VP.

reflexive within VP. Indeed this appears to be a serious problem because in the pronoun case the subject NP needs to be outside the binding category allowing co-reference under Principle B, whereas in the reflexive case the subject NP needs to be inside the binding category in order to satisfy Principle A. In essence, then, the normal complementary distribution of pronouns and anaphors is contradicted in the comprehension data from Grodzinsky et al.'s (1993) study, in which the subject NP appears to bind either a pronoun or an anaphor in the same environment.

(9) Is [$_{IP}$ Mama Bear$_\#$ [$_{VP}$ t$_\#$ touching herself]]? (# = disrupted chain)

As it turns out, a parallel, noncomplementary distribution of pronouns and anaphors is found in some normal English constructions, and it seems that the solution proposed for such cases is applicable to the agrammatic comprehension of (5) and (6). Consider the following pair from Chomsky (1986b; indices denote co-reference).

(10) *The children$_i$ heard [stories about them$_i$]*

(11) *The children$_i$ heard [stories about each other$_i$]*

The pronoun *them* and the anaphor *each other* can both be bound by *the children* in these examples (cf. *the children heard Mary tell stories about them/*each other*). Analogous to (8), (10) is unproblematic because *the children* is outside the (bracketed) binding domain of the pronoun, as required by Principle B. However, (11) should violate Principle A because the NP *the children* is outside the binding category of *each other*, yet the sentence is well-formed, analogous to (9). Chomsky's (1986b) solution to the problem turns on the observation that in (11), the binding category does not contain a possible binder (antecedent) for *each other*, and therefore Principle A can never be satisfied in that binding category. Intuitively then, we must allow the binding category to be expanded when such a case arises. Accordingly, Chomsky (1986b) proposes that ". . . the relevant [binding] category of β [pronoun or anaphor] is the minimal one in which the Binding Theory could have been satisfied by some indexing" (p. 172). In (11), then, the binding category is expanded to IP which contains the NP *the children*. Note that this proposal has no consequences for the binding category of the pronoun since a pronoun must be free in its binding category, a requirement that is satisfied when there is no potential binder in the binding category of a pronoun. In the agrammatic representation (9), we can apply a similar solution. Because there is no potential binder in the binding domain of the reflexive the binding domain must be expanded to IP which contains the NP *Mama Bear;* co-reference between *herself* and *Mama Bear* will thus satisfy Principle A.

Grodzinsky et al. (1993) tested one additional type of sentence involving binding relations; an example is given below in (12).

(12) Is every bear touching her?

Despite the involvement of pronouns, performance on these sentences was quite good in their group of agrammatics, and this pattern held for RD and FC (see Appendix). This appears to be problematic for the account of pronoun comprehension outlined above because the subject *every bear* should be outside the binding domain of the pronoun (allowing co-reference) and yet agrammatics reject this reading. We will return to this finding in the next section.

Wh-QUESTIONS

Hickok and Avrutin (1995) tested comprehension of Wh-questions in two agrammatics, RD and FC, and found a different pattern of performance dependent on the type of Wh-phrase. Wh-questions headed by *which-N* yielded, in both patients, the typical subject–object asymmetry in comprehension with subject-extracted questions (13a) being comprehended significantly better than object-extracted questions (13b) (see the Appendix). This result is consistent with all of the chain-based accounts of agrammatic comprehension and can be accounted for in the same manner as other cases of subject–object asymmetries in Wh-movement constructions such as in relative clauses. Comprehension of Wh-questions headed by *who* did not produce a subject–object asymmetry in either patient. Performance on subject-extracted *who* questions (14a) was, as expected, quite good, but object-extracted *who* questions (14b) were comprehended equally well, contrary to the predictions of *all* of the chain-based accounts.

(13) (a) Which psychologist attacked the linguist?
      (b) Which psychologist did the linguist attack?

(14) (a) Who attacked the linguist?
      (b) Who did the psychologist attack?

Hickok and Avrutin suggested that this set of findings might be explained in terms of the type of chain that is formed by movement of the two types of questions. Rizzi (1990) has argued for two types of operator/variable relations: Binding, formed by movement of a referential element, and Government, formed by movement of a nonreferential element. Following up on work by Pesetsky (1987), Cinque (1990) has proposed that there is a typology of wh-phrases that break down along these lines. *Which-N* phrases are referential and hence give rise to Binding chains; *who* phrases are nonreferential and give rise to Government chains. If we hypothesize that chain-disruption is specific to Binding chains, with Government chains preserved, then the data in (13) and (14) can be accounted for. This more restrictive generalization does not impact the account of *which-N* questions since these involve Binding chains. However, it does enable us to explain preserved comprehension of (13b): because of the assumption that NP-movement yields a Binding chain (Hickok & Avrutin, 1995; see below, however) the subject NP will still not receive its role grammatically, but because movement of *who* yields a Government chain it will receive the patient role in the agrammatic representation. As Hickok has argued in the case of actives and subject-gap constructions the assignment of at least one role in one-verb sentences provides sufficient information to make the correct response.

Data from all of the other sentence types discussed thus far can receive the same analysis under Hickok and Avrutin's more restrictive proposal since on their assumptions all these involve Binding chains. We now return to sentence (12) from Grodzinsky et al.'s (1993) experiment in which contrary to the prediction of Hickok's account, performance on these constructions was significantly better than performance on non-quantified sentences with pronouns [i.e., the agrammatics correctly rejected reflexive interpretations of (12)]. With Hickok and Avrutin's restrictive chain–disruption account, we now have a potential solution. Quantified NPs, like *who* phrases, are nonreferential and therefore enter into Government chains (Cinque, 1990). If Government chains are intact, then in (12) the quantified subject *will* be linked, via a chain, to the VP-internal position and therefore the subject NP will be in the Binding category of the pronoun. Co-reference is then ruled out by Principle B, and correct performance results, as desired. (See Avrutin & Hickok (1992) for further evidence supporting this proposal.)

Finally, a restrictive Binding-chain-disruption hypothesis can account for preserved verb movement in agrammatic patients (Lonzi & Luzzatti, 1993) because verb movement also gives rise to Government chains (Chomsky, 1986a; Cinque, 1990; Rizzi, 1990).

SOME ALTERNATIVE PROPOSALS

While Hickok and Avrutin's (1995) proposal provides considerable coverage of the data, there is a technical problem which at this point limits its appeal. Recall that Hickok and Avrutin assume that NP-movement yields Binding chains. This is crucial to their analysis because if NP-movement gave rise to Government chains, the chains associated with movement of a subject out of VP and in movement in passives would be intact, by hypothesis, and this would by familiar reasoning provide enough information to the agrammatic comprehender to give a correct response in comprehension of passives and object extracted sentences. However, some authors have hypothesized that NP-movement creates Government chains, contrary to Hickok and Avrutin's assumption, because NP-movement is subject to strict locality constraints, a prominent feature of Government chains (Rizzi, 1990).[5] It is possible that the local nature of NP-movement could be derived in some other fashion as has been proposed previously [e.g., Generalized Binding Theory (Aoun, 1986)], but this remains an outstanding problem for Hickok and Avrutin's restrictive account.

None of the proposed representational models of agrammatic comprehension, then, provides a fully satisfactory account of the range of data discussed here. However, if one steps back from the details of the syntactic analyses and looks at the data, a fairly clear pattern seems to emerge. It appears that there is an interaction between two variables, the position from which movement occurs and whether the element that is moved is referential. This is seen most clearly in the data from Wh-questions in which movement from object position causes comprehension problems but only when the moved element is referential (*which-N*) and not when it is nonreferential (*who*). The interaction can also be seen in the pronoun sentences in which the contrast is between definite NP-antecedents (5) which are referential and yield poor performance versus quantified NP-antecedents (12) which are nonreferential and are comprehended well. The work of Saady (this volume) may represent another example of an interaction between syntactic movement and referentiality. This apparent interaction was not previously noticed because all of the constructions used to probe agrammatic comprehension—actives, passives, relative clauses—involved movement of referential NPs.

Hickok and Avrutin (1995) attempted to cash in this interaction with referentiality in terms of a syntactic distinction in the type of chain involved, but as noted above, there is the potential problem of the type of chain created by NP-movement. However, because NP-movement in passives and with VP-internal subjects is still movement of a referential element (in the sentences studied thus far), this problem can be avoided if the generalization could be stated in terms of movement of a referential element rather than in terms of the type of chain.[6] Rizzi (1990) proposes

---

[5] There appears to be some tension between referentiality and Government chains with respect to NP-movement. On the one hand, there is the proposal that referential elements can enter into Binding relations, and clearly the moved NPs in passive and VP-internal subject constructions discussed above are referential. On the other hand, there is the claim that NP-movement (even with referential NPs) gives rise to Government chains. Rizzi (1990) suggests that the locality requirements on A-dependencies are enforced as a result of the Theta Criterion which requires a local chain in the case of A-movement. (See Rizzi 1990, pp. 92–94.)

[6] Grodzinsky (this volume) attempts to capture the referential/nonreferential distinction via a reformulation of his Default Principle, proposing that default thematic role assignment applies only to referential elements. While this captures the data in regard to referentiality, as noted above, it is not clear how the Default Principle can be maintained together with the VP-Internal Subjects Hypothesis when sentences with only referential elements are considered. See footnote 1.

one possible syntactic distinction that turns on referentiality alone. He argues, following Chomsky (1965), that the use of referential indices should be restricted to referential elements. He suggests further that such an element, ". . . if moved, can carry its index along. No other position [i.e., nonreferential elements] can a carry a referential index" (p. 86). Although it is not fully clear exactly how this idea might play out at the level of interpretation, one might argue that interpretation of referential dependencies is supported by referential indices, whereas interpretation of nonreferential dependencies is not. A deficit in the establishment of referential indices, which is essentially Mauner et al.'s proposal but with a more literal interpretation of "referential," may then capture the range of agrammatic comprehension facts.

Here, too, however there are potential pitfalls. One is that if interpretation of nonreferential dependencies is possible without indices (presumably because the localness of the relation restricts alternative interpretations), why can't nonindexed referential dependencies in the agrammatic representation be interpreted in the same manner when such a relation happens to be local (and presumably involves Government chains) as in NP-movement? Another problem is that Cinque (1990) has argued that restricting referential indices to referential elements is incorrect; to the extent that he is correct a deficit involving referential indices in agrammatism will be inadequate.

Perhaps the appropriate level at which to make a representational generalization is not the level of syntax, but rather at a higher level of representation, for example at the level of referential interpretation itself. This seems a priori plausible given that in the normal parsing literature, referential context has been shown to have a dramatic impact on parsing decisions. It has been claimed that certain linguistic structures carry with them referential presuppositions in the discourse model (Altmann, Garnham, & Dennis, 1992; Altmann & Steedman, 1988; Crain & Steedman, 1985). For example, the use of a definite NP such as *the psychologist* presupposes that there is a psychologist in the discourse context to which the definite NP refers. It is argued further that the use of contextually unsupported linguistic structures—as is typically the case in agrammatic comprehension studies (but see Hickok et al., 1993)—creates an additional load on the processor because an appropriate discourse representation must be *created* in order to support the referential presuppositions of the linguistic structure. As support for their position, they cite evidence from ambiguous sentences in which readers consistently prefer the structural analysis that is best supported by the discourse context in terms of referential presuppositions. Further evidence along these lines and with particular relevance to this discussion comes from a number of studies: Crain and Ni (1991) have shown that the above-noted parsing effects also hold for ambiguities involving definite versus quantified NPs;

Avrutin (1994) has proposed that children's patterns of comprehension of sentences involving binding relations, which show similarities to agrammatic comprehension, can be explained in discourse referential terms; and De Vincenzi (1991) has found processing differences between *who* and *which-N* questions in normal speakers of Italian.

What we are suggesting, then, is that the difference between referential and nonreferential elements in agrammatic comprehension may be traceable to differences in the processing of these two types of elements in the normal case. Referential NPs require interpretive links to discourse representations, and in situations in which referential presuppositions are not satisfied, appropriate discourse representations must be created. Nonreferential NPs do not require links to preestablished discourse referents; thus they may impose less processing demands leading to better performance. Admittedly, our suggestion is somewhat vague and needs to be worked out in much more detail—primarily because the theory of reference is not worked out to the same level of detail as syntactic theory—but in our view the proposal looks sufficiently promising to warrant further investigation.

CONCLUSIONS

We have reviewed three major proposals aimed at providing a representational description of agrammatic comprehension and have considered how these proposals fare in light of a set of new data gathered from two agrammatic aphasics. The following conclusions can be drawn. First, the complete pattern of performance claimed to hold of agrammatic comprehension does in fact exist in at least two patients. We can therefore put to rest concerns that the representational accounts discussed above are vacuous theories, describing a range of deficits that do not exist except in the abstract. Second, none of the proposals, including our own earlier restrictive refinements (Hickok & Avrutin, 1995), characterizes, in a fully satisfactory way, the data found in the patients presented here. Some fail on grounds of empirical coverage while others incorporate potentially incorrect linguistic assumptions. Perhaps advances in basic linguistic research will improve this situation—much as the VP-Internal Subjects Hypothesis has—and indeed some of the work discussed above may motivate a reconsideration of linguistic analyses in the normal case.

The principal contribution of this work, however, is to stress the importance of referentiality in the description of agrammatic comprehension and the potential role of performance in contributing to the observed pattern of deficit and sparing. The idea that processing limitations may contribute to agrammatic comprehension is far from new and is not inconsistent with representational generalizations. What is new, as far as we are aware, is the proposal that differing processing demands dependent on the referential properties of linguistic elements may play a role in the agrammatic pattern of comprehension.

Finally, some may question the use of rather top-heavy linguistic theories to account for data from a relatively small number of sentences. While acknowledging that overinterpretation is a distinct risk in this situation, we are heartened by the fact that a number of researchers are converging on a small set of analyses that are covering a widening range of data, and that from these analyses comes a collection of highly specific predictions that are easily testable and thus falsifiable. Even if a unitary representational description of agrammatic comprehension proves untenable, our understanding of these issues will benefit.

APPENDIX
RD and FC's Comprehension Performance in a Sentence Verification Paradigm Given in Percentage Correct

	RD	FC
Actives	93 ($n = 30$)[a]	90 ($n = 30$)[a]
Subject relatives	93 ($n = 70$)[b]	90 ($n = 30$)[a]
Passives	58 ($n = 40$)[b]	57 ($n = 30$)[a]
Object relatives	36 ($n = 70$)[b]	40 ($n = 30$)[a]
Matrix of relative	31 ($n = 70$)[b]	60 ($n = 20$)[a]
Pronouns	42 ($n = 12$)[c]	58 ($n = 12$)[c]
Reflexives	100 ($n = 12$)[c]	83 ($n = 12$)[c]
Quantified pronouns	83 ($n = 12$)[c]	100 ($n = 12$)[c]
Which subject	87 ($n = 15$)[d]	87 ($n = 15$)[d]
Which object	47 ($n = 15$)[d]	47 ($n = 15$)[d]
Who subject	80 ($n = 15$)[d]	93 ($n = 15$)[d]
Who object	87 ($n = 15$)[d]	87 ($n = 15$)[d]

[a] Unpublished data (G. Hickok, 1992).

[b] Data reported in Hickok et al. (1993); cells with $n = 70$ represent pooled data from two experiments, one using a sentence-to-picture matching paradigm and the other using a sentence-verification paradigm. No task differences were found.

[c] Data from Grodzinsky et al. (1993).

[d] Data from Hickok and Avrutin (1995).

REFERENCES

Altmann, G., Garnham, A., & Dennis, Y. 1992. Avoiding the garden path: Eye movements in context. *Journal of Memory and Language,* **31,** 685–712.

Altmann, G., & Steedman, M. 1988. Interaction with context during human sentence processing. *Cognition,* **30,** 191–238.

Aoun, J. 1986. *Generalized binding.* Dordrecht: Foris.

Avrutin, S. 1994. *Psycholinguistic investigations in the theory of reference.* Unpublished Ph.D. thesis, MIT.

Avrutin, S., & Hickok, G. 1992. *Operator/variable relations, referentiality, and agrammatic comprehension.* Unpublished manuscript, MIT.

Baker, M., Johnson, K., & Roberts, I. 1989. Passive arguments raised. *Linguistic Inquiry,* **20,** 219–252.

Caplan, D., & Futter, C. 1986. Assignment of thematic roles by an agrammatic aphasic patient. *Brain and Language,* **27,** 117–135.

Caramazza, A., & Badecker, W. 1989. Patient classification in neuropsychological research. *Brain and Cognition,* **10,** 256–295.

Caramazza, A., & Zurif, E. B. 1976. Dissociation of algorithmic and heuristic processes in sentence comprehension: Evidence from aphasia. *Brain and Language,* **3,** 572–582.

Chomsky, N. 1965. *Aspects of the theory of syntax.* Cambridge, MA: MIT Press.

Chomsky, N. 1986a. *Barriers.* Cambridge, MA: MIT Press.

Chomsky, N. 1986b. *Knowledge of language: Its nature, origin, and use.* New York: Praeger.

Cinque, G. 1990. *Types of A' dependencies.* Cambridge, MA: MIT Press.

Crain, S., & Ni, W. 1991. Parsermony. In *Current issues in natural language processing.* Austin: University of Texas.

Crain S., & Steedman, M. 1985. On not being led up the garden path: The use of context by the psychological syntax processor. In D. R. Dowty, L. Karttunen, & A. M. Zwicky (Eds.), *Natural language parsing: Psychological, computational, and theoretical perspectives.* New York: Cambridge University Press.

De Vincenzi, M. 1991. *Syntactic parsing strategies in Italian.* Boston, MA: Kluwer Academic Publisher.

Gibson, E. 1991. *A computational theory of human linguistic processing: Memory limitations and processing breakdown.* Unpublished Ph.D. thesis, Carnegie Mellon University.

Gibson, E., & Hickok, G. 1993. Sentence processing with empty categories. *Language and Cognitive Processes,* **8,** 147–161.

Goodall, G. 1993. On case and the passive morpheme. *Natural Language and Linguistic Theory,* **11,** 31–44.

Goodglass, H., & Kaplan, E. 1976. *The assessment of aphasia and related disorders.* Philadelphia, PA: Lea & Febiger.

Grimshaw, J. 1990. *Argument structure.* Cambridge, MA: MIT Press.

Grodzinsky, Y. 1986. Language deficits and the theory of syntax. *Brain and Language,* **27,** 135–159.

Grodzinsky, Y. 1989. Agrammatic comprehension of relative clauses. *Brain and Language,* **31,** 480–499.

Grodzinsky, Y. 1990. *Theoretical perspectives on language deficits.* Cambridge, MA: MIT Press.

Grodzinsky, Y., Wexler, K., Chien, Y.-C., Marakovitz, S., & Solomon, J. 1993. The breakdown of binding relations. *Brain and Language,* **45,** 396–422.

Hickok, G. 1992. *Agrammatic comprehension and the trace-deletion hypothesis.* Occasional Paper No. 45, MIT Center for Cognitive Science.

Hickok, G., & Avrutin, S. 1995. Comprehension of Wh-questions in two Broca's aphasics. *Brain and Language,* in press.

Hickok, G., Zurif, E., & Canseco-Gonzalez, E. 1993. Structural description of agrammatic comprehension. *Brain and Language,* **45,** 371–395.

Kitagawa, Y. 1986. *Subjects in Japanese and English.* Unpublished Ph.D thesis. University of Massachusetts, Amherst.

Koopman, H., & Sportiche, D. 1988. *Subjects.* Unpublished manuscript, UCLA.

Linebarger, M. C., Schwartz, M., & Saffran, E. 1983. Sensitivity to grammatical structure in so-called agrammatic aphasics. *Cognition,* **13,** 361–393.

Lonzi, L., & Luzzatti, C. 1993. Relevance of adverb distribution for the analysis of sentence representation in agrammatic patients. *Brain and Language*, **45**, 306–317.

Mauner, G., Fromkin, V. A., & Cornell, T. L. 1993. Comprehension and acceptability judgments in agrammatism: Disruptions in the syntax of referential dependency. *Brain and Language*, **45**, 340–370.

Miyake, A., Carpenter, P. A., & Just, M. A. 1993. *Normal adults' syntactic comprehension under strong temporal constraints: Implications for theories of syntactic comprehension disorders.* Tucson, AZ: Academy of Aphasia.

Pesetsky, D. 1987. Wh-in-situ: Movement and unselective binding. In E. J. Reuland & A. G. B. T. Meulen (Eds.), *The representation of (in)definiteness.* Cambridge, MA: MIT Press.

Rizzi, L. 1990. *Relativized minimality.* Cambridge, MA: MIT Press.

Schwartz, M. E., Saffran, E., & Marin, O. 1980. The word-order problem in agrammatism. 1. Comprehension. *Brain and Language*, **10**, 249–262.

Shankweiler, D., Crain, S., Gorrell, P., & Tuller, B. 1989. Reception of language in Broca's aphasia. *Language and Cognitive Processes*. **4**, 1–33.

Sherman, J., & Schweickert, J. 1989. Syntactic and semantic contributions to sentence comprehension in agrammatism. *Brain and Language*, **37**, 419–439.

Wulfeck, B., Bates, E., & Capasso, R. 1991. A cross-linguistic study of grammaticality judgments in Broca's aphasia. *Brain and Language*, **41**, 311–336.

Zurif, E., Swinney, D., Prather, P., Solomon, J., & Bushell, C. 1993. An on-line analysis of syntactic processing in Broca's and Wernicke's aphasia. *Brain and Language*, **45**, 448–464.

BRAIN AND LANGUAGE **50,** 27–51 (1995)

A Restrictive Theory of Agrammatic Comprehension

YOSEF GRODZINSKY

Tel Aviv University, Israel, and Aphasia Research Center, Department of Neurology, Boston University School of Medicine

In this paper I propose a new, restrictive theory of Trace-Deletion in agrammatism. This theory subsumes the Trace-Deletion Hypothesis (TDH; Grodzinsky, 1984a,b, 1986, 1990), which maintains that traces are deleted from agrammatic representations and that a cognitive strategy augments the patients' performance. This claim accounts for the pattern of loss and sparing observed in these patients' comprehension of a wide variety of syntactic constructions and is thus important for our understanding of the neural representation of syntax. Yet there are reasons for revising the account and making it more precise, stemming from both recent empirical findings and new developments in the theory of syntax. The original TDH was based on observations of agrammatic comprehension of structures containing traces resulting from either NP- or Wh-movement. Nevertheless, heads (as opposed to phrasal projections) also move and leave traces behind. Head movement (of verbs, for instance) has come to play a central role in linguistic theory (which currently postulates a wider variety of empty categories than any previous theoretical framework). Recent findings suggest that verb movement is retained in agrammatism, indicating that a sweeping claim regarding the deletion of all empty categories is too strong. This motivates the first restrictive move, resulting in a theory that picks out a restricted set of traces—only those for which deficient performance is indeed observed. All other empty categories are left intact. Trace-Deletion is tied to Θ-positions. The second restrictive move is motivated by two types of surprising asymmetries that have recently been discovered for agrammatic comprehenders: First, agrammatic comprehension on passives of psychological predicates provides an error pattern that distinguishes this construction from agentive passive, indicating that the deficit is tied to the thematic properties of the predicate; Second, asymmetries have been observed in agrammatic comprehension of questions and quantifiers. These findings motivate a modification of the augmentative strategy, whose domain of application is restricted to referential NPs. Thus, the new account amounts to the claim that only traces in Θ-positions are deleted, and that the strategy applies to referential NPs alone. This, I argue, not only derives all the data precisely but is also conceptually superior to any previous account of agrammatism. Finally, I discuss the consequences of this account to linguistic theory, and to theories of brain/language relations. © 1995 Academic Press, Inc.

This paper was supported by NIH Grant NIDCD 00081 to the Aphasia Research Center, Department of Neurology, Boston University School of Medicine. Address correspondence and reprint requests to Yosef Grodzinsky, Department of Psychology, Tel Aviv University, Tel Aviv 69978, Israel. E-mail: yosef1@freud.tau.ac.il.

202

INTRODUCTORY REMARKS

In this paper I revise the Trace-Deletion Hypothesis (TDH), according to which all traces are deleted from S-structure representations in agrammatism (Grodzinsky, 1984a,b, 1986, 1990). Doing aphasia research is getting to be a difficult trade, as the issues are becoming increasingly subtle. This has happened due to developments that have been both empirical and theoretical in nature. Indeed, new empirical evidence has been recently accumulating, giving further indications as to the fine nature of the syntactically selective deficit in this syndrome and making such a revision necessary. New theoretical developments in linguistics force reconsideration as well. A revision, aimed at refining the account and making it more precise, will thus advance our understanding of brain/language relation and, in particular, of the neural substrate of the human syntactic capacity.

One recent development concerns verb movement, which has come to play a rather central role in linguistic theory (cf. Pollock, 1989; Chomsky, 1992) and which appears to be preserved in agrammatism (cf. Lonzi & Luzzatti, 1993, and below). This development motivates a restrictive move, which limits trace-deletion to Θ-positions. A second development concerns two types of surprising asymmetries that have been recently discovered in the comprehension performance of agrammatic aphasics. The first comes from contrasts in performance on passive constructions that contain predicates of different thematic types (Grodzinsky, 1995a). Briefly, the finding is that while on passives of agentive predicates agrammatic comprehension is at chance level in tasks involving Θ-role assignment, when the predicate is a psych-verb, comprehension levels of passive go down to below-chance (i.e., systematic reversals of Θ-roles).

The second asymmetry is from agrammatic differential performance on constructions with moved constituents (i.e., antecedents of deleted traces) with different referential properties (cf. Hickok & Avrutin and Saddy, this issue). It was found that while agrammatics perform at chance when presented with object *Which* questions (as the TDH predicts), they surprisingly give a virtually normal performance on *Who* questions. In addition, they comprehend normally (above-chance) when presented with passives containing quantified subjects, although they fail in passives, whose subjects are referential.

These two types of findings thus motivate a natural reformulation of the TDH in a second respect: the nonlinguistic, cognitive strategy that augments the deficient abilities of the patients is restricted to referential expressions.

The TDH is thus restated restrictively: only traces in Θ-positions are deleted, and NPs lacking a Θ-role receive one strategically iff they are referential.

The reformulation has surprising implications regarding the proper view of agrammatism, as it casts the disturbance in terms that contradict accepted ideas. Most importantly, it has the consequence that in agrammatic comprehension the deficit is limited to lexical categories and their phrasal projections, whereas functional categories are intact. This conclusion is diametrically opposed to the standard view of the deficit in this syndrome, according to which functional elements are impaired, whereas lexical ones are not.

Finally, this reformulation has important implications to linguistic theory: It strengthens the view that passive constructions contain traces in object position [cf. also Grodzinsky, Pierce, & Marakovitz (1991), for an earlier neuropsychological argument] and provides a new neurologically based diagnostic method for long Wh-movement.

This paper is structured as follows: The first three sections present the basic data and conceptual background that originally motivated the Trace-Deletion Hypothesis. Sections 4 and 5 discuss the TDH in the context of current Chain Theory and in light of recent neurological evidence regarding chain types. Section 6 proposes a reformulation of the TDH along the lines suggested above, and section 7 discusses the reformulation in light of recently discovered comprehension asymmetries. Section 8 draws some general conclusions regarding the significance of the account to various theoretical domains.

1. PAST VIEWS

Within the many studies carried out in the past 20 years on agrammatic aphasia, one can identify roughly three views of the agrammatic comprehension limitation. The first two views postulate a deficit whose range is very broad:

A. Complete syntactic loss—"asyntactic comprehension," according to which agrammatic patients have lost all ability to represent syntactic structure (e.g., Caramazza & Zurif, 1976; Berndt & Caramazza, 1980; Caplan, 1985; Caplan & Futter, 1986, and many others).

B. An interpretive deficit—"the mapping hypothesis," according to which agrammatics have lost all abilities involved in mapping grammatical functions onto semantic roles (cf. Schwartz, Saffran, & Marin, 1980; Linebarger, Schwartz, & Saffran, 1983a,b; Schwartz, Linebarger, Saffran, & Pate, 1987).

These early views have had, for the most part, similar empirical consequences and, given the paucity of data at the time, could not be easily distinguished from one another. Yet as experimental evidence was pouring in, it turned out that they were both too strong and that the deficit they argued for was far too wide in scope. Thus, a third view was put forth, viewing the deficit in terms that are more restricted:

C. Partial syntactic deficit—"impaired closed-class" (Bradley, Garrett, & Zurif, 1980), "Trace-Deletion Hypothesis" (e.g., Grodzinsky,

1984a,b, 1986, 1990; Mauner, Fromkin, & Cornell, 1993; Hickok, Zurif, & Canseco-Gonzales, 1993, and many others), "Θ-constrained deficit" (Rizzi, 1985).

The trend, then, has been toward more restrictive accounts. Recent findings, however, suggest that even the narrowly defined partial syntactic deficit that the TDH postulated is too wide, and a new, restrictive theory of agrammatic comprehension needs to be constructed.

2. THE CENTRALITY OF MOVEMENT

On testing, it seems that constructions governed by most of the modules of grammar are intact in agrammatism. The one clear exception, which has stood out virtually since the beginning of the experimental investigations in the late 1960s, is syntactic movement, as indicated by marked comprehension deficiencies on movement-derived structures. The limited evidence that was available consisted mostly of patients' scores on "sentence-to-picture matching" tests, which assessed the subjects' ability to assign Θ-roles to NPs. The range of constructions investigated was also narrow: Actives, passives, subject and object clefts, and object relative clauses (cf. Goodglass, 1968; Caramazza & Zurif, 1976; Schwartz et al., 1980a,b; Ansell & Flowers, 1982). Auxiliary evidence also existed from agrammatics' grammaticality judgment on assorted violations of grammaticality (Gardner & Zurif, 1975; Grossman & Haberman, 1982; Linebarger et al., 1983; Goodenough, Zurif, & Weintraub, 1977) and from hierarchical clustering (Zurif & Caramazza, 1976).

In light of this, and given that the main issue debated in the early 1980s was whether agrammatism is "overarching" comprehension and production, an initial attempt was made to capture all aspects of agrammatic grammatical aberrations in one descriptive generalization that would span over all the modalities. The hope was that patterns of impairment and sparing in speaking, listening, reading, and writing would all fall under the same generalization. Thus labor was invested in obtaining such a generalization—a unified deficit analysis of agrammatism. The initial proposal was, then, that all nonlexical terminals at S-structure (which were to include empty categories, as well as φ-features—gender, person, and number agreement) are underspecified in syntactic representations of agrammatic aphasics, and hence, the deficits in production (substitution and omission of inflectional and other nonlexical elements) and in comprehension (problems with moved constituents that could be viewed as deletion of empty categories and their indices) are accounted for uniformly (Grodzinsky, 1984a,b; Zurif & Grodzinsky, 1983).

However, it quickly turned out that this conclusion had been too optimistic. The account turned out to be both too weak and too strong: Too weak, since the idea to create S-structure representations in which all nonlexical terminals are underspecified excludes certain impaired elements (e.g., Friederici, 1982, 1985). Too strong, because the attempt to generalize over modalities (i.e., production and comprehension) could be successful only if some data, as well as certain important linguistic distinctions, were glossed over. The pattern of selective impairment thus turned out to be more intricate and severe than this account could allow and hence, the second stage separated the modalities and proposed two descriptive statements, one for production, and the other for comprehension (Grodzinsky, 1986; and more explicitly in Grodzinsky, 1990). The consequence of this move was, quite naturally, to abandon (at least for the time being) the claim that agrammatism is an "overarching" deficit and attempt to construct separate accounts for the deficit in each modality.

Since that time, numerous empirical studies have been published, producing new evidence regarding the grammatical basis of aphasic performance by both extending the range of grammatical structures on which agrammatic patients were tested and varying the tasks with which the patients were faced. This evidence underscores the centrality of movement in the agrammatic comprehension deficit in that it documents, with very few exceptions, a rather overwhelming near-normal performance in most other domains of syntax. The state of the evidence is roughly the following, presented according to the various syntactic modules:

A. *Phrase structure:* Agrammatic patients have intact abilities in this domain (in both comprehension and production). In production they appear to construct sentences that do not violate basic sentence structure (see Lapointe, 1985), and more importantly in the present context, in comprehension they have no problem in building tree structure for sentences that do not contain intrasentential dependency relations, such as actives, for instance. They are also able to construct syntactic representations that respect the argument structure of predicates (Shapiro & Levin, 1990; Shapiro, Gordon, Hack, & Killackey, 1993) and are near-normal in detecting violations of phrase structure rules (Linebarger et al., 1983).[1]

B. *Lexical properties:* Agrammatics have no lexical impairment in comprehension. They detect violations of subcategorization (Linebarger et al., 1983) and demonstrate a normal time-course of lexical processing when argument structure is at issue (Shapiro & Levin, 1990; Shapiro et al., 1993). They are also virtually normal on tasks that involve lexical processing (Swinney, Zurif, & Nicol, 1989).

C. Θ-*assignment:* Agrammatics have intact abilities in this domain. This is evident from their normal performance in comprehension tasks that involve Θ-role assignment in simple structures (cf. for instance,

---

[1] One potential exception is the recent claim by Hagiwara (1994) that CP is impaired. At the time of writing, this claim could not yet be incorporated into the discussion.

Schwartz et al., 1987). In addition, they never violate the Θ-criterion when they construct syntactic representations (Lapointe, 1985).

D. *Case assignment:* Agrammatics have virtually intact abilities in this domain. This has been shown time and again in judgment and comprehension studies in several languages (cf. Lukatela, Crain, & Shankweiler, 1988; Crain, Shankweiler, Gorell, & Tuller, 1989; Linebarger et al., 1983).

It would appear, then, that on every aspect of basic sentence structure the comprehension of these patients is virtually intact. This conclusion, coupled with the fact that agrammatics have little, if any, deficit in other linguistic domains in comprehension, is the reason, perhaps, that for almost 50 years students of agrammatism believed that there was no comprehension impairment in this syndrome. Yet when one takes dependency relations into account, the picture changes. Next, a survey of such relations is in order.

E. *Binding:* The formal aspects of binding relations are intact in agrammatism (cf. Grodzinsky, Wexler, Chien, Marakovitz, & Solomon, 1993; see also Crain & Shankweiler, 1985; and Avrutin, 1994). To the extent that certain relations among pronouns, reflexives, and their antecedents are impaired, they have to do with discourse-related aspects of pronominal reference and not with binding theory (cf. Grodzinsky & Reinhart, 1993; Avrutin, 1994).[2]

F. *Other syntactic domains:* Other than the list above (and movement which is discussed below), no other domains (e.g., Bounding, Control) have ever been tested systematically; hence, no data are available.

G. *Movement:* In sharp contrast with the above findings that indicate intactness of comprehension abilities we see a rather severe deficit in movement-derived constructions, as evidenced through the following familiar patterns:

(1) Above-chance performance
   a. The girl pushed the boy
   b. The girl who pushed the boy was tall
   c. Show me the girl who pushed the boy
   d. It is the girl who pushed the boy
   e. The boy was interested in the girl
   f. The woman was uninspired by the man

(2) Chance performance
   a. The boy was pushed by the girl

---

[2] Grodzinsky and Reinhart discuss children and agrammatics' deficit in executing coreference relations in language comprehension and claim that the deficit (identical in both groups) is not related to syntax per se, but rather to a processing component that is responsible for holding two representations concurrently and carrying out computations over them. Avrutin attempts to recast this claim in terms of the Discourse Representation Theory.

b. The boy who the girl pushed was tall
c. Show me the boy who the girl pushed
d. It is the boy who the girl pushed
e. The woman was unmasked by the man

It has also been found that the time-course of language processing in movement derived structures is impaired (Shapiro et al., 1993) and that other time-constrained tasks also reveal a deficit in this type of syntactic construction (Zurif, Swinney, Prather, Solomon, & Bushell, 1993).

It thus appears that every aspect of syntax, whether pertaining to basic relations or to the more intricate dependencies, is intact in agrammatism, with one salient exception: syntactic movement.

3. THE ESSENCE OF THE TDH

3.1. Trace Deletion

To accommodate these findings, it was assumed that in agrammatism, all traces of movement are deleted from S-structure representation. As a consequence, Θ-role transmission to moved constituents, normally mediated by the chain that the trace and its antecedent constitute (and potentially, intermediate traces as well), cannot take place. A moved NP thus lacks a Θ-role, and the hypothesis thus provides a formal means to partition the data, by saying that structures containing traces are impaired, and the rest preserved. Yet it was obvious that mere partitioning was insufficient, because it lacked explanatory force: While it pointed to the structures that gave the patients trouble, the patients' actual performance rates were not derived deductively from just trace-deletion. The deletion of traces explains why the transmission of Θ-roles to a moved constituent is impossible, yet it does not indicate why this, in itself, prevents the patient from inferring the missing role from the rest of the information that is available to him (i.e., the Θ-grid of the predicate, the fact that another NP is assigned a Θ-role directly; cf. Grodzinsky, 1990, Chap. 5). Further, as we will see below, if current theory is assumed, the TDH does not even partition the data accurately.

3.2. The Default Strategy

To remedy this situation, an auxiliary assumption was deemed necessary in order to derive chance performance on passive, object-gap relatives, and clefts. A nonlinguistic, general cognitive strategy (reminiscent of Bever's (1970) influential proposal or of Pinker's (1984) learning procedure for children) assigns such NPs a default role, by their linear position in the sentence, which, for the cases tested, was always Agent. The idea was that since the moved constituents lack a Θ-role, and since NPs must have some role in interpretation, the strategy assigns them a role by linear considerations, which for the cases discussed was always Agent. As a consequence, the thematic representation the patient has in such cases contains two Agents (one assigned grammatically and the other strategically), and the observed chance performance is deduced. For example, in the passive construction, which generates chance performance by agrammatics, the external argument of the verb (namely, the subject of the active) is assigned the Agent role. This means that in passive the oblique object (the NP argument of the *by*-phrase) gets this role. Crucially, no syntactic movement is involved here; hence, no chain mediates the assignment of this role. The subject of the passive, by contrast, being derived by movement, is linked to a trace in object position, and this link is the channel for Θ-role transmission. In agrammatism this cannot take place, and hence the subject of a passive sentence receives no Θ-role grammatically. It is at this point where the strategy kicks in, assigning Agent to this NP, with the result of a thematic representation with two Agents. The patient is incapable of determining the Agent of the action uniquely, and he is forced to guess, performing at chance. The unimpaired constructions contain no traces and therefore create no comprehension problem, precisely as the data indicate.

In sum, the derivation of the agrammatic performance rates on all constructions is done by assuming trace-deletion and a strategy. Performance is thus deduced through either thematic *competition* or *compensation:* The strategy always assigns an Agent label to clause-initial NPs. Thus, if a moved constituent is linked to a different Θ-role normally (as is the case in passive, object-gap relatives, object clefts, and the like), this constituent now becomes Agent, and since there is another, grammatically assigned Agent in the thematic representation, the two Agents compete, thereby inducing chance performance by agrammatics. In cases where the moved NP was supposed to be Agent (such as subject-gap relatives, subject clefts, or actives under the VP-Internal Subject Hypothesis), this role is not assigned normally through the trace due to Trace-Deletion, yet the strategy correctly compensates by assigning that NP the Agent role by default.

Direct evidence to the validity of this strategy comes from an experiment with psych-verbs (Grodzinsky, 1995a). In an experiment conducted on one type of psychological predicates, it was found that agrammatics perform below-chance on passives of psychological predicates such as in (3), below (even though they perform normally on their active counterparts). This contrasts sharply with the chance-level performance rate that patients exhibit on movement-derived structures in which the predicate is agentive.[3]

---

[3] An additional study to be considered in this context is Hagiwara (1993), in which psych-predicates in Japanese are discussed, and their comprehension in agrammatism is investi-

(3) Below-chance performance:
     The girl was admired by the boy

This finding has been used to rule out certain variants of the TDH
which have attempted to formulate it without making reference to the
default strategy (Hickock et al., 1993; Mauner et al., 1993). The surprising
contrast between agentive and psychological passive is explained only if
the patients indeed use an agent-first strategy, which leads to differences
in the thematic representations available to them. Below, normal and
agrammatic Θ-representations are given for several construction types:

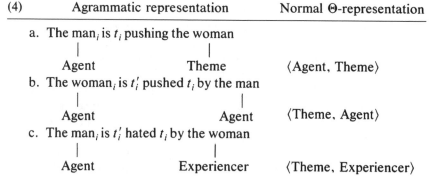

(4)   Agrammatic representation   Normal Θ-representation

a. The man$_i$ is t_i pushing the woman

   Agent   Theme   ⟨Agent, Theme⟩

b. The woman$_i$ is t_i' pushed t_i by the man

   Agent   Agent   ⟨Theme, Agent⟩

c. The man$_i$ is t_i' hated t_i by the woman

   Agent   Experiencer   ⟨Theme, Experiencer⟩

(4a) is an active sentence, in which the VP Internal Subject had moved
to the Specifier of IP, leaving a trace behind (see Koopman & Sportiche,
1988; Kuroda, 1986; Kitagawa, 1986, and much related literature for arguments in favor of this hypothesis, which amounts to the claim that subjects are base-generated VP internally and are then moved to Spec of IP,
leaving a trace behind as in (4a)). Given the TDH, the subject cannot
receive its Θ-role normally, yet we can see that the strategy correctly
compensates for this deficit, since the NP in question is clause-initial.
The normal Θ-representation and the agrammatic one are thus identical.
In (4b), however, the situation is different: here, we have the chain
⟨woman, t', t⟩, where t is the original position of the subject, and t' is
the VP Internal Subject position to which the subject moves first before
ending up in subject position (see Burton & Grimshaw (1992) for arguments from VP-ellipsis to that effect). By hypothesis, these two traces
are deleted, leaving the subject without a Θ-role, and under the scope of

gated. The results, while not exactly parallel to the English ones, must be viewed in relation
to the structural differences between English and Japanese and the possibility that the
strategy operates differently in the two languages. Similarly, the interesting results obtained
by Beretta, Harford, Patterson, and Pinango (1994), who studied movement-derived and
base-generated passives in Spanish, should be looked at, opening the way to a comparative
study of aphasic syndromes (cf. Grodzinsky (1995b)).

the default strategy. The strategy assigns the subject the Agent role, which interacts with the remains of the Θ-representation (i.e., an Agent in *by*-phrase) in a way that leads to guessing—the standard result on passive. In (4c) there is yet another situation, because the Θ-role in the *by*-phrase is different from Agent, and in fact, lower on the thematic hierarchy. This results in a Θ-representation that has an Agent (by default) and an Experiencer. Given the hierarchical nature of thematic relations this leads to a Θ-representation in which the subject of the passive is more salient; hence, patients reverse the Θ-roles, rather than guess, giving further empirical support to the validity of this extremely local strategy, applying only to NPs at an interpretive stage.[4]

4. THE TDH AND CHAIN TYPES

The TDH was a sweeping generalization. It claimed that any trace, in any position, is deleted in agrammatism. What follows is that every structure containing a (nontrivial) chain would bring about aberrant comprehension performance in agrammatism.

Yet there are reasons to suppose that this formulation is too strong and that the trend toward more restrictive accounts of agrammatic comprehension must continue. First, empirical evidence currently available speaks against this formulation. Second, recent developments in the theory of syntactic chains (Chomsky, 1992; Rizzi, 1985, 1990; Cinque, 1991; Snyder, 1992, for example) and the extension of the ECP to cover verb movement (Pollock, 1989; Chomsky, 1991, 1992), as well as the development of economy principles in linguistic theory (Chomsky, 1991, 1992), have had implications to the description of aphasic syndromes. A rough typology of syntactic chains is thus in order. These are composed of three types:

4.1. X^0-Chains

A lexical category—a head—is moved, leaving a trace behind. This type of movement is distinct from others in that it is subject to the Head Movement Constraint (Travis, 1984; Chomsky, 1986), according to which a head cannot skip an intervening head between its base position and its landing site. A typical case is verb movement:

(5) a. They could have left
   b. Could they *t* have left?
   c. *Have they could *t* left?

---

[4] An additional finding is that on adjectival passives, which presumably are not derived transformationally, agrammatic patients perform rather successfully (cf. Grodzinsky, Pierce, & Marakovitz, 1991).

This case, as well as others (relating to constraints on negation, placement of adverbs in certain languages, Subject-Aux inversion, Do-support, the movement of main verbs in Germanic languages, etc.), falls under Relativized Minimality (RM; cf. Rizzi, 1990), which is an attempt to unify the relation between empty categories and their antecedents, while preserving certain distinctions among chain types.

4.2. A-Chains

Covering movement resulting in chains headed by an element in A-position. This includes passive, unaccusatives (including Raising), and Psychological predicates (cf. Belletti & Rizzi, 1988). Here movement is again constrained by RM, which blocks, among other things, cases like (6):

(6) *Mary seems that it is likely [t to win]

4.3. A'-Chains

Headed by an element in A'-position, including questions, relative clauses, and the like. Here, RM blocks cases like (7):

(7) *How do you wonder [which problems to solve t t']
     (where How relates to the solution)

While each chain type is different from the others in certain respects, the three groups do not constitute totally distinct formal objects. Rizzi's Relativized Minimality is an attempt to unify the conditions that govern the relations among links in a chain and determine whether a particular link can be part of a legitimate formal object. Yet each of these chain types is distinct from others in important ways (most prominently, the "relativized" part of Relativized Minimality). With this in mind, we can proceed to examine the relevant facts regarding agrammatism. The TDH as stated, it will be recalled, claims that all traces are deleted. The implications of this hypothesis, then, are far reaching. It also leaves many questions open: for instance, while we know that if a trace of a Θ-assigned category is deleted, the main consequence would be an inability to transmit this role properly through the chain, we do not know what would happen in chains headed by categories that are not Θ-recipients, namely, head or X^0-chains.

5. A TYPOLOGY OF THE RELEVANT NEUROPSYCHOLOGICAL FACTS

Following the typology sketched above, we can now look at the empirical evidence from agrammatism, which breaks down into two general types:

5.1. XP Movement (A- and A'-Chains)

For those standard cases presented above we have empirical evidence in support of the claim that traces are deleted.

5.2 X⁰ (Head) Movement

There are several sources of evidence which suggest that X^0-chains are intact in agrammatics in comprehension (other results suggest intactness in production as well).

5.2.1. Linebarger et al. (1983) present a relevant experimental condition (their condition 3, "Subject-Aux inversion"), in which they found that all their four agrammatics were sensitive to violations of the following types, performing at near-normal levels:

(8) a. *Is the old boy is having a good time?
    b. Is the old boy having a good time?

(9) a. *Did the old man enjoying the view?
    b. Did the old man enjoy the view?

5.2.2. Lonzi and Luzzatti (1993) have presented an experiment that demonstrates the same phenomenon through an investigation of agrammatics' ability to place adverbs properly in Italian. In Italian verbs move around adverbial expressions, depending on their finiteness properties. Agrammatics were shown to be able to place adverbs correctly around the verb, an ability that indicates the availability of verb movement for them.

If this is the case, and verb movement is intact, then there are two logical possibilities: First, it could be that verbs move in agrammatism and their traces are deleted but, given that these traces have no consequences to Θ-role assignment, the deficit caused by trace deletion is simply undetected. Were this to be the case, we would not have had data such as these just reviewed, for these data come from judgment, not interpretation, and the presence of traces in both Linebarger et al.'s and Lonzi and Luzzatti's data is crucial for correct performance. We are thus led in another direction, which is that the TDH does not cover verb movement, and that, contrary to the TDH, traces of such movement are not deleted.

Before continuing, it is worthwhile to observe an immediate, important corollary that this conclusion has:

(10) Wh-elements are fully intact in agrammatic comprehension.

Such a corollary is important to our understanding of the nature of the agrammatic deficit in Wh-movement, so here is how it is derived. Rizzi (1991) argues for the Wh-criterion, which requires, roughly, that each

Wh-expression be in Spec-head relation with a head of the right kind and vice versa. It is this principle that accounts for, among other things, subject/object asymmetries in the English rule of Do-support (an instantiation of SAI), as in (11):

(11) a. What did John buy?
     b. *What John bought?
     c. Who bought junk?
     d. *Who did buy junk?

According to Rizzi, Do-support is applied only to achieve the required congruence between the Wh-expression in Spec and a lexical head. Auxiliaries thus head-move to be in a position that they can agree with a Wh-element in Spec of CP. This explains, according to Rizzi, the presence of Do-support in object questions and its absence in subject questions, because in the latter the verb is already in the appropriate head position relative to the Wh-element in Spec position, whereas in the former it must move in order to be close enough to the Wh-expression.

Consider agrammatic comprehension now. If head movement in all its variants is intact, as the evidence suggests, and if it is triggered in general solely to satisfy the Wh-criterion, then the patients are capable of applying this criterion. But in order to do so they must be aware of the existence of a Wh-expression in Spec of CP, so that congruence between it and a lexical head would force the auxiliary to move (or Do to be inserted). Hence, they must be aware of the properties of Wh-expression, and, in particular, of Wh-words like "what" and "who." This means that in Wh-constructions on which agrammatic comprehension is deficient, the reason for the deficiency cannot be lexical, namely an inability to detect the Wh-antecedent. Rather, any deficit that will be postulated for these constructions must implicate either the link between the Wh-word and the trace or the trace itself. Following, we will see the significance of this corollary. At this stage, it is appropriate to reexamine the TDH in light of these conclusions and try to make it more precise and general.

6. A RESTRICTIVE MOVE—A NEW GENERALIZATION

The TDH must be reformulated in a restrictive way to account for the new facts from head movement. Structures containing traces which tail A-chains and A'-chains yield erroneous performance, whereas traces of head movement (X^0-chains) do not. It thus follows that this statement is descriptively correct:

(12) *Restrictive TDH (rough version I):*
     Traces of XP movement are deleted.

Namely deleted are traces of movement of whole phrases (as opposed to traces of heads that are retained). But this is not the only imaginable descriptive statement which may cover our data. Moreover, it is most likely that, for this description to be explained, it must be cast in other terms. For instance, if the deficit is to some processing mechanism, it will have to be stated in terms other than those in (12). Such terms are readily available. Traces of NP- and Wh-movement in the data are also in argument position, in Θ-position, and have some other, less central, properties, which distinguish them from traces of head movement. Thus, there are several ways to restrict the TDH so that it account for the data, of which we focus on two:

(13) *Restrictive TDH (variants):*
   a. Traces in Θ-positions are deleted.
   b. Traces in A-positions are deleted.

Note that the fact that an account can be cast in more than one way points to a gap in our understanding. If we seek a causal explanation to the generalization, it is advisable to distinguish these accounts, whether empirically or conceptually. These proposals are not easily distinguishable, but we can get some initial clues as to which one may be correct. We thus turn to the issue of whether the deleted traces are those in Θ-positions or A-positions. To distinguish these empirically we have to test agrammatic comprehension on structures containing traces in A-positions which are not Θ-positions. There are several such structures, those containing pleonastic elements (existential sentences and sentences containing weather verbs) and structures with quasiarguments (e.g., idiom chunks or measure phrases; cf. Rizzi, 1990). None of these have been tested in agrammatism, to the best of my knowledge. Empirical data bearing on this question may be hard to come by, but there are good conceptual reasons to believe that only one of these is the generalization of choice. They have to do with the following question: Are traces truly deleted from agrammatic representation? Once raised, this question opens the way to conceptual considerations that point to the Θ-based account as the correct one.

Recall that the available data come almost exclusively from interpretive tasks, which require Θ-role assignment. Does the pattern of impairment and sparing force a claim as strong as the TDH or is it, rather, consistent with weaker claims? The latter possibility appears more plausible. The involvement of traces in the agrammatic deficit (as far as is known) is with respect only to Θ-role assignment. This opens the way to another possible view of the status of traces in agrammatism, somewhat reminiscent of the Visibility Hypothesis of Chomsky (1981). In this view, traces are intact, but are invisible to Θ-role assignment. This view would mean that every aspect of the construct trace is intact, except its involvement in Θ-role assignment. To distinguish between complete deletion and invisibility, other experimental tasks are necessary, for instance, an examination of agrammatic sensitivity to violations of grammaticality that crucially rely on traces (e.g., ECP violations). There are no available data that bear on this issue at this point, but experiments are currently underway. In the new account, then, one would like to leave room for nondeleted, yet thematically invisible, traces. Crucially, these considerations are unstatable if an account based on A-positions is chosen, which leads us to exclude (13b) and stay with a restrictive Trace-Based Account as follows:

(14) *Trace-Based Account (TBA)*
Traces in Θ-positions are deleted from agrammatic representation (or are invisible to Θ-role assignment).

7. ASYMMETRIES IN QUESTIONS AND QUANTIFIERS AND A REFORMULATED STRATEGY

7.1. Questions

Hickok and Avrutin (1994) have recently tested agrammatic comprehension on four types of questions, along two dimensions: questions pertaining to subject (15b,d) vs. object (15a,c) position, and those expressed by *who* (15a,b) vs. *which* (15c,d):

(15) a. Who did the girl push *t*?
 b. Who pushed the girl?
 c. Which boy did the girl push *t*?
 d. Which boy pushed the girl?[5]

They obtained a surprising finding. The two patients they tested were above-chance on subject questions (15a,d), and at chance on the object question beginning with *Which* (15c) as consistent with the TBA, as well as with previous data on subject–object asymmetries (cf. Ansell & Flowers, 1982, Caplan & Futter, 1986 for cleft sentences, and Grodzinsky, 1989 for relative clauses). Yet on (15b), namely on the *who* object question, the patients were, unexpectedly, above-chance, in apparent violation of the TBA.

Hickok and Avrutin observe that there is a linguistic difference between *which* phrases and *who* phrases. *Which* phrases are "Discourse-linked," requiring reference to previous discourse (cf. Pesetsky, 1987).

---

[5] Traces in subject position were not annotated here, because their presence or absence from the representation has no empirical consequences in the present cases (cf. Grodzinsky, 1990, p. 170).

The question in (15c), for instance, presupposes the existence of a set of boys, already mentioned in the discourse, from which one boy will be picked. It is pragmatically odd (although syntactically well-formed) to ask questions (15c,d) if there are no boys around. Thus, the interpretation of *which* questions requires both syntactic and contextual information. By contrast, no such requirements exist for *who* questions. Questions (15a,b) can be asked without presupposition, and the answer does not pick an element from a previously established set. Their interpretation is based only on intrasentential (syntactic and lexical) information. This difference, noted by Pesetsky, had led Cinque (1990) to propose a refinement to Rizzi's RM and argue in favor of the existence of two types of chains: Government (covering (15a,b) in the present context) and binding (15c,d) chains, in which only the latter are D-linked. This distinction helps Hickok and Avrutin to claim that in agrammatism only the latter type is disrupted, which presumably explains the asymmetry in the data.

Yet theirs is far from being an adequate explanation. Suppose, first and foremost, that only binding chains are disrupted. Does that account for the data from agrammatism? According to this claim, government chains are intact, which is why (15a,b) yield above-chance performance. If one makes the (rather dubious) assumption that there is no movement from subject position (i.e., no vacuous movement), then the near-normal performance on (15d) follows as well. But what about (15c)? This, indeed, is the critical case for Hickok and Avrutin. It is a case of a disrupted binding chain. Given that Θ-roles are transmitted through the chain, and given the disruption, it follows that no Θ-role is assigned in the wh-phrase (i.e., to *the boy*). However, the subject (i.e., *the girl*) does receive an Agent Θ-role. Given that the patient knows the thematic structure of the verb, what then would stop him from inferring the missing role? It is precisely for this reason that the default strategy was initially assumed. Hickok and Avrutin's proposal thus does not predict their data correctly.

Second, the distinction between Government and Binding chains does not cover all the available data on agrammatism. For example, one of the most basic findings on agrammatic comprehension, namely the chance performance on passive, is not predicted. For it to be accounted for, the A-chain in passive needs to be (exclusively) a binding chain, yet as Cinque (1990, pp. 17–18) acknowledges, it is not at all clear whether his analysis assumes that. Similarly, the status of adjectival passives vis-à-vis this analysis is not clear.

It is thus advisable to seek an alternative explanation for the interesting puzzle Hickok and Avrutin have documented. It is also appropriate to ask whether the new TBA can account for this new set of data. A restrictive strategy to account for these data, as well as data on agrammatic comprehension of structures containing quantified NPs, is proposed below.

7.2. A Solution through the TBA

7.2.1. The empirical problem. At issue are asymmetries concerning agrammatic comprehension of questions, as evident from the data in (15). There are several ways to look at this data set, yet from the perspective of the TBA (and the (unmodified) Default strategy), the subject–object asymmetry (between (15c) and (15d)) is expected. What is not expected is the difference between the two types of questions, or, more accurately, unexplained is why the patients perform above-chance on (15a). As is, the TBA's prediction is incorrect for this data point: The trace is in a Θ-position; hence, it is invisible. As a consequence, the NP *who* lacks a Θ-role, and the strategy assigns it with Agent. Yet there is already another Agent in the representation (the subject *the girl*); hence, chance performance is predicted. How, then, can the TBA be reconciled with this result?

7.2.2. Agrammatic knowledge of the referential properties of Wh-phrases. Recall, first of all, the corollary derived above from Rizzi's Wh-criterion and its interaction with the results from agrammatism concerning Do-support: Given that this criterion requires a lexical head for a Wh-element in Spec of CP, Do-support in object questions, but not subject questions, was forced. In agrammatism, sensitivity to violations of Do-support has been demonstrated; hence, it follows that this group of patients is sensitive to the Wh-criterion. However, in order to be sensitive to it, one must have the Wh-element represented. It thus follows that patients are aware of the lexical properties of Wh-words, as stated in (10):

(10) Wh-elements are fully intact in agrammatic comprehension.

Now, this conclusion entails knowledge of the referential properties of Wh-elements by the patients. But what are these properties? As Pesetsky (1987) points out, there are important differences between *who* and *which* questions, in terms of the necessity to connect to previous discourse. *Who* questions do not presuppose a set in discourse; hence, they are not D(iscourse)-linked. *Which* questions are D-linked. Moreover, other syntactic differences (with respect to Superiority) lead to the following conclusions:

(16) a. Non-D-linked phrases are quantifiers and adjoin to S' (Pesetsky's (33))
     b. D-linked wh-phrases are not quantifiers (Pesetsky's (34))

This conclusion means that non-D-linked phrases (*who*) are not referential (since quantifiers never are), whereas D-linked phrases (*which*-NP) are referential and we have seen that this is a distinction agrammatics are aware of, since they must be aware of the Wh-criterion.

7.3. A Reformulated Strategy

Consider, now, the Default strategy. As is, it assigns a Θ-role to a thematically lacking NP according to linear considerations. It does so indiscriminately, namely, regardless of whatever properties these NPs have. But why should that be? Consider the nature of cognitive strategies. They are, as is commonly held, results of inductive inferences over experience. As such, they fit words denoting entities with some semantic attribute, and critically, they do so in the absence of linguistic knowledge (since by hypothesis, when such knowledge is present, strategies are not operative). In this view, one would not expect cognitive strategies to apply to nonreferential elements.[6] Thus, a strategy effectively matches semantic roles to referential expressions on the basis of nonlinguistic knowledge. This is the most natural view of cognitive strategies that apply in the language domain. The strategy can thus be reformulated as follows:

(17) *R(eferential)-Strategy*
Assign a referential NP a role by its linear position iff it has no Θ-role.

Nonreferential NPs are exempt from the strategy. In particular, quantifier-like, nonreferential Wh-expressions are outside its scope. Consider, now, the findings by Hickok and Avrutin, repeated below once again:

(15) a. Who did the girl push *t*? (above chance)
    b. Who pushed the girl? (above chance)
    c. Which boy did the girl push *t*? (chance)
    d. Which boy pushed the girl? (above chance)

The interaction between the TBA and the R-strategy gives precisely the desired results. (15c–d) are accounted for as before. In (15c) the strategy-assigned role on the NP [which boy] conflicts with that assigned to the subject NP [the girl], yielding chance performance. (15d) is a subject question; thus, if there is movement, it is correctly compensated for by the R-strategy. But consider (15a–b) now. Since *Who* is a nonreferential expression, it is exempt from the R-strategy. Thus in both cases, no role is assigned strategically to the wh-word. As a result, only one role is assigned (to the subject in (15a) and to the object in (15b)), and, given the intactness of lexical knowledge in agrammatism, the correct semantic

---

[6] Referentiality is used here in the manner common in linguistics, namely, in a sense that does not require reference in the world, but rather, in the universe of discourse. An element is thus used referentially when it refers to a member of a set that has been preestablished in discourse (cf. Chomsky, 1981; Pesetsky, 1987; Rizzi, 1990; Cinque, 1990).

role of the thematically dangling NP can be easily inferred.[7] Hence above-chance performance is predicted, fitting the data—old and new— precisely.

7.4. Passives with Quantified Antecedents

What are the empirical consequences of the TBA? There are many, but a notable result is this: in movement-derived structures, with agentive predicates, one would expect chance performance if the moved constituent is extracted from object position and is referential. However, a change in one of these properties changes the prediction, along the following lines: (a) when agentive verbs are replaced by psych-predicates, performance goes down to below chance (as confirmed experimentally in Grodzinsky, 1995a); (b) when the trace is in subject position, performance goes up to normal (confirmed by many studies, e.g., Hickok & Avrutin, 1994; Grodzinsky, 1989); and (c) when the antecedent of the trace is nonreferential, performance should go up to normal levels, even though it contains an agentive predicate and a trace in object position, as we saw in (15a).

This last prediction is rather counterintuitive, yet surprisingly, there is an additional recent finding from an independent domain, precisely to that effect. This is a study by Saddy (this issue), conducted independent of the TBA, in which he shows that while Broca's patients perform at chance on passives, their performance level goes up to virtually normal if the subject of the passive is a quantified expression, even though the latter is ostensibly more "complex."[8]

(18) a. The man is pushed by the boy (chance)
b. Every man is pushed by a boy (above chance)[9]

---

[7] As Na'ama Friedmann correctly points out, an additional assumption is necessary here: that the language processing device be capable of carrying out this inference in a way that has access to all the data structures that are required, namely the syntax as well as the argument structure. This is a nontrivial, yet a rather plausible, assumption.

[8] The result discussed here is one of several experimental results Saddy reports, mostly concerning the phenomenon of "quantifier spreading" in agrammatic comprehension, similar to children. These other effects, while interesting in their own right, are irrelevant in the present context.

[9] In such a sentence, when given to the patients in a sentence-to-picture matching task, as Saddy did, there can be several imaginable foils. Saddy reports having used the correct ones, namely, those involving reversal of Θ-role. Thus, the patient had to choose between a picture in which every man pushed a woman and one in which a woman was pushing every man.

This contrast is predicted by the TBA precisely: in (18a) chance performance is predicted, as we have seen above; in (18b), however, the subject *every man* is not referential and is thus exempt from the strategy. The agent role is assigned normally and transmitted to the oblique object (perhaps through clitic doubling),[10] yet unlike (18a), the R-strategy is blocked, and no Θ-role is assigned to the quantified subject. As a result, its role can be easily inferred from the (available) knowledge of the lexical entry of the verb, and normal performance follows. The new restrictive account thus generalizes over the asymmetries in agrammatic performance in both questions and quantifiers.

8. A SHORT SUMMARY AND A FEW CONSEQUENCES

Let me summarize the claims made in this paper very briefly, before some general conclusions are drawn. The TDH has been modified, to account for the new data and to accommodate theoretical innovations in linguistics. The restrictive theory of agrammatic comprehension is this:

(19) a. TBA: Traces in Θ-positions are deleted from agrammatic representation (or are invisible to Θ-assignment).
   b. R-strategy: Assign a referential NP a role by its linear position iff it has no Θ-role.

8.1. The TBA and the Standard View of Agrammatism

Reflect for a moment on this account. It contradicts most traditional beliefs about agrammatic aphasia: The impairment is restricted to Θ-positions, and the strategy applies to referential expressions only, whereas functional categories are preserved. This is almost exactly the reverse of the common belief that the comprehension impairment in this syndrome involves the minor categories, and not the major ones; that the "closed class" is disrupted, whereas "open class" is intact (Bradley et al., 1980); that Θ-assigners and assignees are intact, whereas the rest are impaired (Rizzi, 1985); and that lexical categories are preserved (Caplan, 1985). The standard conception of agrammatism has not made the necessary distinction between phrasal projections and heads in this syndrome, and it is perhaps for this reason that the accounts proposed to the deficit were incorrect. I hope to have convinced the reader of the necessity of a conceptual shift and that the data from comprehension require a

---

[10] In this respect, agrammatic comprehension is contrasted to children's abilities; as in the latter case, clitic doubling seems to be the problem (cf. Fox, 1993; Fox, Grodzinsky, & Crain, 1995).

characterization that restricts the deficit to Θ-positions, even though this claim goes against a long tradition that should now be abandoned.

8.2. Agrammatic Comprehension, Referentiality, and Long Wh-Movement

Consider the R-strategy now. If it is restricted to referential expressions (referentiality being defined relative to a discourse), then it provides us with a powerful test for the referentiality of antecedents and of linguistic accounts that make use of this concept. Specifically, the distinction between long and successive cyclic wh-movement has been linked to referentiality (Rizzi, 1990, with further refinements in Cinque, 1990). The validity of such a claim can thus be readily tested in agrammatic aphasia: Just as we saw a distinction in the agrammatic comprehension system between *Which* and *Who* questions, we expect each case involving long wh-movement to result in impaired performance (to the extent that the strategy would compensate incorrectly for the loss of one Θ-role). We also expect every case of cyclic movement to remain intact in agrammatism. We thus provide another instance in which evidence from aphasia can be used for a direct evaluation of the biological feasibility of grammatical theory.

8.3. Agrammatic Comprehension and the Syntactic Analysis of Passive

The proper analysis of the passive construction has long been a subject of an unresolved debate. In previous work (Grodzinsky et al., 1991), arguments were given for a movement-based analysis, in that a distinction between the patients' performance on adjectival vs. verbal passive was observed, in which the latter patterned with Wh-movement cases, generating erroneous performance, and adjectival passive yielded normal performance. We now observe another piece of data that leads to a similar conclusion: the contrast between passives with and without quantified subjects cannot be explained unless one assumed that the subject binds a trace (and that the R-strategy operates the way it does). We thus find ourselves in the interesting situation in which different types of passive generate virtually every possible performance type in agrammatism, as can be observed in (20):

(20) a. verbal passive: The man is pushed by the woman   (chance)
     b. adjectival passive: The man is interested in the woman   (above chance)
     c. psych passive: The man is loved by the woman   (below chance)
     d. quantified passive: Every man is pushed by a woman   (above chance)

This rich pattern and the theory that accounts for it argue quite strongly for traces in the post-participial position in passive.

8.4. Simplicity, Canonicity, and the Neural Representation of Grammatical Processes

For several years there has been an intuitive suggestion floating around, according to which any deviation from canonical ordering of constituents is bound to cause comprehension problems to agrammatic patients. The notion underlying this idea is that brain damage results in a difficulty to analyze complex constructions, and given that canonically ordered sentences are simple and hence the easiest, we would expect our patients to succeed there and fail elsewhere. The current status of the data shows rather decisively that this view is incorrect: First, there are noncanonical arrangements that yield normal performance—*who* questions in which extraction is from object position and passives with quantified antecedents (which seem, in fact, to be more complex than regular passives which yield chance performance). Second, head movement, which sometimes results in surface noncanonical ordering, is intact. We can thus reject this type of account and direct our attention to another, according to which the problem in agrammatism is one of indirect projection of thematic structure. In this view (first proposed in Grodzinsky, 1984b, and now refined and substantiated), Broca's area and its vicinity are the loci of processes responsible for projecting lexical material onto sentence structure and linking Θ-roles to NPs. It is this type of process, and nothing else, that is disrupted in agrammatic comprehension. Given the rich database that is currently available (for instance, the intactness of binding relations, of head movement, etc.) such a localizing statement can be confidently made.[11]

8.5. Cognitive Strategies

Nongrammatical guidelines for analysis of input strings have occupied psycholinguists for a long time. Bever's (1970) well-known proposals generated a huge literature on strategies for linguistic analysis. These strategies, as is well-recognized by now, divide into those which help the parser to choose among grammatical representations (such as right association, for instance) and those which presumably compete with the parser (such as first NP = agent, etc.). With the former type linguists have no quarrel, for it is clear that in states of uncertainty (whether temporary or not) there must be some principles that direct the parser in its action. Yet the latter case, namely, when strategies come to direct conflict with the pars-

---

[11] This statement opens the way to a whole host of new questions: What is the nature of this grammatical process? How is its disruption related to other language-deficient populations, like children (normal and dysphasic)? What is the relation between this evidence and evidence from other measures of cerebral activity in language comprehension (e.g., ERP and PET)? Obviously, none of these questions can be handled in one pass.

ing device, is problematic, for it casts doubts on the necessity of such strategies, as well as their mode of operation.

In the present case, however, the proposal is much more restricted: A nonlinguistic, cognitive strategy operates just in case the parsing mechanism is under duress. This, in fact, is a rather natural assumption: that the deficient language faculty, for want of more information, would do anything it can to get at the analysis of the input string and that it would do so systematically. In particular, it is bound to use whatever information is available to it that is related to its past experiences, for instance, that words appearing sentence-initially are usually agents. It is also quite plausible that since the strategy is not linguistically motivated and operates over content, it would be restricted to elements that are referential.

8.6. A Final Word

The linguistic investigation of aphasia is maturing rapidly. One can only hope that this development will bring with it harder problems, and lots of intellectual challenges that will attract young, adventurous investigators to come and study the neural representation of grammar.

REFERENCES

Ansell, B., & Flowers, C. 1982. Aphasic adults' use of heuristic and structural linguistic cues for analysis. *Brain and Language,* **16,** 61–72.

Avrutin, S. 1994. *Psycholinguistic aspects of establishing reference.* Ph.D. thesis, Department of Brain and Cognitive Sciences, MIT.

Belletti, A., & Rizzi, L. 1988. Psych-verbs and th-theory. *Natural Language and Linguistic Theory,* **6,** 291–352.

Beretta, A., Harford, C., Patterson, J., & Pinango, M. 1994. *The proper description of comprehension deficits in agrammatic aphasia.* Paper presented at TENNET V, Montreal.

Berndt, R. S., & Caramazza, A. 1980. A redefinition of the syndrome of Broca's aphasia: Implications for a neuropsychological model of language. *Applied Psycholinguistics,* **1,** 225–278.

Bever, T. G. 1970. The cognitive basis of linguistic structures. In J. R. Hayes (Ed.), *Cognition and the development of language.* New York: Wiley.

Bradley, D. C., Garrett, M. F., & Zurif, E. B. 1980. Syntactic deficits in Broca's aphasia. In D. Caplan (Ed.), *Biological studies of mental processes.* Cambridge, MA: MIT Press.

Burton, S., & Grimshaw, J. 1992. Coordination and VP-internal subjects. *Linguistic Inquiry,* **23,** 305–313.

Caplan, D. 1985. Syntactic and semantic structures in agrammatism. In M.-L. Kean (Ed.), *Agrammatism.* New York: Academic Press.

Caplan, D., & Futter, C. 1986. Assignment of thematic roles by an agrammatic aphasic patient. *Brain and Language,* **27,** 117–135.

Caramazza, A., & Zurif, E. B. 1976. Dissociation of algorithmic and heuristic processes in sentence comprehension: Evidence from aphasia. *Brain and Language,* **3,** 572–582.

Cinque, G. 1990. *Types of A'-dependencies.* Cambridge, MA: MIT Press.

Chomsky, N. 1981. *Lectures on government and binding.* Dordrecht: Foris Publications.

Chomsky, N. 1986. *Barriers*. Cambridge, MA: MIT Press.

Chomsky, N. 1991. Some notes on the economy of derivation and representation. In A. Kasher (Ed.), The Chomskyan turn. Cambridge, MA: Blackwell.

Chomsky, N. 1992. A minimalist program for linguistic theory. MITWPL 1.

Crain, S., & Shankweiler, D. 1985. *Comprehension of relative clauses and reflexive pronouns by agrammatic aphasics*. Paper presented at the Academy of Aphasia, Pittsburgh.

Crain, S., Shankweiler, D., Gorrell, P., & Tuller, B. 1989. Reception of language in Broca's asphasia. *Language and Cognitive Processes*, **4**, 1–33.

Fox, D. 1993. *The get-passive, implicit arguments and passive acquisition*. M.A. thesis, Tel Aviv University.

Fox, D., Grodzinsky, Y., & Crain, S. Forthcoming.

Friederici, A. 1982. Syntactic and semantic processes in aphasic deficits: The availability of prepositions. *Brain and Language*, **15**, 249–258.

Friederici, A. 1985. Levels of processing and vocabulary types: Evidence from on-line processing in normals and agrammatics. *Cognition*, **19**, 133–166.

Gardner, H., & Zurif, E. B. 1975. Critical reading at the sentence level in aphasia. *Cortex*, **11**, 60–72.

Goodenough, C., Zurif, E. B., & Weintraub, S. 1977. Aphasics' attention to grammatical morphemes. *Language and Speech*, **20**, 11–19.

Goodglass, H. 1968. Studies in the grammar of aphasics. In S. Rosenberg & J. Koplin, (Eds.), *Developments in applied psycholinguistics research*. New York: Macmillan.

Grodzinsky, Y. 1984a. The syntactic characterization of agrammatism. *Cognition*, **16**, 99–120.

Grodzinsky, Y. 1984b. *Language deficits and linguistic theory*. Doctoral dissertation, Brandeis University.

Grodzinsky, Y. 1986. Language deficits and the theory of syntax. *Brain and Language*, **27**, 135–159.

Grodzinsky, Y. 1990. *Theoretical perspectives on language deficits*. Cambridge, MA: MIT Press.

Grodzinsky, Y. 1995a. Trace-deletion, Θ-roles, and cognitive strategies. *Brain and Language*, in press.

Grodzinsky, Y. 1995b. Comparative aphasiology. Paper presented at RUG-SAN-VKL Conference on Aphasiology, Groningen.

Grodzinsky, Y., Pierce, A., & Marakovitz, S. 1991. Neuropsychological reasons for a transformational derivation of syntactic passive. *Natural Language & Linguistic Theory*, **9**, 431–453.

Grodzinsky, Y., & Reinhart, T. 1993. The innateness of binding and coreference. *Linguistic Inquiry*, **24**, 69–102.

Grodzinsky, Y., Wexler, K., Chien, Y. C., Marakovitz, S., & Solomon, J. 1993. The breakdown of binding relations. *Brain and Language*, **45**, 396–422.

Grossman, M., & Haberman, S. 1982. Aphasics' selective deficits in appreciating grammatical agreements. *Brain and Language*, **16**, 109–120.

Hagiwara, H. 1993. Nonagentive predicates and agrammatic comprehension. *Metropolitan Linguistics*, **13**, 127–142.

Hickok, G., Zurif, E. B., & Canseco-Gonzales, E. 1993. Structural description of agrammatic comprehension. *Brain and Language*, **45**, 371–395.

Kitagawa, Y. 1986. *Subjects in English and Japanese*. Doctoral dissertation, University of Massachusetts at Amherst.

Koopman, H., & Sportiche, D. 1988. *Subjects*. Unpublished manuscript, UCLA.

Kuroda, S.-Y. 1986. *Whether we agree or not*. Unpublished manuscript, UCSD.

Lapointe, S. G. 1985. A theory of verb form use in agrammatism. *Brain and Language*, **24**, 100–155.

Linebarger, M. C., Schwartz, M., & Saffran, E. 1983. Sensitivity to grammatical structure in so-called agrammatic aphasics. *Cognition,* **13,** 361–393.

Lonzi, L., & Luzzatti, C. 1993. Relevance of adverb distribution for the analysis of sentence representation in agrammatic patients. *Brain and Language,* **45,** 306–317.

Lukatela, K., Crain, S., & Shankweiler, D. 1988. Sensitivity to closed-class items in Serbo-Croat agrammatics. *Brain and Language,* **13,** 1–15.

Mauner, G., Fromkin, V., & Cornell, T. 1993. Comprehension and acceptability judgments in agrammatism: Disruption in the syntax of referential dependency. *Brain and Language,* **45,** 340–370.

Pesetsky, D. 1987. *Wh*-in situ: Movement and unselective binding. In E. Reuland & A. ter Meulen (Eds.), *The representation of (in)definiteness.* Cambridge, MA: MIT Press.

Pinker, S. 1984. *Language learnability and language development.* Cambridge, MA: Harvard University Press.

Pollock, J.-Y. 1989. Verb movement, universal grammar and the structure of IP. *Linguistic Inquiry,* **20,** 365–424.

Rizzi, L. 1985. Two notes on the linguistic interpretation of aphasia. In M.-L. Kean (Ed.), *Agrammatism.* New York: Academic Press.

Rizzi, L. 1990. *Relativized minimality.* Cambridge, MA: MIT Press.

Rizzi, L. 1991. Residual verb second and the Wh-criterion. Unpublished manuscript, University of Geneva.

Schwartz, M., Saffran, E., & Marin, O. 1980a. The word-order problem in agrammatism. I. Comprehension. *Brain and Language,* **10,** 249–262.

Schwartz, M., Saffran, E., & Marin, O. 1980b. The word-order problem in agrammatism. II. Comprehension. *Brain and Language,* **10,** 263–280.

Schwartz, M. F., Linebarger, M. C., Saffran, E. M., & Pate, D. C. 1987. Syntactic transparency and sentence interpretation in aphasia. *Language and Cognitive Processes,* **2,** 85–113.

Shapiro, L. P., & Levin, B. A. 1990. Verb processing during sentence comprehension in aphasia. *Brain and Language,* **38,** 21–47.

Shapiro, L. P., Gordon, B., Hack, N., & Killackey, J. 1993. Verb-argument structure processing in complex sentences in Broca's and Wernicke's aphasia. *Brain and Language,* **45,** 423–447.

Snyder, W. 1992. *Chain formation and crossover.* Unpublished manuscript, MIT.

Swinney, D., E. B. Zurif, & J. Nicol. 1989. The effects of focal brain damage on sentence processing. An examination of the neurological organization of a mental module. *Journal of Cognitive Neuroscience,* **1,** 25–37.

Travis, L. 1984. *Parameters and effects of word order variation.* Ph.D. dissertation, MIT.

Zurif, E. B., & Caramazza, A. 1976. Linguistic structures in aphasia: Studies in syntax and semantics. In H. Whitaker & H. H. Whitaker (Eds.), *Studies in neurolinguistics.* New York: Academic Press. Vol. 2.

Zurif, E. B., & Grodzinsky, Y. 1983. Sensitivity to grammatical structure in agrammatism: A reply to Linebarger *et al. Cognition,* **15,** 207–213.

Zurif, E. B., Swinney, D., Prather, P., Solomon, J., & Bushell, C. 1993. An on-line analysis of syntactic processing in Broca's and Wernicke's aphasia. *Brain and Language,* **45,** 448–464.

BRAIN AND LANGUAGE **50**, 52–91 (1993)

Agrammatism as Evidence about Grammar

Marcia C. Linebarger

Unisys Corporation

A variety of experimental paradigms has yielded surprisingly fine-grained evidence about the kinds of syntactic information to which agrammatic aphasics are sensitive. This paper contrasts three accounts of agrammatism which draw quite different conclusions about the implications of this disorder for normal function: the *chain-disruption, trade-off,* and *mapping* hypotheses. Counterarguments to the chain disruption and trade-off hypotheses are presented, and it is argued that agrammatism provides considerable support for the modularity of syntax but provides no evidence more specific than that regarding the psychological reality of government binding theory vis-à-vis other current theories of grammar. © 1995 Academic Press, Inc.

1. INTRODUCTION

Since the late 1970s, research on agrammatism has been driven by a series of strong, testable, and theoretically focused claims put forth by linguistically sophisticated researchers. The work of Kean (e.g., 1977, 1981) illuminated the important if still-mysterious role of closed class elements in sentence processing and educated both linguists and neuropsychologists about the power of linguistic theory to project hypothesized deficits onto testable nonobvious predictions. The very questions that researchers ask about agrammatism have come into sharper linguistic focus as a result of the claim of Grodzinsky (e.g., 1986, 1990) that the agrammatic data provide evidence in support of one particular theory of grammar, government binding theory (Chomsky, 1981).

My purpose here is to examine this interesting claim and a larger claim which it presupposes: that agrammatic comprehension is, at base, a syn-

I acknowledge with gratitude useful discussions with David Caplan, Greg Hickok, Judy Kegl, Herman Kolk, Gail Mauner, Myrna Schwartz, Eleanor Saffran, Lew Shapiro, and the members of the Spring 1993 aphasia seminar at the University of Delaware. Address correspondence and reprint requests to the author at R&D, Valley Forge Engineering Center, Unisys Corporation, P.O. Box 517, Paoli, PA 19301. Internet: marcia@VFL.paramax.com.

tactic deficit. I will contrast three accounts of aggramatism which differ in the extent to which they invoke representational failure as the source of the comprehension difficulties in these patients.

The *chain-disruption hypotheses* (Grodzinsky, 1986, 1990; Hickok, 1992; Hickok, Zurif, & Canseco-Gonzales, 1993; Mauner, Fromkin, & Cornell, 1993) claim that agrammatic comprehension is caused by the underrepresentation of traces (and, in Mauner et al.'s proposal, other referentially dependent elements) in the syntactic representations constructed by these subjects.

The *trade-off hypothesis*, which has recently received a careful articulation in Frazier and Friederici (1991), also attributes agrammatic comprehension failures to impaired parsing. In this account, resource competition between parsing and semantic interpretation underlies agrammatic comprehension failures by degrading syntactic analysis in all but the least demanding tasks.

The *mapping hypothesis* (Linebarger, Schwartz, & Saffran, 1983a; Saffran, Schwartz, & Marin, 1980) claims that agrammatics perform a normal "first-pass parse" but fail to exploit it for further interpretive processes. The mapping hypothesis and the chain-disruption accounts attribute similar (and in some variants identical) syntactic capabilities to agrammatics, but differ in their views about whether inadequacies in the structural representations computed by agrammatics are the cause of agrammatic comprehension.

Despite their differences, these three accounts share the assumption that agrammatism does not represent a complete loss of all syntactic ability under all circumstances. Since agrammatic sentence interpretation is unquestionably "asyntactic" in certain respects, they share the expectation that agrammatism can provide evidence about the interface between syntactic and semantic processing unavailable from normal speakers in whom parsing and interpretation are seamlessly integrated. They differ, however, in their claims about the nature of this evidence. The chain-disruption accounts pinpoint an impairment underlying agrammatic comprehension which can be described most parsimoniously in the vocabulary of government binding theory, thereby providing evidence for the psychological reality of this theory. The mapping hypothesis takes the agrammatic data as evidence for the modularity of syntactic processing, because of the disparity between subjects' ability to parse certain structures and their impaired interpretation of these same structures. The trade-off hypothesis is the most conservative of the three hypotheses with regard to this question because it argues that agrammatic parsing varies quite significantly across different tasks.

These differences may be expressed in terms of a distinction between two types of arguments from neuropsychological data (Marin, Saffran, & Schwartz, 1976). The argument from *selective loss* points to a set of impaired structures which can be demarcated only, or most parsimoni-ously, in terms of a particular theory, thereby providing evidence for the psychological reality of that theory. The chain-disruption accounts may be seen as a selective loss argument, although they carefully eschew heavy-handed appeals to a "trace box." The argument from *exposed encoding* arises when an impairment to process X reveals intermediate representations which are normally "overwritten" by a later process Y. The mapping hypothesis—for which I will argue below—looks to the preserved syntactic functionality exposed by the failure of semantic inter-pretative processes as evidence for syntactic modularity. I argue below that agrammatism has not yet provided a convincing selective loss argu-ment in support of any specific theory of grammar, but that it provides surprisingly fine-grained exposed encoding evidence about the implemen-tation of grammar in sentence processing.

The purest selective loss argument from agrammatism is proposed in Caramazza & Zurif (1976): agrammatism represents a catastrophic "syn-tactectomy" and hence provides compelling evidence for syntax as a psychologically distinct information type. This proposal was based upon the finding (cf. also Heilman & Scholes, 1976; Schwartz, Saffran, & Marin, 1980) that an agrammatic comprehension impairment (henceforth, "asyntactic comprehension") frequently co-occurs with agrammatic pro-duction. Asyntactic comprehenders experience difficulty with reversible sentences, especially when they are syntactically complex, with pre-served comprehension of nonreversible sentences attributed to the use of heuristics based upon lexical content rather than grammatical structure. I argue below for the correctness of two of the claims made in Caramazza & Zurif (1976); that agrammatism reveals syntactic modularity and that sentence interpretation in agrammatic patients crucially involves not only algorithmic, grammar-driven processes but also extragrammatical heuris-tics of one sort or another. What I will argue against is the claim that agrammatic comprehension derives primarily from inadequate represen-tations of syntactic structure.

Given the reported dissociations between agrammatic comprehension and production (Goodglass & Menn, 1985; Marin, Wetzel, Blossom-Stach, & Leher, 1989; Miceli, Mazzuchi, Menn & Goodglass, 1983), the discussion here will be restricted to receptive language processing. Fur-thermore, I will focus almost exclusively upon the classic pattern of asyn-tactic comprehension which has served as the basis for all three accounts of agrammatism to be discussed below. The core data of this pattern include good performance on comprehension tasks involving simple ac-tives and subject gaps and poor performance on comprehension tasks involving passives and object gaps. Although agrammatic performance reveals far more individual variation than this oversimplified formula sug-gest, the question to be raised. here is: can these theories adequately explain even the core data over which they have been developed and articulated?

2. THE PARADOX OF PRESERVED GRAMMATICAL SENSITIVITY

2.1 Evidence for Preserved Parsing Ability

One major counterexample to the "selected loss of syntax" account is the evidence that some agrammatic patients with severe asyntactic comprehension and production are nevertheless quite sensitive to grammatical structure. Such evidence has come from the grammaticality judgment paradigm (Linebarger et al., 1983a; Berndt, Salasoo, Mitchum, & Blumstein, 1988; Lukatela, Crain, & Shankweiler, 1988; replicated on-line in Shankweiler, Crain, Gorrell, & Tuller, 1989) and from a variety of on-line paradigms (e.g., Friederici & Kilborn, 1989). Below I summarize those constructions upon which subjects performed well in grammaticality judgment tasks [with average raw scores of 85% or higher unless otherwise indicated; see Linebarger et al. (1983a,b) and Linebarger (1989, 1990) for more detailed discussion].

(1) *Subject-aux Inversion*
    (a) Was the girl enjoying the show?
    (b) *Was the girl enjoy the show?
(2) *Passive*
    (a) John has finally kissed Louise.
    (b) *John was finally kissed Louise.
(3) *Incomplete extraction*
    (a) How many birds did you see_in the park?
    (b) *How many did you see_birds in the park?
(4) *Empty elements* (83.7%)
    (a) Frank thought he was going to get the job.
    (b) *Frank thought_was going to get the job.
    (c) Who_thought he was going to get the job?
    (d) *Who_thought_was going to get the job?
(5) *Gapless relatives* (84.2%)
    (a) Bill dropped a plate that_was too hot.
    (b) *Bill dropped a plate that the stove was too hot.
(6) *Wh-moved subcategorization* (83.1%)
    (a) Why did the principal frown_?
    (b) *Who did the principal frown_?
    (c) What did the furniture company send_?
    (d) *Why did the furniture company send_?
(7) *Particle movement*
    (a) They stood in the line very patiently
    (b) *They stood the line in very patiently
    (c) We broke in the engine very patiently
    (d) We broke the engine in very patiently
(8) *Phrase structure* (mostly case violations)
    (a) The photograph of my mother was very nice.
    (b) *The photograph my mother was very nice.

(9) *Subcategorization*
    (a) The man sat on the new sofa.
    (b) *The man sat the new sofa.
(10) *Pronoun case* (see also Grossman & Harberman, 1982)
    (a) John gave her a new dress.
    (b) *John gave she a new dress.
(11) *Pronoun case, SAI*
    (a) Can they speak German very well?
    (b) *Can them speak German very well?

The contrast between this good performance and the same subjects' agrammatic comprehension is quite striking; the six subjects who performed with 85–100% accuracy on passive sentences such as those in (2) performed at-chance in comprehension tasks involving passive sentences. Similarly, agrammatic comprehension difficulties with *wh*-moved object gap sentences are widely reported (Caramazza & Zurif, 1976; Caplan & Futter, 1986; Grodzinsky, 1989; Sherman & Schweickert, 1989; but see Hickok & Avrutin, this issue) and yet subjects' performance on the *wh*-moved subcategorization,[1] gapless relative, empty elements, and incomplete extraction conditions was far above-chance. The arguments that extragrammatical strategies would not have sufficed to perform this task are detailed in Linebarger et al. (1983b) and Linebarger (1990); I take note here of a subsequent proposal regarding such a strategy. Caplan and Hildebrandt (1988) and Caplan (1995) have argued that the grammaticality judgment task could be performed without parsing in some cases, by means of a strategy based upon preserved appreciation of the thematic requirements of the verb or other predicate. Their examples focus upon *wh*-constructions. In their account, subjects could reject a gapless relative such as (5b) without parsing this structure on the basis of knowledge that the predicate *hot* takes only a single argument, and hence that *plate* is an extra argument; the *wh*-moved subcategorization violation (6d) could be rejected on the basis of the missing obligatory NP argument; and (6b) could be rejected on the basis of the unincorporatable NP argument; and so forth.

It is certainly true that the sentences in (3)–(6) all result in structures which do not satisfy the verb's thematic requirements. However, *the inventory of argument NPs upon which the hypothesized strategy relies cannot be performed without the very sorts of parsing operations that this strategy is supposed to circumvent.* For example, the fact that subjects accepted sentences like (5a) and (6c), in which an obligatory subject or

---

[1] The mean level of performance on the *wh*-subcategorization condition was lowered here by one subject (FM) who, importantly, performed exactly as poorly on a baseline subcategorization condition involving violations such as *The teacher smiled the boy.* Thus we cannot attribute FM's poor performance here to any impairment specific to the processing of *wh* gaps.

object is missing from its canonical position as a result of *wh*-movement, but rejected sentences like (4b), in which the same elements are missing in a structure without *wh*-movement, would seem to require that we grant them an appreciation that *wh*-structures license such gaps. Furthermore, the same subjects' ability to perform the judgments in (6) indicates that they recognize a fronted *wh*-word as syntactically linked to a postverbal gap, since they rejected sentences in which the syntactic category of the fronted *wh*-word conflicted with the verb's subcategorization requirements. Finally, consider the incomplete extraction condition. Sentences such as (3b) were presented in order to provide a somewhat trickier case of gapless relatives, because a subject insensitive to the constraints on extraction might accept (3b) by construing *how many . . . birds* as a single NP. Now of course we have no way of determining which analyses these patients consider and reject, and it is quite likely that such an illegal reconstitution of the NP is not entertained at any point in the attempt to parse this sentence, in which case (3b) represents another case of gapless relatives like (5b). But even then the agrammatics' performance on this condition provides important additional support for the claim that the judgment task requires parsing. Why?—Because we know from their good performance on the sentences in (1) and (7) that they do make such links between nonadjacent sentence elements, and the fact that they did not similarly "reconstitute" the NP in (3b) demonstrates that they do not link nonadjacent sentence elements blindly. Thus their good performance on condition (3) provides additional support for the claim that their judgments in (1) and (7) are truly derived from parsing and that they do not approach sentences as unordered anagrams to be reconstructed without regard for linear order and the constraints on movement. Thus, *contra* Caplan and Hildebrandt (1988), I see no way to account for subjects' good performance on the *wh*-sentences *taken as a whole* without granting to them the ability to detect gaps in phrase structure, to recognize that these gaps are permitted only in *wh*-structures, and to recognize that the syntactic category of the fronted *wh*-word must correspond to the syntactic category of the gap: in sum, to parse.

If subjects are able to parse structures such as *wh*-gaps and passives, why do they perform so poorly on comprehension tasks involving these structures? One clue about the source of this disparity comes from patterns of performance within the grammaticality judgment task itself.

2.2 Patterns of Performance within the Grammaticality Judgment Task

Linebarger et al. (1983a) and Linebarger (1989, 1990) report a number of constructions which the same agrammatic patients were not able to judge reliably. These "difficult" conditions are summarized in (12)–(18)

below; subjects performed with average raw scores of below 65% unless indicated otherwise.[2]

(12) *Reflexives*
    (a) The girl fixed herself a sandwich.
    (b) *The girl fixed himself a sandwich.
    (c) The old man himself will be at the ceremony.
    (d) *The old man itself will be at the ceremony.

(13) *Flagged reflexives*
    (a) Pouring himself coffee, the old man sat down.
    (b) *Pouring herself coffee, the old man sat down.

(14) *Tag questions: Pronouns*
    (a) The blonde woman laughed, didn't she?
    (b) *The blonde woman laughed, didn't it?

(15) *Wh-head agreement*
    (a) The pencil which you brought is nice.
    (b) *The pencil who you brought is nice.

(16) *VP ellipsis (69%)*
    (a) John is here, and so is Bill.
    (b) *John is here, and so does Bill.

(17) *Tag questions: Auxiliaries*
    (a) John is very tall, isn't he?
    (b) *John is very tall, doesn't he?

(18) Negative polarity, complex (Ladusaw, 1983; Linebarger, 1987, 1992)
    (a) No one who we met knew any French.
    (b) *The people who we met knew any French.
    (c) *The people who we didn't meet knew any French.
    (d) The people who we didn't meet knew French.

(19) *Quantifier float*
    (a) The boys will all be here.
    (b) *The boy will all be here.

One striking feature of this pattern is that, in many cases, the same lexical elements figure in both the easy and difficult conditions: *auxiliaries* are crucial to the easy conditions (1) and (2) and also to the difficult conditions (16) and (17); the easy conditions (3)–(6) and the difficult condition (15) all turn on *wh-words;* and *pronouns* occur in both the easy conditions (10) and (11) and the difficult conditions (12), (13), and (14). It is argued in Linebarger (1989, 1990) and also in Mauner et al. (1993) that this pattern of easy and difficult conditions reveals a preserved ability

---

[2] Two number agreement conditions elicited such a wide range of performance in these same patients that we leave them both unclassified. Four subjects (AT, FM, VS, LS) were tested on subject–verb agreement (e.g., *The child are laughing aloud*) and intra-NP number agreement (e.g., *This children can read almost anything*). Subjects' raw percentage scores on the former condition were 55, 80, 77.5, and 95, respectively; on the latter, they were 55, 70, 70, 97. LS's excellent performance on these conditions (95 and 97% correct) provides an interesting contrast to her poor performance (57% correct) on the semantically similar quantifier float condition exemplified in (19).

to recover constituent structure (including, notably, syntactic linkage of moved elements and gaps) but an impaired processing of various kinds of anaphoric relationships among sentence elements. This same insensitivity presumably underlies the poor comprehension of sentences like *The boy watching the chef bandages himself* reported in Blumstein, Goodglass, Statlender, and Biber (1983). An apparently contradictory report of agrammatic sensitivity to reflexive–antecedent relations is provided in Grodzinsky, Wexler, Chien, Marakovitz, & Solomon (1993), who found virtually error-free performance by agrammatic subjects on a comprehension task involving sentences like *Mama Bear touches herself*. However, Hickok (1992) observes that since the sentences used in this study contained only one potential antecedent, the agrammatics' good performance could be attributed to the "limited solution space"; one might invoke a nearest NP strategy (Blumstein et al., 1983) linking the reflexive pronoun to the only available antecedent in the sentence. Such a strategy would also account for the tendency of Grodzinsky et al.'s subjects to erroneously interpret *Mama bear is touching her* as reflexive.[3]

The contrast between the easy and difficult conditions involving *wh*-words is of particular interest, as it suggests that a certain granularity will be required in any account of the processing of these structures. As argued above, the fact that agrammatics rejected sentences like (6d) in which the fronted *wh*-elements fail to meet the verb's subcategorization requirements virtually compels us to say that these subjects are able to make this link between the *wh*-element and the trace. Let us represent this link for (6c) as in (20) below, abstracting away from all unnecessary detail. I follow Mauner et al. (1993) in using angled brackets to represent the fact that two elements are involved in a chain.

(20) [NP What]$_i$ did the furniture company send [NP e]$_j$?
     $<NP_i, NP_j>$

The indices i and j are used to indicate that the information that the two positions form a chain is distinct from the information that they must have the same referential index (that $i=j$), a point argued persuasively in Mauner et al. (1993).

---

[3] One intriguing finding of Grodzinsky et al. (1993) is not addressed by these alternative explanations: the fact that agrammatic patients correctly interpreted sentences like *Every bear touches her* as nonreflexive. Hickok (1992) suggests that subjects reject the incorrect reflexive reading because it requires a distributed reading of *every bear* in order to co-occur with the singular pronoun and that the disruption in trace relations prevents the quantifier phrase from properly binding the pronoun *her*, as it must be in order to get this distributed reading. However, any claim that the distributed reading of *every bear* is unavailable to these subjects would seem to predict, incorrectly, that they would fail to arrive at the (correct) reflexive interpretation of sentences like *Every Bear washes herself* in which *every bear* must also be linked with a singular pronoun.

In order to interpret a sentence like (6c), much more is required than simply the establishment of the chain. The listener must retrieve the actual lexical items associated with this higher position and/or the meanings of the lexical items occupying this position; he must appreciate the semantic implications of coindexation, among which is the fact that co-indexed elements must all refer to the same entity and hence must not involve contradictory properties; and, in order to detect violations such as (15b), he must notice that the coindexation results in the assignment of contradictory semantic features. Thus the representation (20) is a necessary starting point for the processing of the chain, but the fact that $i = j$ represents, basically, an IOU which may not be cashed until the point of semantic interpretation.

In normals, a large body of evidence (e.g., Stowe, 1986; Frazier & Clifton, 1989) indicates that subjects actively attempt to carry out some of these further interpretive operations at the point at which the gap is encountered. There are some indications that agrammatics may not. Zurif, Swinney, Prather, Solomon, and Bushnell (1993) report a study utilizing the cross-modal lexical priming paradigm in which Broca's aphasics, in contrast to normals and Wernicke's aphasics, failed to show priming at the site of a gap for semantic associates of the most plausible antecedent. Although some questions have been raised about these findings (cf. Mauner, 1995), they do suggest that (20) may represent the cutoff point for agrammatic processing of traces, a possibility that is suggested by the pattern of performance within the grammaticality judgment task as well.

Thus the disparity between impaired comprehension and preserved judgment of grammaticality is echoed within the judgment task itself by the pattern of easy and difficult conditions. I have argued that this pattern demonstrates sensitivity to grammatical properties of sentences relevant to the recovery of phrase structure and insensitivity to more semantic properties such as anaphoric relations. We turn now to three accounts of agrammatism—the chain-disruption, trade-off, and mapping hypotheses—which come to quite distinct conclusions about the implications of these disparities and the nature of the impairment underlying this disorder.

3. CHAIN-DISRUPTION ACCOUNTS OF AGRAMMATIC COMPREHENSION

The three chain-disruption accounts to be examined here attribute agrammatic comprehension to a specific deficiency in these patients' representations of syntactic structure. The argument from agrammatism they employ is what we have termed the selective-loss argument: the linguistic structures which present difficulty for agrammatics form a natural class only within one theory of grammar, GB theory, and hence agrammatism provides evidence for the psychological reality of this theory. We begin with a brief synopsis of the three chain-disruption accounts.

3.1 Three Chain-Disruption Accounts

Grodzinsky's trace-deletion hypothesis (TDH). Grodzinsky (1984, 1986, 1990) proposes that the agrammatic comprehension pattern derives *in toto* from two sources: a representational deficit involving traces and an extragrammatical heuristic which applies obligatorily, and often counterproductively, to associate NPs with thematic roles in the event that they are not grammatically theta-marked. In some formulations of the TDH, the representational deficit involves the outright absence of empty categories from agrammatic representations (e.g., Grodzinsky et al., 1993, p. 415), while in others (e.g., Grodzinsky, 1984) it involves what we will term their "referential stranding," the loss of information about their co-indexation with other positions in the sentence.

For each of the theories to be considered here, we may ask: does this theory explain why agrammatics generally perform well on actives and subject gaps, as in (21), while also explaining their poor performance on passives and object gaps, as in (22)? (I will argue in Section 3.2.1 that none of the chain-disruption accounts provides an adequate explanation for agrammatic difficulties with the passive, so discussion of this construction is deferred.) Under the TDH, actives do not involve syntactic movement and so present no problem to agrammatics. However, both subject gap and object gap sentences contain only one moved element under the linguistic assumptions of Grodzinsky's account, so an additional mechanism is required to differentiate between them.

Grodzinsky recognizes that the representational deficit involving traces does not in itself predict agrammatics' poor comprehension of sentences with object gaps. This is because, in each case, listeners should be able to infer the correct thematic assignments from the fact that there remains a sentence-initial NP to which a thematic role has not been assigned, along with one unassigned thematic role. In (22a), for example, the only unassigned role is that of Patient, assigned to the object of *kiss*. Since Grodzinsky proposes that agrammatics are unimpaired in all respects save their inability to represent traces, an explanation is required for the fact that they do not use the information that is available even in these (*ex hypothese*) impoverished representations.

(21) (a) The boy kissed the girl. (Simple active)
    (b) It was the boy who [NP e] kissed the girl. (Subject gap)
(22) (a) It was the girl who the boy kissed (NP e]. (Object gap)
    (b) The girl was kissed [NP e] by the boy. (Full passive)
    (c) The girl was kissed [NP e]. (Truncated passive)

Therefore Grodzinsky hypothesizes that agrammatic processing is subject to an obligatory and in some cases counterproductive heuristic known as the default principle (DP). The DP comes into play whenever an NP which has not been assigned a thematic role is encountered. The DP as formulated in Grodzinsky (1990, p. 95) assigns this un-theta-marked NP the role canonically associated with the position it occupies.[4] This most frequently means that the NP is assigned the role of Agent if it occurs clause-initially. In full passives like (22b) this heuristic assignment conflicts with the syntax-based assignment of Agent to the NP in the *by*-phrase, *the boy;* the result of this conflicting assignment is the chance performance on such sentences that is widely, although not universally, reported for agrammatics. Subject gaps as in (21b) trigger the same strategy, but this time the strategy results in a correct interpretation since, in its original location, the moved NP was in fact the subject, and for this verb grammatical processes also assign the subject the role of Agent.

Grodzinsky's invocation of the DP—and his appeal to its sometimes destructive effect upon comprehension—has been criticized by some as a *deus ex machina,* but I find these objections unwarranted in the light of the overwhelming evidence that extragrammatical processes play a role in normal language processing. I will, however, take issue below with the claim (e.g., Grodzinsky, 1995) that such processes are operative only when grammatically based operations fail.

Hickok's revised trace-deletion hypothesis (RTDH). The revised trace-deletion hypothesis (Hickok, 1992; Hickok et al., 1993) differs from the TDH in how it claims sentences are represented in normals. Under the VP-internal subject hypothesis (Burton & Grimshaw, 1992; Kitigawa,

---

[4] For the sake of exposition, the working of the DP has been simplified. If the role canonically associated with a given sentence position is intrinsically incompatible with that NP (if the NP is, for example, an inanimate), then the next compatible thematic role in the Thematic Hierarchy is assigned to that NP. Also, Caplan and Hildebrandt (1968) note that object–object relatives would be predicted to present no problem to agrammatics if the DP is formulated as in Grodzinsky (1986): the role assigned to the NP occurring postverbally in the matrix clause would be the correct role in the relative clause as well. But, as reported in Grodzinsky (1984, 1989), object–object relatives are equally difficult for agrammatics. One possibility, as Caplan and Hildebrandt also observe, is to revert to the formulation of the DP in Grodzinsky (1984), in which the Agent role is always assigned to NPs lacking theta roles, unless it conflicts with the semantic properties of the NP. This reformulation, as far as I can tell, removes this counterexample without creating new ones, as in all other cases the DP virtually always assigns the Agent role (or the role associated with the subject). Caplan and Hildebrandt (1986) observe that further assumptions about representation must be made in order to apply the TDH to relative clauses, since in these cases there is no overt NP lacking a theta role, as required to trigger the DP. Rather, the DP must be triggered by the subjects' appreciation (perhaps because of preserved appreciation of the predicative relationship between the head NP and the relative clause) that the head NP must also be linked to an argument position with respect to the embedded verb.

1986; Koopman & Sportiche, 1988; Woolford, 1991), the subject of a sentence is linked to a trace in the specifier position of VP, where it is base-generated and receives its thematic role. Like the TDH, the RTDH proposes that traces are somehow underrepresented at S-structure, leaving open a wide range of psycholinguistic implementations. But now, under the VP-internal subject hypothesis, the subject NP is linked to its theta position via a trace; thus, under the RTDH, in the agrammatic representation it does not receive a grammatically mediated theta role either. The only lexical NP that gets a theta role *in situ* is an unmoved direct object or other internal argument. Hickok represents this information in a thematic assignment representation (TAR), defined in Hickok (1992) as "what the grammatical system makes available to the general cognitive system with respect to theta-role assignments." The asterisk represents unassigned arguments; elements following the semicolon represent NPs which are available as arguments of that predicate.

(23) TAR for simple active (21a) and embedded clause of subject gap (21b)
    kiss (*(*girl*)); *boy*

As for the TDH, we may ask: does this theory explain why agrammatics generally perform well on actives and subject gaps, as in (21), while also explaining their poor performance on object gaps, as in (22a)? Under the RTDH, the thematic role of the subject NP is never grammatically assigned by these patients since the NP in surface subject position is not linked to the VP-internal subject position. Therefore, every English sentence is given an impoverished syntactic representation by these patients. Why, then, do subjects perform well on simple actives and subject gaps?

Hickok et al. (1993, pp. 388–389) account for agrammatic patients' preserved comprehension of simple actives as follows:

> Although not represented in the TAR, it is assumed that the patient has access to the lexical semantics of the items that do not receive thematic roles grammatically; thus, for [*The tiger chased the lion*], the patient would know that the lion was chased and also that a tiger was mentioned in the string.

This account of agrammatics' good performance on subject gaps and actives despite the disruption of the subject trace attributes to these patients the ability to make reasonable inferences based upon the underspecified TAR in conjunction with lexical semantic information. This inferencing allows for relatively unimpaired performance as long as the TAR is unambiguous, that is, as long as there is only one unfilled slot and one unassigned NP.

In this account, poor comprehension arises from an ambiguous TAR. The TAR for the embedded clause in the object-gap sentence (22a) is given in (24) below; note that it contains two unfilled positions because both the subject and the object remain unassigned.

(24) TAR for embedded clause in (22a)
     kiss(*(*)); boy,girl

Unlike the TDH, the RTDH captures the difference between subject gaps and object gaps on the basis of the representational deficit alone: given the VP-internal subject hypothesis, the TARs for the latter, but not for the former, are ambiguous. However, TAR ambiguity does not suffice to account for agrammatics' difficulties with an additional structure, S-S relatives. Hickok et al. (1993) (see also Caramazza & Zurif, 1976; Grodzinsky & Marek, 1988; Sherman & Schweickert, 1989) report significantly impaired performance by agrammatics on sentences such as (25) below, with a tendency to take *the lion* rather than *the tiger* as the entity of which *big* is predicated.

(25) The tiger$_i$ that [NP e]$_i$ chased the lion is big.

This requires Hickok to make some additional claims about agrammatic sentence processing. Although *lion* is theta-marked with respect to the embedded predicate, Hickok represents it as "available" with respect to the matrix predicate and claims that the agrammatic is actually faced with two available fillers for the single argument slot of *is big*. From this ambiguity, chance performance ensues.

(26) TAR for (25)
     is big(*); tiger, lion

Observe that (26) contains only one unfilled argument position (the sole argument of *is big*) and only one NP clausemate of *is big,* viz. *the tiger.* The second NP in (26), *the lion,* occurs embedded in the relative clause and is grammatically enjoined from being theta-marked by the matrix predicate, a fact which should allow agrammatics impaired only in the representation of traces (recall that their good performance on actives is attributed to their ability to deduce the correct assignment despite an imperfect TAR) to similarly deduce the appropriate assignment of thematic roles. Thus the presence of *the lion* as "available" in (26) represents a strong claim, to which I return below: that agrammatics faced with an unfilled slot in a TAR do not use all of the linguistic resources at their disposal—including presumably unimpaired ability to recover phrase structure—to arrive at an interpretation.

Mauner et al.'s double dependency hypothesis (DDH). Of the three chain-disruption accounts examined here, the DDH is the only one that turns entirely upon a representational deficit. Mauner et al. (1993) propose that agrammatics are able to establish chains but are impaired in appreciating or enforcing the obligatory coindexation between the links

of a chain and between other elements linked together in the S-structure
of the sentence, e.g., reflexives, traces, and their antecedents. They refer
to this as a disruption of the "coindexation condition." The coindexation
condition is the requirement that there be a common index assigned to
R-dependent elements, i.e., elements linked in chains or anaphoric relationships of one sort or another. They argue that it is this condition, and
nothing in the machinery of "move alpha" per se, that requires that $i=j$
in (20) above; that the fact that two elements are involved in a chain need
not be represented by the same grammatical machinery that enforces
their ultimate coreference in the interpretation of the sentence. Thus a
subject with a deficient appreciation or enforcement of the coindexation
condition would be expected to make the relevant links between positions
in a chain; but, at the point of semantic interpretation, nothing would
ensure that the antecedent NP and its trace share a common R index.
They argue that "the pattern of asyntactic comprehension follows
straightforwardly if we inhibit the Coindexation Condition and do nothing else" (Mauner et al., 1993, p. 361). This is spelled out in the DDH,
which predicts poor performance in sentences containing more than one
syntactic referential dependency.

As with the TDH and the RTDH, we may ask: does this theory explain
why agrammatics generally perform well on actives and subject gaps, as
in (21), while also explaining their poor performance on object gaps, as
in (22a)?

Like the RTDH, the DDH accounts for poor performance on object
gaps like (22a) on the basis of the disconnection of both subject and object
NPs from the feet of their respective chains. Like the TDH, it does not
provide an account of agrammatic difficulties with S-S relatives such as
(25). Of some interest here is the account it provides for agrammatics'
good performance on subject gap sentences.

Under the RTDH, the agrammatic parser generates two representations for a sentence such as *The boy is chasing the girl*. In one, *the boy*
is correctly linked to the subject trace; in the other, this trace is associated with *the girl*. Mauner et al. (1993, pp. 359–360) argue that agrammatics are able to reject this latter, deviantly coindexed, structure because
it contains two unintegratable subparts: an "orphaned" NP, *the boy,*
denoting an individual; and a meaning fragment paraphraseable as *x is
the girl and x chases x:*

> There is no way to combine an individual with a closed sentence to yield another
> closed sentence. Hence, under widely shared assumptions about natural language
> semantics, the interpretation of [*The boy is chasing the girl*] required by the [devi-
> antly coindexed structure] is deviant on semantic grounds.

Thus the deviant coindexation is rejected and the correctly indexed structure is accepted. Notice that the deviance of the structure arises out of

the yoking of a particular meaning with a particular linguistic structure, rather than out of the deviance of the meaning per se. This is because there is nothing deviant about the utterance of an isolated NP, as in exclamations, telegraphic language, or book titles; nor is the linkage of an isolated NP and a proposition in itself anomalous, as in a telegraphic newspaper title such as *War! US arming itself.* What is deviant is the expression of these two meaning fragments within a single clause. Thus the processing operations by which agrammatics reject the deviant indexing must have access both to the semantic representation and the linguistic structure from which this representation is derived; the rejection is based upon the inappropriateness of the latter as an expression of the former. We return to this point below.

3.2 Empirical and Conceptual Shortcomings of the Chain-Disruption Hypotheses

I believe that two major difficulties arise in connection with the chain-disruption accounts. First, the claimed impoverishment of agrammatics' syntactic representations does not suffice in and of itself to predict the agrammatic comprehension data. Therefore the representational deficit is augumented, in the TDH and the RTDH, by extralinguistic heuristics and/or counterintuitive and in some cases contradictory claims about the unavailability of linguistic information to general cognitive systems. This additional machinery threatens the "argument from aphasia" advanced by the chain-disruption accounts, since it is only the representational deficit that provides the link to government binding theory. The only way to prevent the representational deficit from becoming moot is to make the problematic claim that the TDH's default principle and the linguistically blind guessing posited by the RTDH are *triggered exclusively by the impoverished syntactic representations.*

The second major difficulty with the chain-disruption accounts is that they appear to be empirically indistinguishable from any number of other accounts of agrammatic sentence processing, e.g., from accounts based upon linear order strategies alone.

3.2.1 Inability of the Representational Deficit to Account for Agrammatic Comprehension

We will consider the first problem in connection with three structures: passives, S-S relatives, and actives.

Passives. The problem with passives is that the loss of traces should not prevent subjects from arriving at the correct interpretation of these sentences. Consider full and truncated passives such as (22b) and (22c) above. Recall that the agrammatic subjects in the grammaticality judgment studies performed at or in one case below chance on comprehension tasks involving passive sentences but achieved a mean score of 91.6% in the passive condition of the grammaticality judgment task. So clearly these agrammatic comprehenders are sensitive to the presence of the passive morphology; the chain disruption hypotheses (unlike the closed class hypotheses of, e.g., Kean, 1977, 1981) posit absolutely no impairment in the processing of passive morphology, only in representing the links between sentence elements. This is important because the passive morphology carries with it the important information that the external argument of the active form need not be expressed in the corresponding passive structure. This fact may be implemented by positing suppression of the external argument in the passive (Grimshaw, 1990) or by altering the thematic expectations associated with the verb in some way that reflects that the thematic role normally assigned to the external argument need not be assigned to any lexical NP. Under either of these formulations, the presence of the passive morphology should serve to narrow the thematic search space considerably in passive sentences, even in patients who fail to link traces correctly with their antecedents: traceless representations of passives are no more ambiguous than traceless representations of subject gaps, because there is only one NP filler and only one *obligatory* slot to be filled.

Consider first a truncated passive like (22c) above. Let us grant to the chain-disruption accounts that the NP here is no longer coindexed with its D-structure position. So what? The passive morphology indicates that the external argument has been suppressed (or, alternatively, that it is now optional) so there is only one *obligatory* argument position (the internal argument) and one available NP. As for full passives like (22b), the second NP comes packaged in an undisrupted *by*-phrase, which ought to allow it to be distinguished from the subject. No disruption to the internal structure of the *by*-phrase itself is claimed, and the lexical content of the preposition itself ought to provide sufficient information to allow for the exploitation of this additional information.

None of the three chain-disruption hypotheses provides an adequate account of agrammatics' failure to use this information.

The TDH and the passive. Grodzinsky's default principle at least provides a mechanism for agrammatic difficulties with the passive. Agrammatics' poor performance on full passives like (22b) is accounted for by saying that the NP in the *by*-phrase is assigned the Agent role, engendering conflict with the DP-assigned agent role of the subject. As Grodzinsky (1990) observes, this predicts worse than chance performance on truncated passives like (22c), since the DP's incorrect role assignment does not conflict with any other role assignments. However, Martin et al. (1989) reported that agrammatics perform no worse on truncated passives than on full passives. This is not a particularly serious problem for the DP, however; Grodzinsky (1990, p. 171) suggests that if the data should turn out this way they could be explained by appealing to the implicit agent role of the passive to provide a second Agent, thereby inducing the two-Agent conflict which, on his account, underlies chance performance.

Thus the DP can be made to work with the passive, but the central question remains unexplained: why do subjects use the DP instead of their (*ex hypothese*) preserved knowledge of verb semantics to interpret passive sentences? Grodzinsky (1990, p. 139) acknowledges this problem with regard to full passives: that subjects do not exploit the information about filled and unfilled thematic roles that is available to them. He responds with the suggestion that the relevant thematic information about the verb is simply unavailable and that this unavailability arises from the modularity of the linguistic system:

> . . . although the thematic properties of predicators are available to the parser at the time it constructs a syntactic analysis for the sentence, this knowledge is unavailable to processes that are outside the parser. . . . The later activity of augmentative processes (that is, the heuristic strategy) is not guided by grammatical knowledge, and in fact these processes do not have access to such knowledge. (1990, p. 139–140)

Note, incidentally, that this suggestion directly contradicts the argument in Zurif and Grodzinsky (1983) that the agrammatic subjects in the Linebarger et al. (1983a) study performed well on grammaticality judgments because they were able to utilize off-line grammatical knowledge. If, as he now argues, the linguistic system is so encapsulated as to render its principles and data structures inaccessible to later interpretive processes, how could agrammatic subjects utilize such knowledge to perform the syntactic analysis required by an off-line grammaticality judgment task, as Zurif and Grodzinsky proposed?

More importantly, Grodzinsky's claim about the subsequent unavailability of linguistic knowledge is both untenable and indispensable to his account. Its untenability seems straightforward. If information about verb arguments is unavailable to processes outside of the parser, how do we account for, e.g., the filling of thematic roles not expressed in the syntax, something which normals do effortlessly in the course of interpreting (27b) in discourses such as (27)?

(27) (a) John cooked Mary a huge supper.
    (b) She sat down and ate greedily. (Theme = the supper)

Furthermore, how can we account for normals' ability to perform off-line judgments such a recognizing that *buy* and *purchase* are synonymous, not to mention the evidence for off-line access to thematic information provided by the vast literature on lexical semantics?

There is also an internal contradiction. Grodzinsky (1995) argues that the DP applies only to referential NPs, in order to explain the performance of two agrammatic subjects who comprehended sentences like

Who did the boy kiss? more accurately than sentences like *Which girl did the boy kiss?* (Hickok & Avrutin, 1994). Following (with Hickok & Avrutin) the analysis of *who* as nonreferential and *which N* as referential, he proposes that the DP only applies to referential expressions. The effect of this is is that *which N* questions are, so to speak, contaminated by the counterproductive DP and rendered uninterpretable, whereas the nonreferential *who* questions retain a "thematically dangling" NP, since they are not subject to the DP. Grodzinsky (1995) asserts that "given the intactness of lexical knowledge in agrammatism, the correct semantic role of the thematically dangling NP can be easily inferred." In this account, then, the lexical semantic information is available outside of sentence grammar (for the interpretation of structures which have escaped the heavy hand of the DP), a direct contradiction to his 1990 modularity claims quoted above.

The RTDH and the passive. The same problem arises here: why can't agrammatics interpret passive sentences despite the chain disruption? Given the suppression of the external argument (cf., e.g., Grimshaw, 1990) which Hickok et al. adopt, the TAR for the truncated passive (22c) must be as follows, where θ represents the suppressed argument.

(28) TAR for (22c)
    kiss (θ(*)); girl

This TAR is not ambiguous. There is one unfilled argument position (the internal argument) and one available NP (given the suppression of the external argument). Why don't agrammatics use this information?

One approach—something of a straw man—would be to treat the Agent role associated with passive verbs as akin to thematic roles which may but need not be overtly expressed with a given predicate, such as the missing theme of unergatives like *eat* in (27b) above. In this approach, the TAR for a given predicate would contain slots for all arguments which that verb can take in any syntactic structure it is subcategorized for. In addition, this variant of the RTDH would have to stipulate that agrammatics do not use information about the obligatoriness of particular arguments in making thematic assignments, although such knowledge is clearly part of linguistic as distinct from real-world knowledge. Adopting this approach would yield an ambiguous TAR for (22c):

(29) Alternative TAR for (22c)
    kiss(*(*)); girl

Given this TAR and the assumption that agrammatics do not use information about obligatoriness of arguments, poor performance would be correctly predicted given that there are two argument positions competing for one NP. However, this is not a very appealing solution. For example, it would make the implausible (albeit untested) prediction that agrammatic subjects would regularly accept sentences like (30) or (31) below in a semantic anomaly task, since *eat* can take (in other sentence positions) a Theme role for which sandwiches are obviously appropriate, and *the radio* could, if it occurred elsewhere, provide a Source argument for *listen*. I am not aware of systematic investigations of such sentences, but it seems most unlikely that this is the case.

(30) The sandwich ate.
(31) The radio is listening.

Mauner (1995) argues that false acceptance of such sentences would not be predicted because "if *sandwich* or *radio* were assigned an Agent role, the resulting interpretation would be rejected because the semantic features of sandwiches and radios are not compatible with the semantic features of an Agent of an eating or listening event." However, the argument here is that acceptance of sentences like (30) and (31) would be predicted from a variant of the RTDH which posits TARs with unfilled slots for all thematic roles which a given predicate can assign. Since *eat* can assign a Theme role and *listen* can assign a Source role (mediated by the preposition *to*) in sentences such as *John ate lunch* and *Mary listened to the radio,* the agrammatic TARs would presumably have open positions for these optionally expressed roles. Since, *ex hypothese,* the sentence-initial NPs in (30) and (31) are not recognized as subjects, they would not be "earmarked" for whatever thematic role the verb assigns to its external argument and ought to be available to express these optional arguments. Thus (30) ought to be accepted with the meaning that some unspecified individual ate the sandwich and (31) with the meaning that some unspecified individual listened to the radio. The question of how agrammatics would in fact perform on such a task remains to be explored, but it seems to be a prediction of this hypothetical variant of the RTDH that they would be insensitive to such violations.

The DDH and the passive. The DDH appears to face the same difficulties with regard to the passive. Agrammatic subjects' unimpaired lexical semantic knowledge along with their preserved appreciation of passive morphology (revealed in the grammaticality judgment studies) ought to render them cognizant that the internal argument of the passive verb must be overtly expressed but that the external argument need not be, with the result that the orphaned subject NP is assigned to fill the role associated with the obligatory *internal* argument.

And even if we argue that agrammatics are not able to infer from the passive morphology that the external argument need to be overtly expressed by a lexical NP but that the internal argument is obligatory, the same kinds of processes by which deviant interpretations for subject gaps are rejected under the DDH ought to suffice for passives as well. Consider first the truncated passive. Under the analysis of the passive adopted in Mauner et al. (1993), the external argument in a normal representation of the truncated passive is assigned to the passive morpheme *en* itself.

This information should suffice for patients to choose correctly among the four possible indexings of *en* and the NP trace in (22c). The first, coindexation of *the girl* with *en* but not with the trace in object position, would presumably be rejected since it results in a deviant interpretation, an open proposition in which the trace is an unbound variable. The second coindexation, in which *the girl, en,* and *t,* are referentially distinct from one another, would presumably be rejected on these same grounds and also because of the orphaning of the NP *the girl* argued for in connection with subject gaps. The third, coindexation of *the girl* with both *t* and *en,* would lead to a reflexive interpretation which ought to be rejected easily in a sentence-picture matching task (cf. Grodzinsky et al., 1993). This would seem to leave as the sole contender the correct coindexation of *the girl* and *t.*

The full passive is also problematic. Mauner et al. (1993, p. 356) adopt an analysis in which the NP in the *by*-phrase is coindexed with the passive *en.* They treat full passives as analogous to object gaps, containing two NPs and two possible elements with which these NPs may be coindexed. But I do not believe that these two structures are analogous. Since subjects' appreciation of phrase structure is (*ex hypothese*) undisturbed, the disruption of the coindexation between the NP in the *by*-phrase and the passive morpheme seems harmless because the preposition *by* signals the possibility that its object may correspond to the external argument. Unlike object gap sentences, in which two NPs compete for two slots, a full passive contains (*ex hypothese*) one uncoindexed NP and one intact *by*-phrase; agrammatic patients' unimpaired knowledge of argument identification ought to allow them to fill the external argument role with the element in the *by*-phrase.

I stress here that I make no claim that the *by*-phrase signals Agency as distinct from any other thematic role that may be associated with the external argument. In (22b), the *by*-phrase is associated with the Agent because the external argument of *kiss* is an Agent; a reference to this association in an earlier version of this paper was understandably taken by Mauner (1994) as a wider claim that *by*-phrases express Agents. As Mauner (1995) points out, the linguistic literature provides ample documentation that the *by*-phrase may express a wide variety of thematic roles in passive sentences, as well as locative adjuncts. The point here is that the *by*-phrase, if it expresses an argument of the verb rather than a locative adjunct, almost invariably expresses the *external argument* of the passive verb.[5] Subjects' *ex hypothese* unimpaired appreciation of argument structure ought to allow them to use that information.

---

[5] In the rare event that it expresses an internal argument, as in *The idea was finally run by the committee,* the role of the preposition in identifying this internal argument is part of speakers' lexical knowledge and the presence of the unimpaired *by*-phrase should suffice for interpretation.

S-S relatives. A similar issue arises in connection with S-S relatives such as (25) above. Hickok et al. (1993) report that such sentences are frequently misinterpreted by agrammatics, with the matrix predicate adjective predicated of the closer by syntactically unavailable NP in the relative clause. (We have seen above that only the RTDH attempts to account for agrammatic performance on such sentences; for the TDH and the DDH, they stand as a counterexample.) Under the RTDH, the matrix subject NP is not grammatically assigned to fill a role of *big,* and so the patient simply guesses, violating the theta criterion freely. Why doesn't the patient use the information that is available from phrase structure, which ought to tell him that only one NP is a grammatically legitimate candidate? Hickok (1992) considers this question and suggests that this is because such information is not available to general problem-solving mechanisms which have been assigned the task of coming up with an interpretation. Like Grodzinsky (1990, but not 1995), then, Hickok seems to be providing the following account: the underrepresentation of traces leads to an interpretation constructed by the general cognitive system which ignores grammatical information that these patients have already computed, and an appeal to modularity is made in order to account for this failure to exploit linguistic information. As noted above, these modularity claims are intrinsically problematic, given, e.g., the ease with which normals interpret deviant and fragmentary input and perform metalinguistic analysis over sentence structures. They also leave unanswered the question of why the interpretation of incomplete syntactic representations for subject gaps—and, for the RTDH, of simple actives as well—is not similarly precluded by these modularity effects.

Furthermore, the RTDH's account of S-S relatives makes some quite testable predictions. It would seem to predict that, given the VP-internal trace hypothesis, the subject of a sentence has no more reason to fill a slot in the TAR of the predicate than any other NP not theta-marked by that predicate. But why, then, don't agrammatics perform at chance when there are other NPs in the vicinity of the subject in filling this slot? There is considerable evidence that they do not choose randomly among preverbal nouns. For example, in the syntactic padding conditions of a semantic plausibility judgment study reported in Schwartz, Linebarger, Saffran, and Pate (1987) there were many NPs which would be available for theta marking by verbs which, under the RTDH, received underspecified TARs. Consider one such sentence:

(32) As the sun rose, the bird in the cool wet grass swallowed the worm quickly and went away.
(33) TAR for (32)
     swallow(*(worm)); sun, bird, grass

In (33), presumably the TAR of the first clause of (32), the subject of *swallow* is unspecified (*ex hypothese*) and there are three "available"

NPs preceding. Agrammatics would be predicted to respond with many false rejections of such sentences, since two of these NPs would represent implausible Agents of *swallow;* but in fact performance was well above chance (81%). Furthermore, the difference between sentences such as (32) and "unpadded" counterparts like *The bird swallowed the worm* was only 4%. Since the unpadded variants have unambiguous TARs with no NP foils, the great majority of the errors that were made cannot be accounted for by the claimed ambiguity of TARs like (33). But if subjects guess when they are faced with an ambiguous TAR, why wasn't performance on sentences like (32) at chance, with subjects rejecting (32) whenever *grass* or *sun* were incorrectly assigned the Agent role of *swallow?*

Hickok (personal communication) suggests, plausibly, that the subjects in the Schwartz et al. (1987) study may have adapted a strategy of accepting any TAR for which there is at least one plausible NP filler available. In this account, sentences like (32) would never be rejected, because there is always at least one plausible NP available. Thus only the implausible sentences could be used to test this alternative explanation, since the plausible sentences always have at least one good reading. The materials employed in Schwartz et al. (1987) do not allow for a test of this possibility because, in the implausible sentences, subject padding virtually never contained an NP which met the selectional restrictions of the matrix verb; sentences like *The worm next to the cat swallowed the bird,* for example, were not used. (The design of this study is detailed in Section 4.2 below.) However, a replication of Schwartz et al. (1987) using the Dutch translation of the same materials (Kolk & Weijts, 1995) does—by virtue of the error patterns of certain subjects—provide some data that bear on Hickok's claim that agrammatics treat all NPs in the subject padding as potential subjects of the matrix verb. In Schwartz et al. (1987), it was argued that subjects would have rejected many plausible padded sentences if they were unable to recover the head noun of the subject NP, because NPs in the padding would have violated selectional restrictions on the matrix verb. However, the positive response bias shown by our subjects in both the semantic plausibility and grammaticality judgment studies makes it difficult to test this hypothesis. Not all of the subjects in Kolk and Weijts (1995), however, showed this bias. Although for the group as a whole there was a bias toward overacceptance, half of the patients in the padded condition responded with false negatives equally or more often than false positives (Kolk, personal communication). These patients could not have adapted the strategy of "accept if there is any plausible reading" suggested by Hickok, and they would therefore be predicted by the RTDH to perform at chance on padded plausible sentences, such as (32) above. In (32), for example, they should have regularly mismapped *grass* to the agent role of *swallow* and falsely rejected the sentence. These subjects, however, were no more adversely affected by the padding manipulation than the subjects who showed a pattern of over-acceptance.

I stress here that errors were made on both the unpadded and the padded condigions of the task, and any theory must ultimately account for these errors. My argument here is that the RTDH makes a very strong claim: that the agrammatics' TARs of sentences like (32) are ambiguous and that subjects' performance on these sentences is the result of guessing, unconstrained by grammatical information about phrase structure. The good peformance of subjects on the padded condition of the two semantic plausibility judgment tasks suggest that this claim is incorrect; although a strategy of overacceptance would account for the data in Schwartz et al. (1987), it does not account for the performance of many patients in the Kolk and Weijts (1994) replication of the study.

Simple actives. Finally, none of the chain disruption accounts is compatible with impaired comprehension of simple active sentences. Although such sentences have been reported to cause difficulty for agrammatics (e.g., Schwartz et al., 1980), many agrammatics perform well above-chance on simple actives. However, a rather surprising pattern of agrammatic performance on a semantic anomaly task (Saffran, Schwartz, & Linebarger, submitted) casts doubt upon the claim that simple active sentences are not affected by the deficit underlying agrammatism. The implausible sentences in this task were of two types. The "global" anomalies, like the syntax-based anomalies in Schwartz et al. (1987), were plausible at the subject–verb and verb–object level; the implausibility arose out of the entire predicate argument structure, as in

(34) (a) The cat carried the mouse.
    (b) #The mouse carried the cat.

The other kind of implausible anomalies, termed "local anomalies," contained one NP which violated the selectional constraints on one of the thematic roles of the verb, as in

(35) (a) The mouse ate the cheese.
    (b) #The cheese ate the mouse.

For both the local and global anomalies, then, the implausibility is "correctible" by reversing the syntactic roles of the two nouns. Normal subjects rated the locals as more anomalous than the globals. On the implausible sentences, however, agrammatics' performance was significantly worse on the locals, even on the simple active sentences. Thus for the implausible versions of simple actives such as these, the agrammatics' means were 8.86 correct (out of 10) on Globals such as (34b) but declined to 5.71 correct on locals such as (35b), a significant effect. We will consider the sources of this effect in more·detail in our discussion of the mapping hypothesis. We note it here only because it represents another example of agrammatic difficulty with sentences in which thematic assignment does not turn on the interpretation of moved elements.

Summary of 3.2.1. I have argued above that the structural impoverishment claimed by the chain-disruption accounts does not suffice to distinguish the impaired from the unimpaired structures in asyntactic comprehension. All three chain-disruption accounts attribute to agrammatics an unimpaired ability to infer the correct interpretation from impoverished syntactic representations in certain cases (subject gaps, simple actives), but cannot explain why the same kinds of interpretive inferencing cannot be employed in other cases (passives, S-S relatives). And none of the three chain disruption accounts addresses the evidence for "pathologic heuristics" in simple actives reported in Saffran et al. (1994); extralinguistic strategies, on the chain-disruption accounts, *must be triggered only by structural impoverishment.* Evidence that such strategies are operative in *ex hypothese* unimpaired constructions like simple actives is problematic because it renders the structural deficit moot; and if we argue that simple actives too are vulnerable as a result of the hypothesized disconnection of the subject trace, then all English sentences containing subjects now fall into the category of impaired structures. We turn now to this issue of whether the claims advanced by the chain-disruption accounts differ empirically from other, nonrepresentational, analyses of agrammatic comprehension.

3.2.2 Empirical Indistinguishability from Other Accounts

For the moment, I will set aside the data that the chain-disruption accounts do not cover and ask the question: can these accounts be empirically distinguished from accounts of agrammatism which partition the comprehension data in other ways? In particular, can they be distinguished from explanations which link comprehension difficulty to structures violating canonical order and "nearest NP" strategies? This is difficult, of course, given that trace theory is motivated by the projection principle: movement is typically postulated to account for the fact that an NP occurs in some location which is not is D-structure theta position. However, it should be possible to find a number of distinguishing cases, and the ultimate persuasiveness of any variant of the chain-disruption hypotheses would seem to require such evidence.

Hickok et al. (1993) acknowledge the difficulty in differentiating between the predictions made by their version of the chain-disruption hypothesis and the "nearest NP" strategy of Blumstein et al. (1983). They point to only one case in which there is evidence to distinguish the two theories: the single patient SP in Caplan and Futter (1986) who performed at chance on sentences like (36):

(36) The goat kicked the frog that kissed the cow.

Caplan and Futter's patient was as likely to select the more distant NP *the goat* rather than the nearer NP *the frog* to be the agent of *kissed*. Assuming, for the moment, that this pattern were to co-occur in other patients, it is not clear how it could be interpreted given that a perfectly acceptable parse is available under which the relative clause has been extraposed, as in (37), suggested by a reviewer of Hickok et al. (1993, p. 387):

(37) The man hit the tree who was driving a new car.

If Caplan and Futter's subject were to assign to (36) in some cases a parse in which the final relative clause actually modifies *the goat,* then, given that parse, the choice of *the goat* as the Agent of *kiss* would, in fact, represent the correct mapping, replaced in a significant number of cases by *the frog,* the latter choice actually an incorrect mapping influenced by the nearest NP strategy. Hickok et al. reply as follows to the reviewer's suggested alternate parse:

> But notice that the extraposed relative clause analysis requires a long-distance association. So in order to maintain the long-distance association hypothesis, one cannot appeal to the extraposed relative clause analysis in explaining away S.P.'s difficulties with OS relatives. (1993, p. 387)

I take note of this mini-debate because it bears on an issue central to the interpretation of agrammatism: the distinctness of parsing and interpretation. There is considerable evidence (from, e.g., grammaticality judgments) that agrammatics can handle long-distance syntactic dependencies, but that need not imply that they are able to handle comparable dependencies in the course of semantic interpretation. Recall Mauner et al.'s distinction between establishment of chains and the coindexation condition. It may be that establishing an extraposed relative clause far from the noun it modifies is much easier than linking that distant NP to a slot in the theta grid associated with this relative clause. No contradiction is involved here. Agrammatics demonstrate considerable ability to set up long-distance dependencies in the course of parsing. A subject who tends to map between the syntax and the theta grid on the basis of surface order is thus presented with a parse in which the syntactically mandated role filler is not "at the top of the stack." There is no contradiction in attributing to agrammatics the ability to handle long-distance parses in the syntax in conjunction with a tendency to (incorrectly) select the "nearest NP" in thematic interpretation.

Thus I can see no empirical basis upon which to distinguish current formulations of the chain-disruption hypotheses from accounts of agrammatism which represent agrammatics as heavily influenced by canonical word order and the proximity of NP antecedents at certain points in sentence processing. In order for agrammatism to provide evidence in support of theories of grammar which posit traces, it must be demonstrated that this grammatical mechanism provides the only—or the most parsimonious—account of agrammatic sentence processing.

4. THE TRADE-OFF HYPOTHESIS

We return to the paradox of agrammatics' ability to judge the grammaticality of certain constructions which they do not interpret reliably. Two possible explanations for this disparity were considered in Linebarger et al. (1983a): the *trade-off hypothesis* and the *mapping hypothesis*. In the trade-off hypothesis the disparity between preserved ability to make grammaticality judgments and asyntactic comprehension follows from a processing impairment which allows parsing or interpretation, but not both simultaneously. On this account, agrammatics' good performance on the grammaticality judgments is not taken as evidence about the syntactic representations available to these patients in comprehension tasks. Rather, it is assumed that parsing degrades under the pressure of tasks more demanding than grammaticality judgments and that, ultimately, the agrammatic comprehension impairment derives from inadequate syntactic analyses rather than from any difficulty in exploiting syntactic representations. In contrast, the mapping hypothesis claims that the syntactic representations computed by agrammatics provide enough information to support interpretation and that the "weak link" in agrammatic sentence processing is the mapping between these representations and meaning, with the process of thematic assignment representing a particularly vulnerable processing operation.

A version of the trade-off hypothesis has recently been proposed by Frazier and Friederici (1991). To a great extent, they argue for the trade-off hypothesis by arguing against the mapping hypothesis, since the trade-off hypothesis might be seen as a more conservative interpretation of the grammaticality judgment data than the mapping hypothesis. Three of their arguments are considered below.

4.1 Frazier and Friederici's Arguments against the Mapping Hypothesis

The theta criterion. Frazier and Friederici (1991, p. 57) argue that the mapping hypothesis predicts that agrammatics should be insensitive to the theta criterion. But, in fact, there is nothing in the mapping hypothesis that requires such a claim. In fact, even in a far stronger variant of the mapping hypothesis than we would argue for, in which agrammatics were hypothesized to be unable to apply even a single mapping rule, the mapping hypothesis would still remain mute on the question of whether the theta criterion, a general principle constraining the linkage between syntactic structures and theta grids, is lost or retained. There is no more reason to assume that an agrammatic subject who fails to access or apply verb-specific mapping rules correctly is unaware of a general constraint on thematic mapping than to believe that, e.g., a severe anomic impaired in the retrieval of specific lexical items is unaware of the phonotactic and morphological constraints of the language. However, the generally good performance of agrammatics on simple active sentences rules out this hypothetical version of the mapping hypothesis under which agrammatics are unable to apply any mapping rules whatever.

Note, incidentally, that it is almost impossible to ascertain from good performance on a task employing natural language sentences whether subjects do or do not appreciate the theta criterion. For example, Frazier and Friederici argue that they have demonstrated an appreciation of this principle in agrammatic patients on the basis of these patients' almost error-free performance of a comprehension task involving stimuli such as *The men take photographs of the boys;* the subjects did not misinterpret the sentences in any way that violated the theta criterion. But since the subjects interpreted the sentences *correctly,* what can we infer? One possibility is that they were simply applying verb-specific mapping rules. Similarly, one might be tempted to infer from agrammatics' good performance on grammaticality judgments that these subjects appreciate the theta criterion (cf. Grodzinsky, 1990, pp. 139–140), since a wide range of ill-formed structures may be seen as violating this principle by containing NPs not associated with a unique theta-marking position. It is possible and in fact likely [cf. the discussion of (20) above] that parsing operations such as the establishment of gaps or the enforcement of subcategorization conditions are psychologically distinct from the thematic interpretation of the same structures.

Grammaticality judgment. A second argument against the mapping hypothesis turns on the disparity between impaired grammaticality judgments and preserved comprehension. Frazier and Friederici (1991, p. 58) appear to believe that the disparity we have reported is between the asyntactic comprehension of the agrammatics described in Saffran et al. (1980) and the good performance of a nonidentical group of agrammatics studied in Linebarger et al. (1983a). However, as reported in Linebarger et al. (1983a), the four agrammatic subjects who performed well on grammaticality judgments in this study were themselves quite severely asyntactic comprehenders: all performed at chance or worse on the comprehension of simple passives, and two performed at chance on simple actives.

Frazier and Friederici (1991, p. 58) also imply that a study reported in Wulfeck (1988) provides counterevidence to the claimed disparity. It does not. Wulfeck examined four basic sentence types, comparing subjects' performance on the same structures in both picture matching and grammaticality judgment tasks, and reported that her agrammatic subjects did not show the striking disparity between grammaticality judgment and comprehension reported in Linebarger et al. (1983a): they performed very well on both tasks, albeit slightly better on the grammaticality judgments. Wulfeck (1988, p. 77) acknowledges that her subjects differ very significantly from those studied in Linebarger et al. (1983a): only the latter were asyntactic comprehenders. But without asyntactic comprehension, how can one test whether asyntactic comprehension co-occurs with preserved judgments of grammaticality? One might also question whether the grammatical constructions selected are relevant to a test of this claim. In order to test the claim that there is a disparity between preserved grammaticality judgments and impaired comprehension, one must base this test on constructions which are claimed to be judged well by agrammatics. Two of the four conditions employed by Wulfeck were reflexives and tag questions, two structures which Linebarger et al. (1983a) listed among the difficult conditions for agrammatics.[6] The idea of using the same stimuli for both comprehension and judgment tasks is an interesting one, however, as long as attention is given to ensuring that the same grammatical information is used in both tasks.[7] Thus the study in question cannot offer usable evidence regarding either the grammaticality judgment–comprehension disparity or the hierarchy of difficulty within the grammaticality judgment task itself.

Length of inferential chain. Frazier and Friederici's hypothesis that parsing is traded off for thematic interpretation is based upon the prediction that "structures involving longer inferential chains will suffer greater degradation than structures involving shorter inferential chains" (1991, p. 55) combined with their belief that "in any sentence, there will be more phrase structure decisions than thematic role decisions" (1991, p. 56). But one might ask: what counts as a thematic role decision? In order to assign a thematic role one must decide, *inter alia,* which sense of the verb is appropriate, if the verb has multiple senses; and whether the

---

[6] As it turned out, the violations in the conditions termed Reflexive and Tag in Wulfeck (1987) turned on quite local number agreement violations in most cases, and so these two conditions were not of the same types that proved difficult for subjects in the Linebarger et al. (1983a) study.

[7] For example, in the center-embedded condition (*The horse that the goat is kicking is dirty*) the comprehension task requires subjects to utilize the trace-antecedent relationship for thematic role assignment, whereas the corresponding grammaticality judgment (**The horse that the goat are kicking is dirty*) turns upon a very local number agreement violation completely orthogonal to the trace or its antecedent. Thus an agrammatic who performed well on the grammaticality judgment task and poorly on the comprehension task might appear to be providing evidence in support of the mapping hypothesis; but, since the grammaticality judgment here requires no appreciation of the *wh* gap relation, the contrast would be spurious.

hypothesized argument satisfies all the semantic and possibly pragmatic constraints associated with this role (if a selectional restriction requires an argument to be, e.g., both edible and liquid, is this one decision or two?). More importantly, the invocation of number of decisions as the critical factor seems a bit suspect. A single decision may require the ruling out of innumerable other possibilities. Counting the number of final decisions made ignores the difficulty of each decision and the number of decisions required to rule out the alternatives. With this logic, deciding who to marry (one decison, given two candidates) is less computationally expensive than deciding what kind of sandwich to make for lunch (two or more distinct decisions being required for bread and filling).

4.2 Counterevidence to the Trade-off Hypothesis

I believe that there is also some empirical counterevidence to the trade-off hypothesis. The Schwartz et al. (1987) study discussed above argues against the claim that parsing is a resource hog or that parsing anything but the simplest structures cannot be maintained in conjunction with sentence interpretation. In this study, simple active ("basic") sentences—(38a) and (39a)—were subjected to a syntactic padding manipulation in which extraneous material was added in the form of NP or adverbial modifiers, as in (38b) and (39b).

(38) (a) #The school was on top of the flag.
(b) #In the photograph, the school—which was in good condition—was on top of the flag and there wasn't a cloud in the sky.
(39) (a) #The chicken killed the famer
(b) #In the early part of the day, the chicken drank some water and then killed and ate the farmer.

Performance on the padded materials was well above chance (81%); furthermore, the difference between "basic" and "padded" sentences was only 4%. Kolk and Weijts (1995) report a significant but still very limited effect of increased syntactic complexity using a Dutch translation of the same materials. Our argument is based upon the conviction that subjects could not have performed the task as accurately as they did unless they were able to extract from these complex parses the arguments of the verbs and prepositions involved in the anomalies. And if they are parsing, then the absence of a syntactic complexity effect is hard to explain under the hypothesis that parsing is a resource hog. Kolk and Weijts (1995) have recently questioned this claim, arguing that the task could be performed on the basis of a nonsyntactic strategy linear order alone: subjects could associate the preverbal noun with the Agent and the role of the Patient or Theme with the postverbal noun. I would like to argue that subjects simply could not have succeeded with such a strategy, for the following reasons.

First, the location of the first noun critical to the anomaly varied considerably: in eight sentences it came first, in six cases it came second, and in 11 cases it occurred at some point thereafter. Second, as Kolk and Weijts observe, it is unclear how such a strategy could apply to locatives, and over half the sentences were locatives such as *The pill is in the drug*. (Additionally, the fact that these anomalies turned on prepositions increases the number of plausible subparts, since a purely linear strategy could not impose any requirements on the noun *preceding* a preposition; the implausibility of *The pill is in the drug* requires an appreciation of the predicative role of the copula; *in the drug* is a perfectly plausible PP in isolation.) Third, consider the sheer logistics of such a strategy for these sentences. There were on average 5.2 nouns and 5.7 verbs or prepositions per sentence. Strategies such as "accept any sentence with at least one plausible N-V-N sequence" would have required subjects to maintain a combinatorial explosion of N-V-N sequences in memory and would in this case have resulted in the gross overacceptance of implausible sentences, virtually all of which contain at least one plausible N-V-N or P-N sequence.

So it appears that the task could not be performed without parsing, and thus our argument would seem to stand: even in long sentences padded with extraneous phrase structure nodes, this basic extraction of the subject, verb, and object (or locative counterparts) proceeded unimpaired. As to whether subjects *subsequently* employed such heuristics as "the syntactic subject must be the agent" we do not know, and the question is not relevant to our argument that the recovery of phrase structure is not prohibitively resource-expensive. Furthermore, our argument is not affected by the absence of what we might call "thematic red herrings," NPs in the padding which might also plausibly be assigned these thematic roles. Such red herrings—which, in Experiment 2 of Kolk and Weijts (1994), did result in degraded performance—would have complicated the mapping process rather than the parsing process, and our intention was to test the *overhead,* so to speak, of syntactic complexity.

5. THE MAPPING HYPOTHESIS

In contrast to the chain-disruption and trade-off hypotheses, the mapping hypothesis claims that asyntactic comprehension arises not from a failure to *compute* syntactic structure but from a failure to *exploit* it. What I have termed the "mapping hypothesis" subsumes a large number of heterogeneous conjectures about the possible antecedents for such a failure. These assorted possibilities, to be discussed in Section 5.2 below, include, *inter alia,* loss of lexical knowledge about predicate argument structure, damage to the psychological mechanism(s) responsible for assigning thematic roles, and nonspecific resource limitations affecting later interpretive processes more severely than early parsing operations.

Thus the mapping hypothesis, taken as a theory of agrammatism, is grossly underspecified, although the more specific conjectures noted above can be restricted so as to make empirically testable claims. But even in its heterogeneity and underspecification, the larger claim of the mapping hypothesis—that agrammatics are impaired not in the recovery of syntactic structure, but in its explotation—may have important ramifications for aphasia therapy. It suggests that the appropriate focus of therapeutic efforts may lie in training patients to make the link between syntactic and semantic information, rather than building fluency in the processing of syntactic information *per se*. It might be argued that the treatment gains reported for "mapping therapy" (Section 5.3) provide support for this approach to the analysis of agrammatism.

5.1 Agrammatic Comprehension

How, then, does the mapping hypothesis—abstracting away from the different variants of this hypothesis to be sketched in the following section—explain the observed patterns of agrammatic comprehension? How does this theory explain why agrammatics generally perform well on actives and subject-gaps, as in (21) above, while also explaining their poor performance on passives and object gaps, as in (22)?

The mapping hypothesis holds that agrammatics are able to recover phrase structure but are impaired in exploiting their syntactically structured representation of the input sentence for interpretive processes. Specifically, sentence types which prove difficult for agrammatics in both comprehension and grammaticality judgment tasks all require the linkage between two positions in the syntactically structured word string or between a position in this structured string and a position in some other structure built up in the course of sentence interpretation. For example, thematic interpretation is often conceptualized as a process of linking up syntactic representations with theta grids (Stowell, 1981). As noted in Mauner et al. (1993), even direct theta assignment of unmoved elements to grid positions can be seen as a process of coindexation between argument positions and grid positions. Under the mapping hypothesis, theta assignment *even for unmoved arguments* is claimed to be a locus of vulnerability in agrammatics, since it involves linking elements in the two structures, the S-structure and the theta grid.

Like the chain-disruption accounts, the mapping hypothesis predicts that syntactic movement further complicates mapping by forcing subjects to process dependencies between elements of the structure as well as between syntactic positions and theta grid slots. The "difficult" conditions of the grammaticality judgment task are thus difficult for the same reason that thematic interpretation of sentences with *wh* gaps is difficult: they require subjects to process relationships between elements in the structured representation of the sentence (Schwartz et al., 1987, p. 105; Mauner et al., 1993).

But, of course, to say that thematic assignment is a point of vulnerability does not explain why structures such as object gaps and passives are more difficult than others such as actives and subject gaps. Under the version of the mapping hypothesis articulated here, the fragility of the mapping process renders it more dependent on, and more vulnerable to, a host of *extragrammatical processes* which are operative in normal as well as aphasic speakers. The difference between these constructions is, on this account, attributed to their differing susceptibility to both the facilitative and the disruptive effects of the extragrammatical processes, which are to be seen not as compensatory mechanisms triggered by representational failure but rather as normal mechanisms which have come to play an abnormally visible role in agrammatism. Three such processes— canonical word order effects, nearest NP effects, and selectionally based role filling—are invoked below to account for the range of comprehension data discussed in connection with the chain-disruption hypotheses.

Canonical word order effects. One frequently invoked explanation for the greater difficulty posed by passives and object gaps is that they violate normal expectations regarding the order in which various thematic roles are introduced (see, e.g., Caplan, Baker, & Dehaut, 1985). An undisputed generalization for English and many other languages is that the most active and controlling argument tends to occur first, the directly affected argument tends to occur next, and other arguments tend to occur after these two. Appreciation of this generalization might faciliate algorithmic mapping onto the theta grid by allowing subjects to make provisional thematic role assignments in parallel with grammatically based processing, thereby laying the conceptual groundwork for the final interpretation. Alternatively, canonical order may be represented in quasi-visual terms, with noncanonical orders such as those in the passive or object-gaps requiring a kind of mental rotation in order to link up the S-structure with canonically ordered positions in the theta grid. Or, finally, it may be that because the canonical mappings are more *frequent* they are more automatized. The range of psychological implementations of these canonical order effects is vast. The claim here is that in agrammatic subjects the fragility of the mapping process renders it abnormally affected by this extralinguistic processing; agrammatics are facilitated in canonical structures and "garden-pathed" in noncanonical structures.

Nearest NP effects. Another facilitating factor in the syntax-based mapping is the proximity of the legitimate role filler (see, e.g., Blumstein et al., 1983): intervening NPs tend to lead to errors even in S-S relatives such as (25) above, in which canonical order is observed—subjects at least precede their verbs—but the subject NP is distanced from the verb by an intervening relative clause. One might visualize an argument stack, so to speak, where argument NPs are stored for insertion into theta grids. If the grammatically-licensed filler is also the NP at the top of this stack, then mapping is enhanced. Again, the mapping hypothesis claims that such effects *enhance or disrupt but do not replace* subjects' attempts to carry out the algorithmic mapping.

Selectionally based role filling. We also assume, following the mass of evidence of on-line semantic and pragmatic processing, that during the parse initial thematic role assignments are also made (cf. Carlson & Tanenhaus, 1988) on the basis of verb-specific selectional information. To the extent that these selectionally based assignments are correct, they facilitate the syntax-based mapping, perhaps reducing it to something more akin to recognition than recall. When they are incorrect, they may degrade performance by creating "thematic garden paths" or perhaps by leading the subject to accept these assignments rather than those of the syntax-based mapping. The data in Saffran et al. (submitted), discussed in Section 3.2.1 above, demonstrate the power of such assignments and also support the mapping hypothesis' claim that thematic role assignment is vulnerable even in simple active sentences.

5.2 Hypotheses about the Source of the Hypothesized Mapping Failure

Explanations for the hypothesized failure to interpret syntactic representations include, but are not limited to, the following.

Loss of verb-specific thematic information. The most straightforward hypothesis is that there is a specific impairment involving the retrieval of thematic role information associated with verbs; see, e.g., Byng (1988). But then, as noted in Schwartz et al. (1987) and Caramazza and Miceli (1991), one must explain why there is a syntactic complexity effect: if the problem is lexical, then for those verbs whose thematic information is intact one would expect to see no degradation of performance in object-gaps and other complex structures. Of course, if only passives were affected one could appeal to a lexical account of that construction (Bresnan, 1982) but this obviously does not account for the difficulty posed by *wh* gaps.

Another source of evidence against this possibility is suggested in Shapiro et al. (1993), where it is argued that the performance of agrammatic Broca's aphasic patients in a cross-modal lexical priming task demonstrates that these patients "exhaustively access the thematic properties of verbs" (1993, p. 423) in the immediate temporal vicinity of the verb. The basis for this claim is that the agrammatics in this study, like the normal subjects, showed a longer latency following verbs which Shapiro et al. judged to be associated with more complex argument structures. Thus subjects responded more quickly following simple transitives than following datives and more quickly following verbs which are associated with two complement types (NP Theme, clausal Proposition) than following verbs which were associated with four complement types (NP Theme, clausal Proposition, clausal Exclamation, clausal Interrogative).

However, it is not clear whether these interesting findings can be shown to reflect sensitivity to argument structure as opposed to subcategorization or other purely structural properties of verbs. They seem equally consistent with a subcategorization-based account because the transitives, which yielded faster reaction times than datives, had an average of 1.5 syntactic object options (NP, Null), whereas the datives were associated with an average of 3 possible syntactic complements (NP, NP-NP, NP-NP-PP). On the other hand, related studies with normals (e.g., Shapiro, Zurif, & Grimshaw, 1987) have revealed no difference between dative verbs which do and do not take the double object construction; if this turns out to be the case for agrammatics as well, then subcategorization could be ruled out as the relevant property. But a greater number of other possibilities remain; for example, it might be that the *number of elements which may occur in the VP* is the relevant factor. Both types of datives take two elements, whereas the transitives take one element in the VP. It might well be that the latency reflects syntactic planning of the VP and hence is affected by the number of elements that the VP will contain.

Similarly, the differing effects of two-complement and four-complement verbs could be seen as reflecting increased syntactic options, since the various types of embedded clauses have different syntactic structures, with only the four-complement verbs licensing embedded *wh*-clauses. A parser actively attempting to predict upcoming structure might well be affected by the difference between verbs which do and do not license embedded *wh*-clauses. And these distinctions among the four complement types seem far too removed from thematic assignment to license the claim that agrammatics have full access to "the thematic properties of verbs" (Shapiro, Gordon, Hack, & Killackey, 1993).

Finally, it is worth emphasizing that quantitive measures of complexity must be distinguished from specific mapping requirements. For example, appreciation that *cover* and *pour* are both associated with the argument structures $x<y>$ and $x<y,Pz>$ must be distinguished from appreciation that y is assigned the Goal role in *cover* (as in *He covered the box*) but the Theme role in *pour* (as in *She poured the wine*) and that z is assigned the Theme role in *cover* (as in *He covered the box with leaves*) but the Goal role in *pour* (as in *She poured the wine into the glass*), not to mention the difference in the prepositions which which z receives it role.

Thus it remains unclear exactly how to interpret Shapiro et al.'s tantalizing findings, but this line of research may ultimately narrow down the theoretical search space considerably.

Specific mapping deficit. One might claim that agrammatics are specifically impaired in the operations which link grammatical functions like subject with thematic roles like Agent. But, obviously, this cannot be correct in its strongest form given the generally good performance of agrammatics on simple active reversible sentences (in the absence of complicating factors such as those discussed in Saffran et al., submitted). However, it may still be the case that these linking operations are a point of particular fragility and that the mapping process is easily disrupted, especially by noncanonical order, additional arguments, reversibility, and linguistic properties of the sentence requiring the linkage of two elements in the structured word string held in memory.

Processing or memory impairments. Accounts based upon STM are complicated by the absence of correlations between verbal span and performance on syntactically complex materials (see, e.g., Martin & Feher, 1990; Saffran, 1990). Working memory impairments (see, e.g., Miyake, Carpenter, & Just, 1994) remain quite plausible but remain to be articulated in sufficiently compelling detail to resolve the issue. Finally, reports of delayed activation and/or rapid decay of syntactic information in agrammatic patients (e.g., Friederici & Kilborn, 1989; Haarmann & Kolk, 1991) represent another potential source for an explanation of the hypothesized failure to exploit an adequate parse; such accounts may combine features of both the mapping and the representational deficit accounts of agrammatism, but I include them under the rubric of the mapping hypothesis because they point to a failure to exploit, rather than a failure to build, representations of syntactic structure.

Closed class deficit. The strongest variants of the closed class hypothesis appear to have been disproved; agrammatic subjects, to cite one source of counterevidence, make very precise distinctions in grammaticality judgments involving function words and inflectional morphology, as detailed above. Nevertheless, it is worth noting that closed class elements are involved in all the "difficult" conditions of the grammaticality judgment task. Of course, this might represent an effect rather than a cause of the impairment: since closed class elements are the vehicle by which agreement and other dependencies between sentence elements are expressed, it is difficult to say whether difficulty with these elements creates or follows from a difficulty in maintaining the dependencies they encode. One might, however, appeal to some difficulty in retaining closed class elements in memory long enough to exploit them for further processing, in both the difficult conditions and in thematic linkage; but Friederici and Frazier (1992) provide evidence (*contra* a related suggestion in Linebarger, 1990) that Broca's aphasics are not significantly more impaired in the retention of function words than other vocabulary types.

5.3 *Evidence in Support of the Mapping Hypothesis*

The evidence in support of the mapping hypothesis has been discussed in previous sections and includes the grammaticality judgment–comprehension disparity—the fact that some agrammatics can judge the grammaticality of structures which they cannot comprehend—and the absence of a syntactic padding effect in the Schwartz et al. (1987) anomaly study. Also relevant to this claim are the preliminary reports of substantial treatment gains in a number of chronic agrammatic aphasics who have undergone a form of treatment known as mapping therapy (Byng, 1988; Byng & Black, 1989; Jones, 1986; Schwartz et al., 1994). Mapping therapy focuses exclusively upon training patients to associate syntactic positions with the thematic roles assigned to that position by a given verb, rather than, e.g., focusing upon the activation of syntactic structure *per se*. Should these encouraging reports be confirmed, for at least some subset of those patients termed agrammatic, they will provide further support for the claim of the mapping hypothesis that it is the relationship between syntax and semantics, rather than the recovery of syntactic structure itself, that is disturbed in these patients.

6. CONCLUSIONS

The agrammatic data reviewed here support the claim that parsing is psychologically distinct from interpretation, since agrammatics are able to parse sentences which they cannot reliably interpret. These data also license surprisingly fine-grained analyses of language processing, such as the distinctions we have been forced to make with regard to the processing of *wh* gaps.

On the basis of such findings, the mapping and the chain-disruption accounts are in agreement that these patients' grammatical representations are frequently impoverished at the level of what we may loosely term the coindexed parse. The two theories differ in their claims as to whether this impoverishment is at the root of the classical agrammatic comprehension impairment. According to the chain-disruption accounts, it is. I have argued against this much more desirable and constrained hypothesis on the following grounds. As Grodzinsky observed early on, the representational deficit by itself does not account for agrammatics' comprehension failures. The range of structures covered by the representational deficit is widened by Hickok and Mauner et al.'s use of the VP-internal subject hypothesis, but at the risk of making the chain-disruption account indistinguishable from other, nonrepresentational accounts, since every sentence in English now contains at least one trace-antecedent relationship. Even with this widening, the representational deficit fails to predict agrammatic comprehension. Therefore extragrammatical processes must be invoked. In order to maintain agrammatism as a structural deficit, the chain-disruption accounts must tie the invocation of these processes to representational failures and are forced into what I believe are unconvincing and contradictory modularity claims about the unavailability of linguistic information to other cognitive processes. Thus, I believe, the agrammatic data remain mute with regard to the choice among current theories of grammar.

REFERENCES

Berndt, R., Salasoo, A., Mitchum, C., & Blumstein, S. 1988. The role of intonation cues in aphasic patients' performance of the grammaticality judgment task. *Brain and Language*, **34**, 65–97.

Blumstein, S., Goodglass, H., Statlender, S., & Biber, C. 1983. Comprehension strategies determining reference in aphasia: A study of reflexivization. *Brain and Language*, **18**, 115–127.

Bresnan, J. 1982. The passive in lexical theory. In J. Bresnan (Ed.), *The mental representation of grammatical relations*. Cambridge, MA: MIT Press. Pp. 3–86.

Burton, S., & Grimshaw, J. 1992. Coordination and VP-internal subjects. *Linguistic Inquiry*, **23**, 305–313.

Byng, S. 1988. Sentence processing deficits: Theory and therapy. *Cognitive Neuropsychology*, **5**, 629–677.

Byng, S., & Black, M. 1989. Some aspects of sentence production in aphasia. *Aphasiology*, **2**, 241–263.

Caplan, D. 1995. Issues arising in contemporary studies of disorders of syntactic processing in sentence comprehension in agrammatic patients. *Brain and Language*, **50**, 324–337.

Caplan, D., & Futter, C. 1986. Assignment of thematic roles to nouns in sentence comprehension by an agrammatic patient. *Brain and Language*, **27**, 117–134.

Caplan, D., & Hildebrandt, N. 1986. Language deficits and the theory of syntax. A reply to Grodzinsky. *Brain and Language*, **27**, 168–177.

Caplan, D., & Hildebrandt, N. 1988. *Disorders of syntactic comprehension*. Cambridge, MA: MIT Press.

Caplan, D., Baker, C., & Dehaut, F. 1985. Syntactic determinants of sentence comprehension in aphasia. *Cognition*, **21**, 117–175.

Caramazza, A., & Miceli, G. 1991. Selective impairment of thematic role assignment in sentence processing. *Brain and Language*, **41**, 402–436.

Caramazza, A., & Zurif, E. 1976. Dissociation of algorithmic and heuristic processes in language comprehension: Evidence from aphasia. *Brain and Language*, **3**, 572–582.

Carlson, G., & Tanenhaus, M. 1988. Thematic roles and language comprehension. In W. Wilkins (Ed.), *Syntax and semantics 21: Thematic relations*. Cambridge, MA: MIT Press.

Chomsky, N. 1981. *Lectures on Government and Binding*. Dordrecht: Foris.

Chomsky, N. 1986. *Knowledge of language: Its nature, origin, and use*. New York: Praeger Publishers.

Frazier, L., & Clifton, C. 1989. Successive cyclicity in the grammar and the parser. *Language and Cognitive Processes*, **4**, 93–126.

Frazier, L., & Friederici, A. 1991. On deriving the properties of agrammatic comprehension: Syntactic structures and task demands. *Brain and Language*, **40**, 51–66.

Friederici, A., & Frazier, L. 1992. Thematic analysis in agrammatic comprehension: Syntactic structures and task demands. *Brain and Language*, **42**, 1–29.

Friederici, A., & Kilborn, K. 1989. Temporal constraints on language processing: Syntactic priming in Broca's aphasia. *Journal of Cognitive Neuroscience*, **1**, 262–272.

Goodglass, H., & Menn, L. 1985. Is agrammatism a unitary phenomenon? In M.-L. Kean (Ed.), *Agrammatism*. New York: Academic Press. Pp. 1–26.

Grimshaw, J. 1990. *Argument structure*. Cambridge, MA: MIT Press.

Grodzinsky, Y. 1984. *Language deficits and linguistic theory*. Ph.D. dissertation, Brandeis University, Waltham, MA.

Grodzinsky, J. 1986. Language deficits and the theory of syntax. *Brain and Language*, **27**, 135–159.

Grodzinsky, Y. 1989. Agrammatic comprehension of relative clauses. *Brain and Language*, **31**, 480–499.

Grodzinsky, Y. 1990. *Theoretical perspectives on language deficits*. Cambridge, MA: MIT Press.

Grodzinsky, Y. 1995. A restrictive theory of agrammatic comprehension. *Brain and Language*, **50**, 27–51.

Grodzinsky, Y., & Marek, A. 1988. Algorithmic and heuristic processes revisited. *Brain and Language*, **33**, 316–325.

Grodzinsky, Y., Wexler, K., Chien, Y.-C., Marakovitz, S., & Solomon, J. 1993. The breakdown of binding relations. *Brain and Language*, **45**, 396–422.

Grossman, M., & Haberman, S. 1982. Aphasics' selective deficits in appreciating grammatical agreements. *Brain and Language*, **161**, 109–120.

Haarmann, H., & Kolk, H. 1991. Syntactic priming in Broca's aphasia: Evidence for slow activation. *Aphasiology*, **5**, 247–263.

Heilman, K., & Scholes, R. 1976. The nature of comprehension errors in Broca's, conduction, and Wernicke's aphasics. *Cortex*, **12**, 258–265.

Hickok, G. 1992. *Agrammatic comprehension and the trace-deletion hypothesis*. Occasional Paper No. 45, MIT Center for Cognitive Science, MIT, Cambridge, MA.

Hickok, G., Zurif, E., & Canseco-Gonzales, E. 1993. Structural description of agrammatic comprehension. *Brain and Language*, **45**, 371–395.

Hickok, G., & Avrutin, S. 1994. *Comprehension of Wh-questions by two agrammatic Broca's aphasics*. Paper presented at the Fifth Annual Conference on Theoretical and Experimental Neuropsychology (TENNET), Montreal, Canada.

Jones, E. 1986. Building the foundations for sentence production in nonfluent aphasic. *British Journal of Disorders of Communication*, **21**, 63–82.

Kean, M.-L. 1977. The linguistic interpretation of aphasic syndromes: Agrammatism in Broca's aphasia, an example. *Cognition*, **5**, 9–46.

Kean, M.-L. 1981. Explanation in neurolinguistics. In N. Hornstein & D. Lightfood (Eds.), *Explanation in Linguistics*. London: Longman. Pp. 174–208.

Kitigawa, Y. 1986. *Subjects in Japanese and English*. Unpublished PhD dissertation, University of Massachusetts, Amherst, MA.

Kolk, H., & Weijts, M. 1995. Judgments of semantic anomaly in agrammatic patients: syntactic complexity, word-order heuristics, and variation over time. *Brain and Language*, in press.

Koopman, H., & Sportiche, D. 1988. *Subjects*. Unpublished manuscipt, UCLA.

Ladusaw, W. 1983. Logical form and conditions on grammaticality. *Linguistics and Philosophy*, **6**, 373–392.

Linebarger, M. 1987. Negative polarity and grammatical representation. *Linguistics & Philosophy*, **10**, 325–387.

Linebarger, M. 1989. Neuropsychological evidence for linguistic modularity. In G. Carlson & M. Tanenhaus (Eds.), *Linguistic Structure in Language Processing*. Dordrecht: Kluwer.

Linebarger, M. 1990. Neuropsychology of sentence parsing. In A. Caramazza (Ed.), *Cognitive neuropsychology and neurolinguistics: advances in models of cognitive function and impairment*. Hillsdale, NJ: Erlbaum. Pp. 55–122.

Linebarger, M. 1992. Negative polarity as linguistic evidence. In L. Dobrin, L. Nichols, & R. Rodriguez (Eds.), *CLS 27-II: Papers from the parasession on negation.* Chicago, IL. Pp. 165–188.

Linebarger, M., Schwartz, M., & Saffran, E. 1983a. Sensitivity to grammatical structure in so-called agrammatic aphasics. *Cognition,* 3, 361–392.

Linebarger, M., Schwartz, M., & Saffran, E. 1983b. Syntactic processing in agrammatism: A reply to Zurif and Grodzinsky. *Cognition,* 15, 207–213.

Lukatela, K., Crain, S., & Shankweiler, D. 1988. Sensitivity to inflectional morphology in agrammatism: Investigation of a highly inflected language. *Brain and Language,* 33, 1–15.

Marin, O., Saffran, E., & Schwartz, M. 1976. Dissociations of language in aphasia: Implications for normal function. *Annals of the New York Academy of Sciences,* 280, 868–884.

Martin, R., & Feher, E. 1990. The consequences of reduced memory span for the comprehension of semantic versus syntactic information. *Brain and Language,* 38, 1–20.

Martin, R., Wetzel, W., Blossom-Stach, C., & Feher, E. 1989. Syntactic loss versus processing deficit: An assessment of two theories of agrammatism and syntactic comprehension deficits. *Cognition,* 32, 57–191.

Mauner, G., Fromkin, V., & Cornell, T. 1993. Comprehension and acceptability judgments in agrammatism: Disruptions in the syntax of referential dependency. *Brain and Language,* 45, 340–370.

Mauner, G. 1995. Examining the empirical and linguistic bases of current theories of agrammatism. *Brain and Language,* 50, 338–367.

Miceli, G., Mazzuchi, A., Menn, L., & Goodglass, H. 1983. Contrasting cases of Italian agrammatic aphasia without comprehension disorder. *Brain and Language,* 19, 65–97.

Miyake, A., Carpenter, P., & Just, M. 1994. A capacity approach to syntactic comprehension disorders: Making normal adults perform like aphasics. *Cognitive Neuropsychology,* 11, 671–717.

Saffran, E. 1990. Short-term memory impairment and language processing. In A. Caramazza (Ed.), *Cognitive neuropsychology and neurolinguistics: Advances in models of cognitive function and impairment.* Hillsdale, NJ: Erlbaum.

Saffran, E., Schwartz, M., & Linebarger, M. *Semantic influences on thematic role assignment: Evidence from normals and aphasics.* Submitted for publication.

Saffran, E., Schwartz, M., & Marin, O. 1980. The word order problem in agrammatism. II. Production. *Brain and Language,* 10, 263–280.

Schwartz, M., Linebarger, M., Saffran, E., & Pate, D. 1987. Syntactic transparency and sentence interpretation in aphasia. *Language and Cognitive Processes,* 2, 85–113.

Schwartz, M., Saffran, E., Fink, R., Myers, J., & Martin, N. 1994. Mapping therapy: A treatment program for agrammatism. *Aphasiology,* 8, 19–54.

Schwartz, M., Saffran, E., & Marin, O. 1980. The word order problem in agrammatism. I. Comprehension. *Brain and Language,* 10, 249–262.

Shankweiler, D., Crain, S., Gorrell, P., & Tuller, B. 1989. Reception of language in Broca's aphasia. *Language and Cognitive Processes,* 4, 1–33.

Shapiro, L., Gordon, B., Hack, N., & Killackey, J. 1993. Verb-argument structure processing in complex sentences in Broca's and Wernicke's aphasia. *Brain and Language,* 45, 423–447.

Shapiro, L., Zurif, E., & Grimshaw, J. 1987. Sentence processing and the mental representation of verbs. *Cognition,* 27, 219–246.

Sherman, J., & Schweickert, J. 1989. Syntactic and semantic contributions to sentence interpretation in agrammatism. *Brain and Language,* 37, 419–439.

Stowe, L. 1986. Parsing WH-constructions: Evidence for on-line gap location. *Language and Cognitive Processes,* 1, 227–245.

Stowell, T. 1981. *Origins of phrase structure.* PhD dissertation, MIT.

Woolford, E. 1991. VP-internal subjects in VSO and nonconfigurational languages. *Linguistic Inquiry*, **2**, 503–540.

Wulfeck, B. 1988. Grammaticality judgments and sentence comprehension in agrammatic aphasia. *Journal of Speech & Hearing Research*, **31**, 72–81.

Zurif, E., & Grodzinsky, Y. 1983. Sensitivity to grammatical structure in agrammatic aphasia: A reply to Linebarger, Schwartz, & Saffran. *Cognition, 15*, 207–213.

Zurif, E., Swinney, D., Prather, P., Solomon, J., & Bushnell, C. 1993. An on-line analysis of syntactic processing in Broca's and Wernicke's aphasia. *Brain and Language*, **45**, 448–464.

BRAIN AND LANGUAGE **50,** 135–150 (1993)

Variables and Events in the Syntax
of Agrammatic Speech

J. Douglas Saddy

*Program in Cognitive Science, Departments of Psychology and English (Linguistics),
University of Queensland, Queensland, Australia*

This paper examines aggrammatics' interpretation of quantificationally ambiguous sentences. Although agrammatics are capable of recognizing quantificational ambiguities, they ascribe nonstandard entailments to those sentences involving universal quantification. Since quantificational ambiguity arises from movement of quantifiers at LF, doubt is cast on accounts of agrammatic behavior that rely on an inability to interpret moved constituents. Furthermore, the agrammatics are seen to improve in their thematic interpretation of arguments in reversible passive constructions and relatives if one of the arguments is universally quantified. The nonstandard entailments and improved performance on passive and relatives are accounted for via an elaboration of event semantics in which we propose that the agrammatic treats the event variable associated with a verb as nominal. © 1995 Academic Press, Inc.

The interpretation of quantificational or scopal dependencies in language impaired individuals is an area that has not received much attention. Much more has been written about the interpretation of thematic dependencies and referential dependencies.

Agrammatic Broca's aphasics are commonly characterized as suffering from a comprehension deficit that renders them unable to reliably determine "who did what to whom" in sentence constructions that involve phrases displaced from their canonical sentence positions. There are three main accounts of this behavior. (a) An interaction between the complexity of the sentence structure and a diminution of computation resources; with reduced resources adaptive strategies are called on in response to structurally complex sentences (see Caplan, Baker, & Dehaut, 1985; Caplan & Futter, 1986; Caplan and Hildebrandt, 1988; Haarman & Kolk 1991; Friederici & Frasier, 1992). (b) An inability to associ-

Address reprint requests to J. Douglas Saddy, Program in Cognitive Science, Departments of Psychology and English (Linguistics), University of Queensland, Queensland 4072, Australia.

267

ate the displaced phrase with its Deep Structure position; a failure to generate or respect the requirements of empty categories and/or chains (see Grodzinsky 1984, 1986, 1989, 1990, 1991; Zurif & Grodzinsky, 1983; Mauner, Fromkin & Cornell, 1993). (c) An inability to assign thematic roles to displaced phrases, although the empty categories are present in the syntactic representation (see Linebarger, Schwartz, & Saffran, 1983a,b; Saffran, Schwartz, & Marin, 1980); Schwartz, Saffran, & Marin, 1980; Schwartz, Linebarger, Saffran & Pate, 1987).

The model of grammar we are assuming here derives the scope of a quantificational operator (negation, quantification, interrogation, relative, etc.) from its c-command domain. The possibility of quantificational scope ambiguity is attributed to the application of movement to quantified expressions in the mapping from S-structure to LF (see Chomsky, 1981, 1986a, 1986b; May, 1977, 1985). Under such a theory the formal properties of the abstract structures associated with scopal sentences will involve displaced phrases and variables bound to the "moved" quantified expressions. Thus the investigation of the comprehension of scopally ambiguous sentences can be relevant to the evaluation of the theories of impaired performance outlined above.

The data reported here are derived from results obtained using a structured test paradigm developed by the author to examine a range of phenomena associated with the processing of the closed class or functional vocabulary. It involves three types of tasks:

1. Sentence picture verification task: This task looks at both traditional comprehension abilities with respect to passive relatives and raising constructions as well as comprehension of quantificationally ambiguous sentences, nominal and verbal agreement phenomena.

2. Insertion task: This task targets the subjects' knowledge of formal properties of lexical items and their ability to integrate such information into a parse tree.

3. Well-formedness judgment task: This task systematically examines the subjects' sensitivity to both S-structure and LF island type effects (i.e., subjacency, ecp, and superiority effects) as well as word order, argument structure, and auxiliary selection. Agreement beyond verbal agreement for person and number and nominal agreement for number is not tested.

Performance on the traditional items in the third task is used to screen subjects for further testing. That is, subjects must perform at chance or worse on reversible passives, object-relatives, and raising to be included as agrammatic subjects for further testing. In addition, subjects must be able to recognize the ambiguity in a simplified sentence picture matching task involving sentences such as "every square touches a circle" and "a square touches every circle."

All subjects tested to date do extremely well on the well-formedness judgment task. All subjects have shown similar performance on the insertion task. That is, they perform well on any insertions involving the nominal or propositional paradigm (i.e., insertion of determiners, demonstratives, quantifiers, and complementizers) but perform very poorly on insertions involving the verbal paradigm (i.e., modals, auxiliaries, and verbal negation).

Testing

This paper will detail only the aspects of the sentence picture verification task relevant to quantificational ambiguities. Details of the well-formedness judgment task and the insertion task can be found in Saddy (1992).

Picture Verification

The subjects are tested using a picture verification task. In this task subjects are presented with the five sentences that represent the possible combinations of indefinite and universal expressions associated with the reversible transitive verbs: photograph, film, call, see, and spray. For example:

A child photographed every man

Every man photographed a child

A man photographed every child

Every child photographed a man

A child photographed a man

In addition sentences using the expressions "touch," "above," and "below" are used in training and screening procedures in association with pictures that involve only geometric shapes. For example, every square is touching a circle, etc.

For each quantificationally ambiguous sentence four picture verifications are employed in order to test the subjects' fundamental appreciation of the ambiguities. Two accurately depict the sentence, one for each scope order. The other two pictures are false to the sentence, one for each scope order. For example, for the sentence "A child photographed every man," there is one picture in which one child is photographing a group of men and another picture in which a different child is photographing each of the men. Both of these pictures are true to the sentence. The first picture represents the reading in which the existential, a child, is interpreted as having wide scope with respect to the universal, every man. The second picture represents the reading in which the universal, every man is interpreted as having wide scope with respect to the existential, a child. The pictures that were false to the sentence also display scopal ambiguity. One false picture shows a child photographing a group of men but there is also a man standing to the side who is not being photographed. This picture partially maintains the wide scope interpretation of the existential but is false to the sentence. The other false picture shows a different child photographing each of the men but again there is a man who is not being photographed. This picture partially maintains the wide scope interpretation of the universal but is false to the sentence.

In addition, for each sentence the subject is presented with the set of four pictures which depict thematically reversed relations, i.e., pictures in which men photographing children are presented with sentences which refer to children photographing men.

Foils

In order to test the subjects' ability to interpret the properties of the individual quantifiers and to examine the interpretation given to the test sentences beyond the level of thematic content, foils were added to the inventory of pictures presented with each sentence. The foils involve adding an activity not mentioned in the test sentence to the picture. The pictures involving foils were always true to the sentence. They are designed to determine how the universally quantified expression is being understood and how the universal affects the interpretation of the sentence as a whole. Part of this information is revealed in the simple sentence picture verification tasks since failure to respect the completeness requirement on the complement to the universal would lead to acceptance of pictures in which "not all x" are involved when the sentence specifies "every x". The foils for sentences with a universally quantified subject differ from the foils for sentences with a universally quantified object.

For example, for a sentence with a universally quantified subject such as "every man filmed a child" the foils would be

1. A woman filming a child who is not being filmed by a man
2. A woman filming a child who is also being filmed by a man
3. A woman filming a potted plant
4. A woman waving
5. An extra child who is not being filmed

1 and 2 above test the subjects' interpretation of the inclusiveness of the verb phrase. 3, 4 and 5 above test for exclusiveness of interpretation of the verbal event.

For a sentence with a universally quantified object such as "a man filmed every child" the foils would be

1. A man filming a potted plant
2. A woman filming a potted plant
3. A woman filming a child who is also being filmed by a man
4. A woman waving
5. A man waving

1, 2, and 3 above test the subjects' interpretation of the inclusiveness of the verb phrase. 4 and 5 above test for exclusiveness of interpretation of the verbal event.

Thus for sentences involving universal quantification there are six false and seven true pictures: four false due to thematic reversal, two false due to incompleteness, two true without foils, and five true with foils.

For sentences involving only existentials there are three false and six true: two false due to thematic reversal and one false due to inappropriate action, one true without foils, and five true with foils.

There are five verbs used giving a total of 175 picture verifications: 100 trues and 75 falses.

The stimuli sentences are presented in both the active and the passive voice; hence, the picture inventory is given twice. In addition a restricted inventory of relative constructions is tested. Six sentences per verb with a total of 100 picture verifications, 50 true, 50 false, with a total of 450 decisions, 250 trues and 200 falses. They are presented in a pseudorandom order in 10 blocks of 45.

Subjects

Three subjects have been investigated in varying depths. Two are currently under study. All show a compatible pattern of performance on the tests reported here. Subject JA, the first investigated, has been most thoroughly documented to date. I will present his performance as representative.

JA suffered a left middle cerebral artery aneurysm at age 40, 5 years prior to testing. He is a right-handed male with no familial history of left handedness. He has a BA in Fine Arts and at the time of his aneurysm was manager of a retail store. JA's extensive lesion involved both Broca's and Wernicke's areas. At the time of the trauma JA was globally aphasic and gradually resolved to an agrammatic Broca's,[1] his present condition.

In screening tests JA performed worse than chance on reversible passives, object-relatives, and raising constructions and had a 30% error rate on subject-relatives.

Basic Findings

(A) JA is capable of recognizing both scope readings associated with quantificationally ambiguous sentences.

The subjects are presented with 230 sentence picture verifications involving quantificationally ambiguous sentences, i.e., "every child films a man", "a woman sprays every child" etc. JA made virtually no errors

---

[1] The diagnosis of agrammatism has been made on the basis of JA's performance on tests of production and comprehension carried out by speech pathologists and his attending neurologist and has been confirmed by our own studies.

(>95% correct) in accepting or rejecting pictures that corresponded or failed to correspond to either scope reading. None of the errors corresponded to thematic reversals.

(B) JA ascribes nonstandard entailments to quantificationally ambiguous sentences involving universal quantification.

JA's responses to pictures involving foils show that both scope readings are available but are systematically accepted or rejected in a way that reflects a nonstandard interpretation of the sentence. Sentences such as "every child films a man" are interpreted as "every child films a man" (either scope order) and "every filmer must be a child" while sentences such as "a child films every man" are interpreted as "a child films every man" (either scope order) and "every filmee must be a man."

(C) JA's comprehension of reversible passives improved when one of the arguments is universally quantified.

In response to reversible passive sentences that contained universally quantified expressions, i.e., "every x", there were *no* errors in thematic reversal while acceptance of thematically reversed pictures was the characteristic error in the nonquantified counterparts. Thus sentences such as (i) resulted in errors of entailment as described in B but improved recognition of the thematic roles played by the actors while sentences such as (ii) resulted in no errors of entailment but apparent lack of sensitivity to thematic roles.

(i) Every man was photographed by a child

(ii) A man was photographed by a child

These results present a challenge for some aspects of current theories of agrammatism. While the traditional approaches make no direct claim with regard to quantificational ambiguities the spirit of their respective approaches would predict that the ability to recognize multiple interpretations would be lost in agrammatism. Moreover, none of the approaches predicts that the introduction of a universally quantified expression to a passive construction will improve an agrammatic's comprehension (however, see Grodzinsky's article in this issue) nor do they suggest a mechanism for explaining the unusual entailment conditions associated with universally quantified expressions.

Characterizing Agrammatism: Sensitivity to Predicate Types

This remarkable pattern of systematic behavior in response to quantificational constructions presents a telling picture of the receptive aspect of agrammatism. It is instructive in both what it reveals about retained abilities in agrammatism and what it reveals about the nature of the agrammatic's comprehension deficit. The fact that JA correctly recognizes and rejects the pictures that correspond to both scope readings associated with the stimuli sentences reveals that the ability to form LF representations involving chains, that is, the ability to respect the grammatical requirement for Quantifier Raising, can be retained. Thus we have additional evidence that (some) analytic linguistic processes are preserved in agrammatism.

The systematic misapprehension of the logical interpretation of sentences involving universal quantifiers provides contrasting evidence of an impairment at the analytic level. The interpretation assigned to such sentences clearly reveals a sensitivity to syntactic analysis since the interpretation reflects whether it is the subject or object that is universally quantified. In addition, the fact that JA's interpretation of reversible passive sentences improved when a universally quantified argument appears in such constructions also provides evidence of the availability of a syntactic analysis of passive constructions. The pattern of behavior seems contradictory. The impaired interpretations are analytic in flavor but they rely on a well-formed syntactic analysis. It appears that a purely syntactic account will be impossible.

In what follows I will try to motivate an account that characterizes the impairment as essentially semantic. I will argue that the agrammatics give a nominal interpretation to verbs. The evidence from scope interpretation, grammaticality judgments, etc., shows that at the syntactic level the agrammatics do not mistake verbs for nouns. However, the pattern of comprehension seen here is compatible with the idea that at the level of analytic compositional semantics the agrammatics treat verbs as having nominal characteristics.

The approach advanced here relies upon the idea that NPs and VPs are similar in that they are both nonreferential predicates and both require "binding" in order to achieve interpretation. This idea is associated with recent elaborations of Davidsonian event semantics, a topic not belabored here (see Davidson, 1966; Higginbotham, 1985; Parsons, 1990). A simple exposition of the relevant properties can be found by considering the consequences of adopting a Determiner Phrase (DP) representation. The Determiner Phrase replaces the traditional notion of a Noun Phrase. It reflects the assertion that what gives a nominal expression its reference is the nominal functor (i.e., determiner, demonstrative, possessive, quantifier, etc.) that is associated with the nominal. The DP consists, minimally, of a D-type head and a complement nominal expression, usually denoted NP. Note that this new NP notation differs from the traditional notion in that the term NP under the Determiner Phrase Hypothesis denotes a phrase headed by a noun and containing the (optional) syntactic expression of the noun's argument structure but does not contain a determiner. This provides a parallelism between NP and VP in that both of these constituents achieve interpretation by being associated with a functor: modals or auxiliaries in the case of VP and determiners or quantifiers in the case of NP. The relation "associated with" is considered to be a type of binding of an event or $<e>$ position (Higginbotham, 1983, 1985) that is associated with all predicates. The binding of such variables in a sentence is obligatory for the sentence to obtain an interpretation (where "obtain an interpretation" usually means be assigned a truth value).

The term "event" is misleading. It was coined in the original discussions of verb interpretations and has been carried over to refer to the abstract referring variable associated with nouns. Perhaps a more perspicuous term would be $<r>$ position. I will use that here since $<e>$ will become confused with a notation for empty category.

The status of a predicate as verbal or nominal depends upon the type of the $<r>$ position. Thus both nouns and verbs are predicted to have associated argument structure with the optionality of syntactically expressing that argument structure dependent upon the type of the referring variable position (syntactic expression of argument structure is optimal with nominal referring variables).

The characterization of the impairment offered here is that the agrammatic treats verbal $<r>$ variables as nominal for the purposes of referential binding. Nominal operators like the universal quantifiers in the sentences under discussion act as proxy binders for the $<r>$ variable associated with verbs. I will argue that the properties outlined above as well as some of the traditional characteristics associated with agrammatism follow from this characterization.

Unusual Entailments

This characterization of the agrammatic's impairment allows an explanatory account of the peculiar performance on sentences involving universal quantification. The interpretation of sentences involving universal quantification is that the universal term is linked to the event. These interpretations are attested by the subjects' systematic rejection and acceptance of various foil constructions.

In the case of sentences with universally quantified subjects such as "every child films a man", which is interpreted as "every child films a man and every filmer must be a child," the agrammatics reject any pictures involving foils in which anything/anyone other than the universally quantified nominal is engaged in filming. Foils such as a woman filming a potted plant or one of the men for example are rejected. In the case of sentences with universally quantified objects such as "a child films every man" which is interpreted as "a child films every man and every filmee must be a man," the agrammatics reject any pictures involving foils in which anything other than the universally quantified nominal is being filmed. Foils such as a woman filming a man or a man filming a man are accepted but a foil such as an extra child filming a plant is rejected.

The "and" in the interpretations is important. The agrammatics understand and respect the scope relations that hold between the universal and the existential. The fact that the interpretation of these sentences reflects whether the universal expression is in subject or object position shows that the interpretation is not adverbial such as "always, a child films a man" or "always, a woman films a child" or "every event is a child filming man event", etc.[2] It is clear from this behavior that the interpretation is consistent with one in which the universally quantified term is used to bind the referring variable associated with the verb. The consequence of this is that the universal operator ranges over both instances of the nominal and instances of the expression of the verb. This gives rise to the following interpretations.

The mechanism by which the $<r>$ variable comes into the scope of the universal is Quantifier Raising (QR). We know from the fact that the agrammatics recognize both scope readings and from their sensitivity to well-formendness judgments involving LF movement that Quantifier Raising (or its equivalent) is available. At Logical Form (LF) after the application of Quantifier Raising, the universal expression will always c-command both its variable and the $<r>$ variable associated with the verb regardless of whether the universal term is subject or object. QR will adjoin the universal expression to a position that has the VP in its scope. In the case of quantified phrases in S-structure subject position LF adjunction is to IP. There are two adjunction positions available to quantified phrases in S-structure object position: adjoined to VP or adjoined to IP. In all cases the QP c-commands the verb.

SS: [[every child] [films $<r>$ [a man]]]
LF: [[every child]$_i$ [e$_i$[films $<r>$ [a man]]]]

SS: [[a woman] [sprays $<r>$ [every child]]]
LF: [[every child]$_i$ [[a woman] [sprays $<r>$ e$_i$]]]
    [[a woman] [[every child]$_i$ [sprays $<r>$ e$_i$]]]

Given that the quantified expression will always c-command the $<r>$ position at LF, what is the nature of the binding relation? If it is the case that agrammatics are treating verbal $<r>$ variables as nominal there is already a mechanism at hand to account for the relation, unselective binding.

Under the extended Davidsonian characterization adopted here both nouns and verbs have an $<r>$ variable position. It has been argued (see Heim, 1982; Higginbotham, 1987) that the $<r>$ variable of indefinite expressions is not bound by the indefinite article; that is, the indefinite

---

[2] This adverbial interpretation has recently been identified in young children's interpretation of quantified sentences by Philip and Crain P.C.

article does not qualify as a "binder." Indefinite expressions therefore may be viewed as containing a free variable. Heim (1982) gives examples like the following:

In every case, if a table has lasted for 50 years, it will last for another 50.

If a person falls from the fifth floor, s/he will very rarely survive.

Heim points to the fact that in the above examples the quantificational force of the indefinite expressions varies with the adverbial expressions. These sentences can be paraphrased as "Every table that has lasted for 50 years will last for another 50." and "Very few people that fall from the fifth floor survive." Thus "a table" is interpreted as "every table" and "a person" is interpreted as "few people" (see Heim, 1982; Lewis, 1975). In Heim's terms, "indefinite expressions resemble variables more than quantifiers." They "have no quantificational force of their own at all, but are rather like variables, which may get bound by whatever quantifier is there to bind them" (Heim 1982, p. 127).

Heim refers to this relation as unselective binding. Heim argues that unselective binding and a related operation, existential closure, which applies if there is no quantificational operator available, provide for the necessary binding of free nominal $<r>$ variables in indefinites in order that an interpretation can be obtained.

This characterization of the quantificational interpretation of indefinites in the normal grammar serves also to characterize the agrammatic's peculiar interpretation of sentences containing universally quantified terms. If the agrammatic treats verbal $<r>$ variables as nominal, then for the agrammatic a VP and an indefinite NP will have the same status with respect to referential binding. Both represent variables that can be bound by an available quantifier. Since the agrammatic treats the verbal $<r>$ variable as nominal, the verbal $<r>$ binders in a syntactic representation do not serve to bind the VP predicate. This means that no interpretation or truth value can be ascribed to the proposition determined by the verbal predicate and its arguments. However, if at the level of Logical Form a quantifier acts as a proxy binder for the verb's predicate argument, a truth value may be assigned to the representation. In the sentences investigated here there is an unusual property associated with the universal expression binding the verbal event predicate; the binder of the $<r>$ variable is also an argument of the verb. Thus in a sentence such as "a man filmed every child", the operator construed as binding the verb's $<r>$ variable is also the operator binding "child." The result of this connection is that the proposition described by the verb and its arguments can be assigned a truth value just in case the events of filming are instances of filming children.

Notice that the mechanisms of thematic role assignment are not disengaged. "Every child" is still the internal argument of "film" and "a man" is still the external argument of "film." Notice also that the scopal ambiguities will still follow. Nothing prevents the existential term from being interpreted as wide with respect to the universal expression.

The interpretation of "every man films a child" follows in the same fashion. Here a truth value can be assigned to the proposition described by the verb and its arguments just in case all filming events are also filming by men events.

We have accounted for the readings the agrammatic assigns to sentences of the form "every x verbs a y" and "a x verbs every y." The account carries over in a straightforward way to the agrammatic's performance on passives. Recall that the agrammatic performs at chance on passives that involve only existential terms but does much better on passives that involve a universal term.

Passives

We can account for the agrammatic's good performance on the passive constructions involving universally quantified terms in the same manner as we dealt with the other universally quantified constructions. After quantifier raising applies to the universally quantified expression unselective binding of the misconstrued <r> variable is possible. Once the event position in the passive construction becomes bound the interpretation of the expression follows. Notice that we are assuming that the assignment of thematic roles proceeds normally in these cases. The chain formed by passive movement is interpreted as bearing the patient role. The event is saturated through its association with the universal operator and hence has a truth value. The adjunct PP determines the optional realization of agent and is incorporated into the meaning of the sentence.

We are lacking, however, an account of why the agrammatic's performance on passives without universals should be as it is. Why should he accept pictures in which the thematic roles are reversed in just these cases?

Heim's analysis demonstrated that existentials can contain free variables; thus we cannot expect an existential expression like "a child" to act as a proxy binder since it needs binding itself in order to be interpreted. If indefinites cannot behave like operators for the agrammatic then his performance on passives involving only indefinite expressions is less puzzling. However, the explanation of the behavior is not entirely transparent.

As we noted above, in order to assign a truth value to a representation all the <r> variables in that representation must be bound. In the case of nominals the <r> variables can be bound internal to the sentence's representation either locally by the appropriate nominal functor or via unselective binding of an indefinite by a c-commanding quantificational operator within the sentential representation or by existential closure which invokes an arbitrary existential interpretation. Existential closure is seen as an operation external to the sentential representation in that it is invoked if a free referring variable remains at interpretation. There is no counterpart to existential closure for the normal verbal paradigm.

For the agrammatic, in the case of passives that do not contain any universal terms, existential closure will be the only option to gain a truth value for the passive construction. By hypothesis, the verbal $<r>$ variable is not bound by the verbal functors internal to the representation and unselective binding of the verbs $<r>$ variable by a c-commanding quantified phrase is not available. Furthermore the nominal $<r>$ variables associated with the indefinite arguments will not be bound internally for the same reasons. Thus, as for normals, existential closure must be invoked for at least one of the indefinites. The difference is that for the agrammatic, existential closure can apply to any or all of three $<r>$ variables:

1. The nominal $<r>$ associated with the noun in subject position
2. The nominal $<r>$ associated with the noun in object position
3. The $<r>$ associated with the verb

The effect of existential closure is to assert the arbitrary reference of the $<r>$ variable. For the agrammatic, applying this to an $<r>$ variable associated with the verb will assert an arbitrary instance. For example, some filming happened or some spraying happened. In the case of existential closure the binding of the $<r>$ variable is not related to the argument structure of the verb. It is external to the sentence altogether. Thus the thematic information associated with the arguments of the verb need not be related to the interpretation of the $<r>$ variable. Therefore an agrammatic facing a reversible passive with no quantified arguments will have two possible interpretations.

For a sentence such as:

a child was filmed by a man,

1. the reading associated with the distribution of thematic roles; child–filmer, man–filmee; or
2. the reading associated with existential closure applying directly to the verb: there was a filming.

The information that filming involves a filmer and a filmee will be available to the agrammatic and the fact that "a man" and "a child" are present in the representation will also be available. The outcome of this is that the agrammatic will know much about the thematic relations relevant to the sentence but will be at doubt as to whether a child being a patient and a man being the agent of "film" is necessarily related to the event of filming portrayed. His performance in the sentence picture matching paradigm is therefore true to his interpretation. It is either the case that a child was filmed by a man or it is the case that there was a filming that involved a man and a child.

In support of this, it has been noted that in grammaticality judgments on implausible passive constructions like 'the boy was eaten by the apple' agrammatics accept the sentences as grammatical but recognize that the sentence is peculiar. This supports the idea that the agrammatic is getting the thematic relations determined by the structure of the sentence but his impairment leads him to an ambiguous interpretation.[3]

SUMMARY AND EPILOGUE

The linguistic analysis of agrammatic comprehension has focused on the problem agrammatics exhibit with displaced arguments. The nature of this behavior suggests some compromise of the mechanisms of chain formation or chain construal. This paper presents some new data relevant to the analysis of agrammatism. It is clearly the case that chain formation and chain construal will play a role in the linguistic characterization of this new data. Chain formation and construal are essential elements of scope interpretation. However, it is not immediately clear that chain formation and/or construal will be adequate to also provide an account of the change in entailment properties associated with sentences involving universal quantification. Does this mean that we should introduce a second area of fundamental impairment? That is, should we propose that agrammatism involves an inability to appropriately deal with chain relations (however they are to be described) plus an inability to correctly determine certain aspects of logical entailment? To do so would be to suggest that these two aspects of behavior are unrelated. The data at hand suggest otherwise.

One of the themes addressed in papers in this volume is the relevance of reference to questions of agrammatic receptive behavior. In this paper an alternative approach is sketched to characterize the comprehension deficit that directly exploits formal notions associated with reference. The conceptual approach advanced here is that agrammatic comprehension involves a kind of nominalization, a notion that can be traced back at least as far as Jakobson (1941). It is clear that a literal interpretation of this hypothesis is untenable. Agrammatics do not behave as if they think that verbs are literally nouns, as their ability to perform grammaticality judgments and their comprehension abilities demonstrate. However, nominalizing behavior is widely observed with agrammatic subjects. In addition, the kinds of receptive behavior found in agrammatism can also

[3] For reasons of brevity the analysis of agrammatic interpretation of relative clauses will not be discussed. The treatment is similar to that of passives; however, interesting questions are raised by the role of the relative operator.

be found mimicked in normal comprehension of complex nominalized constructions. For example, in nominalized verb constructions the expression of the verb's argument structure is optional and when it is partially expressed the thematic role is ambiguous, i.e., in the complex nominal *the vandals' destruction* the interpretation of "the vandals" is either as the agent or the patient of the nominalized "destroy." Complex nominals do not support relativization nor do complex nominals support referential Wh-extraction (of course nonreferential Wh-extraction is not good either).

The normal interpretation of gerundive or acc -ing noun phrases containing universally quantified expressions also supports the claim that nominalization is in part responsible for the agrammatics' unusual entailments. Such complex nominal constructions contain a free variable which is seen to interact with universal quantifiers in a systematic way. If the sentence picture verification stimuli sentences are changed to acc -ing gerundive noun phrases containing universally quantified expressions, undergraduate psychology students show a pattern of interpretation that is very close to that of the agrammatics. For a sentential stimulus such as *in this picture, a child photographs every man* the undergraduates accept all of the foil pictures described above including those rejected by the agrammatics. However, if the stimulus is changed to a nominalized form as in *this is a picture of a child photographing every man* the undergraduates tend to reject the same pictures involving foils that the agrammatics reject. Thus the entailments associated with the normal interpretation of complex nominals involving universal quantification correspond to the agrammatics' comprehension of full clauses involving universal quantification.

The above observations suggest that some aspect of nominalization may be relevant to the range of receptive impairments found in agrammatism. This implies that the centrality of chain phenomena to the characterization of agrammatics' receptive behavior is a consequence of a deeper semantic confusion. The approach proposed here claims that it is in the domain of analytic semantics that the notion of nominalization is relevant: the agrammatic treats verbal event variables as nominal when deriving the compositional semantics of a syntactic representation. As a result the unusual entailments presented here and the interpretation of sentences involving displaced arguments are seen to follow.

REFERENCES

Caplan, D., Baker, C., & Dehaut, F. 1985. Syntactic determinants of sentence comprehension in aphasia. In M. L. Kean (Ed.), *Agrammatism*. New York: Academic Press.
Caplan, D., & Futter, C. 1986. Assignment of thematic roles to nouns in sentence comprehension by an agrammatic patient. *Brain and Language, 27,* 117–134.

Caplan, D., & Hildebrandt, N. 1988. *Disorders of syntactic comprehension,* Cambridge, MA: MIT Press.

Chomsky, N. 1986a. *Knowledge of language.* Praeger: Convergence.

Chomsky, N. 1986b. *Barriers.* Linguistic Inquiry Monograph 13, MIT Press.

Chomsky, N. 1981. *Lectures on Government and Binding.* Dordrecht: Foris.

Davidson, D. 1967. The logical form of action sentences. In N. Rescher (Ed.), *The logic of decision and action.* Pittsburgh: University of Pittsburgh Press. Pp. 105–122.

Friederici, A., & Frazier, L. 1992. Thematic analysis in agrammatic comprehension: Syntactic structures and task demands. *Brain and Language,* **42,** 1–29.

Grodzinsky, Y. 1984. The syntactic characterization of agrammatism. *Cognition,* 16, 99–120.

Grodzinsky, Y. 1986. Language deficits and the theory of syntax. *Brain and Language,* **27,** 135–159.

Grodzinsky, Y. 1989. Agrammatic comprehension of relative clauses. *Brain and Language,* **34,** 480–499.

Grodzinsky Y. 1990. *Theoretical perspectives on language deficits.* Cambridge, MA: MIT Press.

Grodzinsky, Y. 1991. Neuropsychological reasons for a transformational analysis of verbal passive. *Natural Language and Linguistic Theory,* **9,** 431–453.

Haarman, H. J., Kolk, H. H. J. 1991. A computer model of the temporal course of agrammatic sentence understanding: The effects of variation in severity and sentence complexity. *Cognitive Science,* **15,** 49–87.

Heim, I. R. 1982. *The semantics of definite and indefinite noun phrases.* Ph.D dissertation, University of Massachusetts, Amherst, MA.

Higginbotham, J. 1983. Logical form, binding, and nominals. *Linguistic Inquiry,* **14,** 3.

Higginbotham, J. 1985. On semantics. *Linguistic Inquiry,* **16,** 4.

Higginbotham, J. 1987. Indefiniteness and predication. In *The representation of indefiniteness.* E. J. Reuland, & A. G. B. ter Meulen (Eds.), MIT Press.

Jakobson, R. 1941. *Kindersprache, Aphasie und Allgemeine Lautgesetze.* Universitets Arsskrift, Uppsala. Translated as *Child Language, Aphasia and Phonological Universals.* Mouton, The Hague, 1968.

Lewis, D. 1975. Adverbs of quantification. In E. Keenan (Ed.), *Formal semantics of natural language.* Cambridge University Press.

Linebarger, M. C., Schwartz, M. F., & Saffran, E. M. 1983a. Sensitivity to grammatical structure in so-called agrammatic aphasics. *Cognition,* **13,** 361–392.

Linebarger, M., Schwartz, M., & Saffran E. 1983b. Syntactic processing in agrammatism: A reply to Zurif and Grodzinsky. *Cognition,* **15,** 207–213.

Linebarger, M. 1989. Neuropsychological evidence for linguistic modularity. In G. Carlson & M. Tanenhaus (Eds.), *Linguistic Structure in Language Processing.* Dordrecht: Kluwer.

Mauner, G., Fromkin, V., and Cornell, T. 1993. Comprehension and acceptability judgments in agrammatism: Disruptions in the syntax of referential dependency. *Brain and Language,* **45,** 340–370.

May, R. C. 1977. *The grammar of quantification.* Ph.D. dissertation, Massachusetts Institute of Technology, Cambridge, MA.

May, R. 1985. *Logical form: Its structure and derivation.* Cambridge, MA: MIT Press.

Parsons, T. 1990. *Events in the semantics of English: A study in subatomic semantics.* Cambridge, MA: MIT Press.

Saddy, J. D. 1990. *Investigations into grammatical knowledge.* PhD dissertation, Massachusetts Institute of Technology, Cambridge, MA.

Saddy, J. D. 1992. Sensitivity to islands in an aphasic individual. In *Island constraints: Theory, acquisition and processing,* H. Goodluck & M. Rochemeont (Eds.), Kluwer Academic Publishers, ISBN 0-7923-1689-4. Pp. 399–417.

Saffran, E. M., Schwartz, M. F., & Marin, O. S. M. 1980. "The word order problem in Agrammatism. I. Comprehension." *Brain and Language,* **7,** 277–306.

Schwartz, M. F., Linebarger, M. C., Saffran, E. M., & Pate, D. S. 1987. Syntactic transparency and sentence interpretation in aphasia. *Language and Cognitive Processes,* **2**(2), 85–113.

Zurif, E., & Grodzinsky, Y. 1983. Sensitivity to grammatical structure in agrammatic aphasia: A reply to Linebarger, Schwartz, & Saffran. *Cognition,* **15,** 207–213.

BRAIN AND LANGUAGE **50,** 225–239 (1993)

Syntactic Processing in Aphasia

DAVID SWINNEY

University of California at San Diego

AND

EDGAR ZURIF

Brandeis University and Boston University School of Medicine

In this report we comment upon subject selection and methodology, and we describe some recent studies of syntactic processing in aphasia. Our data show that, like neurologically intact subjects, Wernicke's patients reactivate moved constituents (instantiate coreference) at the site of their extraction (even for sentences that they do not understand). Broca's patients, by contrast, are shown not to create such syntactically governed links (even for sentences that they do understand). These data isolate the processing bottleneck in Broca's aphasia and more generally suggest that syntactic comprehension limitations can be traced to changes in cortically localizable resources that sustain lexical processing. © 1995 Academic Press, Inc.

METHODOLOGICAL CONSIDERATIONS

Issues of Subject Selection

The focus of the first major book on agrammatism (Kean, 1984) was on the claim of "overarching" agrammatism, that is, on the claim that Broca's patients were as syntactically limited in comprehension as in production. Even then the claim was challenged. Exceptions were noted: not all agrammatic speakers were agrammatic listeners (Goodglass & Menn, 1984; Kolk, van Grunsven, & Keyser, 1984).

Partly because of these exceptions, very few if any researchers still carry out inquiries concerning this "overarching" hypothesis. However, there is also another reason for the current lack of interest in this hypothe-

This paper and some of the research reported in it were supported by NIH Grants AG 10496 and DC 00081 and by AFOSR-91-0225. We also gratefully acknowledge the support of the Alexander Von Humboldt & W. M. Keck Foundations. Address correspondence and reprint requests to David Swinney, Dept. of Psychology—0109, University of California at San Diego, La Jolla, CA 92093.

sis: there is currently no theoretical focus to any such inquiry. The simple notion of a loss of syntactic competence in Broca's aphasia—a loss that is necessarily equally manifest in all activities—is no longer tenable. And, there is no processing perspective to take its place—nothing to guide us concerning a possible *functional* overlap of production and comprehension systems. Mostly, the ingredients from the production side of the equation are missing. This is especially true at the level of syntax. Whereas aspects of representational formats specified in generative grammar seem to constitute precisely the targets that real-time to be gauged for production (Bock, 1991), the paradigms for doing so have yet to be developed.

In the face of all this, Broca's aphasia is currently being mined for answers to different questions. For the most part, it is being examined for information bearing on the comprehension system on its own, occasionally, for information bearing on the production systems alone, but, again, hardly ever for answers concerning parallelism. In effect, Broca's aphasia exists apart from what is made of it at any given time.

Yet, although Broca's aphasia continues to serve research—including the research efforts of the participants at the TENNET symposium which gave rise to this volume—some of these participants appeared rather tentative about accepting clinical categorization. Two examples among several: In her preconference paper circulated among the participants, Marcia Linebarger entered ". . . the usual disclaimers . . . regarding the heterogeneity of agrammatic performance and the assumptions underlying all neuropsychological research," and during the conference, David Caplan questioned whether there was any empirical basis at all for linguistically characterizable syndrome-specific deficits.

We examine some of Caplan's specific criticisms at a later point—in the context of our work. Here we enter only some general considerations: namely that any empirical challenge to a theoretical claim must always be taken seriously and that the existence of exceptional cases—of Broca's patients who do not show interpretable comprehension problems or even any comprehension problems at all—justifies gingerness concerning classification. However, disagreeable data are not unique to psychology (see Zurif, Swinney, & Fodor (1991) on this matter); also the exceptions have to be put in perspective. Several of the most highly touted ones (Miceli, Mazzucchi, Menn, & Goodglass, 1983; Kolk et al., 1984) are likely not even Broca's patients to begin with: one of Micelli et al.'s (1983) cases was able to repeat and read aloud without any agrammatic limitation and, like Kolk et al.'s (1984) patient, another showed normal fluency and normal phrase length. The risks that we take in seeking generalizations based on analyses of the agrammatism associated with Broca's aphasia are worrisome enough without incorporating patients that do not belong in the category. After all, however variable output is in Broca's aphasia, the patients all share a recognizable nonfluency—one of the important features upon which identification rests in the first instance. Moreover, even given the vagaries of clinical judgment, the Broca's patients who do show comprehension breakdowns far outnumber those Broca's who do not. Were this not the case, there would have been no basis for the TENNET Conference.

Off-Line and On-Line Measurements

Our second methodological concern is with a distinction that has rightly become quite important in the evaluation of theoretical claims: the off-line–on-line distinction.

By off-line measurements we refer to those that reveal aspects of the aphasic limitation measured after comprehension and expressed as a final product—as an inability to comprehend a particular construction or to judge its grammaticality. Typical off-line techniques are sentence enactment, sentence-picture matching, truth-value judgment, and grammaticality judgment. Their worth in helping us think about representational limitations is indisputable. However, they have not been overly valuable in helping us explain these limitations in processing terms.

Linebarger, Schwartz, and Saffran's (1983) interpretation of their grammatical-judgment data illustrates this last point. Their finding is that Broca's patients carry out quite complex syntactic judgments, showing in this respect a sensitivity to structure and to grammatical categories (e.g., empty categories) that they are unable to exploit for comprehension. Linebarger et al. (1983) take this to indicate that the Broca's comprehension problem is not at the level of syntactic processing, but at a later processing stage—at the stage of thematic role assignment or mapping. However, these off-line grammatical judgment data do not compellingly support this interpretation. It is one thing to notice the absence of an empty (trace) position in a deformed sentence and quite another to link the trace with its antecedent in real-time—to fill the gap indexed by the trace during the strict time constraints imposed on the structure-building process. It is entirely possible that sensitivity in the first (off-line) instance is based on a local "checking" procedure—a post-sentence problem solving process in which locally available antecedents are checked against any open (unfilled) verb arguments. This kind of top-down, strategic intervention is likely to be far removed from gap-filling—from the normal reflexive linking of an antecedent and its trace. Thus, although the off-line judgments charted by Linebarger et al. (1983) indicate the Broca's patient's sensitivity to empty categories, the data do not help us fill in details from a real-time processing perspective. In particular, they do not help us distinguish processing at the syntactic level from processing at a later stage.

To isolate such stages we need to apply on-line techniques—techniques that can be brought to bear on ongoing processes at any time. In what follows we describe how we've already used such techniques to study sentence processing in aphasia. First, however, we provide the context for their application.

REPRESENTATIONAL LIMITATIONS AND PROCESSING DISRUPTIONS

As can be seen elsewhere in this issue (e.g., Grodzinsky, Hickok & Avrutin), efforts to characterize Broca's comprehension limitations at the sentence level turn, for the most part, on the notion of trace-deletion or, for current purposes, on the extensionally equivalent notion of chain disruption and a resultant failure of thematic role transmission. Details aside, there remains a relatively uncontroversial observation driving these claims: namely, that Broca's patients have noticeable problems understanding movement-derived structures. It is to this limitation—and the implied failure to form syntactically licensed dependency relations— that processing accounts have been directed.

Syntactic Processing vs. Mapping: A First Pass

As already alluded to in our discussion of grammatical judgments, two options concerning the processing bottleneck have been suggested. One option is that it occurs during the construction of a syntactic representation—the system is unable to establish dependency relations in real time (Zurif, Swinney, Prather, Solomon, & Bushell, 1993). The second option is that the problem is at a later stage—at the stage of thematic mapping (Linebarger et al., 1993; Linebarger, this issue).

As stated here, the two options are evenly matched. In the literature, however, the playing field is invariably less level. Those who support mapping (e.g., Linebarger, this issue)—even some who do not (Kolk & Weijts, this issue)—generally pit their work against the trace-deletion hypothesis (e.g., Grodzinsky, 1986, 1990) or its progeny (e.g., Hickok, Zurif, & Canseco-Gonzalez, 1993; Mauner, Fromkin, & Cornell, 1993) as if these "trace-based" hypotheses were claims about processing. However, they are not about processing. They try to capture the Broca's limitation along structural lines; they do not try to account for the source of the limitation along processing lines. It is immaterial to the trace-deletion notion (in any of its manifestations) whether traces are absent from a syntactic representation or (as the mapping hypothesis has it) present but unusable.

The point here is that the source of the comprehension limitation has to be investigated on independent grounds. Without data to isolate a processing level in terms of its unique operating characteristics, there is no basis for distinguishing one intermediate processing stage from another. More directly to the current concern, without such data the mapping hypothesis remains an unsupported stipulation. As it happens, with such data the hypothesis will be seen to fail.

Lexical Activation in Aphasia

The on-line analyses presented in this section are based on measures of lexical activation in particular syntactic environments. They widen the focus to include Wernicke's aphasic patients as well as Broca's patients, and they build upon earlier observations—data from lexical priming experiments—that Wernicke's patients, but not Broca's patients, show roughly normal lexical activation characteristics in circumstances that support automatic processing (e.g., Milberg & Blumstein, 1981; Milberg, Blumstein, & Dworetsky, 1987; Prather, Zurif, & Love, 1992; Prather, Zurif, Stern, & Rosen, 1992; Swinney, Zurif, & Nicol, 1989). Priming in this case refers to the finding that processing a lexical item (for example, deciding whether a string of letters forms a word) is faster for target words when these are immediately preceded by semantically associated words than when preceded by unrelated words (e.g., Meyer, Schvaneveldt, & Ruddy, 1975; Neely, 1977). In effect, activation of the first, or prime, word aids recognition of the target. Thus, to state the matter directly in terms of the data, Wernicke's patients, but not Broca's, show the normal pattern of faster word recognition (lexical decision) in semantically facilitating contexts.

That noted, we hasten to add that the Wernicke's patients are not likely to be entirely normal in accessing word meaning. To be sure, the priming data for this group ought to be interpreted as reflecting lexical activation (the point of interest here), but these data do not rule out "coarse-coding" and, therefore, ultimate imprecision with the semantic network. Contrariwise, the abnormal priming pattern for Broca's patients should not be taken to indicate that these patients are disbarred from activating word meanings. In fact, they are not completely insensitive to prime-target relations. Rather, for the Broca's patients, automatic priming seems to be only temporally protracted: automatic lexical activation seems still to be present, but to operate under a slower-than-normal time course (Friederici & Kilborn, 1989; Prather et al., 1992a,b; Swinney et al., 1989).

Not all investigators agree with this last assessment of lexical activation in Broca's aphasia. In particular, Ostrin and Tyler (1993) and Hagoort, Brown, and Swaab (1994) claim that Brocas' patients can carry out lexical access in a normally rapid automatic manner. In Hagoort et al.'s (1994) words, automatic activation in Brocas' aphasia is ". . . just fine."

Evaluation of the relative merit of these opposing claims requires an analysis of the on-line paradigms to which the evidence is rooted. In this respect, the most direct evidence of slowing in Broca's patients stems from the two Prather et al. studies (Prather et al., 1992a,b). In these two studies the patients were presented with words in the form of continuous lists. This roughly mimics the unbroken succession of words in sentences, but more than this, this list technique has been independently shown to yield automatic (as opposed to strategy-driven) activation in neurologically intact subjects (Shelton & Martin, 1992). The same cannot be said for the techniques used by Ostrin and Tyler (1993) and by Hagoort et al. (1994). Both used a word-pair paradigm that incorporated neither a distraction manipulation nor relatedness variations. Without the former they most likely elicited controlled or strategy-driven processing and without the latter, they had no way of checking this possibility. Setting words together in pairs (or in triplets) seems to suggest to subjects that the words somehow belong together, and it thereby fosters both expectations of relatedness and a postlexical checking strategy (e.g., Shelton & Martin, 1992). Neither is likely to be relevant to sentence processing. So at least for the present, it remains a reasonable bet that initial lexical activation is not normally rapid in Broca's aphasia. Indeed, as we show below, the payoff on this bet has already had considerable heuristic value.

Gap-Filling in Aphasia

Empty categories have processing consequences. We refer here to gap-filling, the demonstration (based on priming) that antecedents and traces are linked during the course of comprehension. (See Swinney & Fodor (1989) and Swinney & Osterhout (1990) for reviews of this work.) This is an operation that is implemented under strict time constraints and one that is unlikely to accommodate slower-than-normal lexical activation. This being so, it seemed reasonable to hypothesize a connection between the Broca's slowed lexical processing and their syntactic limitation. Specifically, it seemed reasonable to view the Broca's inability to interpret antecedent-trace relations as a failure to reactivate moved lexical items at the normal time in the processing sequence—in time, that is, to fill gaps left by their movement.

We have examined this suggestion by assessing gap-filling in Broca's patients and Wernicke's patients in two experiments (Zurif et al., 1993; Swinney, Zurif, Prather, & Love, 1993).[1]

In the first experiment (Zurif et al., 1993) we used subject-relative constructions of the sort, "The man liked the tailor$_i$ with the British accent

---

[1] We have also assessed gap-filling in age-matched neurologically intact subjects. In fact, the normal subjects were used to pretest the different sentence types for the two experiments.

who $(t)_i$ claimed to know the queen." As shown in this example by co-indexation, movement from subject position is hypothesized.[2]

We chose this construction because of the perspective it offered both within and across aphasic groups. As described elsewhere in this issue (e.g., Grodzinsky), Broca's patients show relatively normal comprehension for this construction. However, Wernicke's patients are unpredictable, more often than not showing chance comprehension. (Grodzinsky, 1984; Shankweiler, personal communication, February, 1992). Thus, for Broca's patients these sentences provided the strongest test of our suggestion that they could not carry out normal syntactic analysis in real time: We could determine if slower-than-normal lexical activation disallowed normal gap-filling even for sentences correctly comprehended, and we could determine if even in such circumstances Broca's were abnormally reliant on nongrammatical strategies. As for Wernicke's patients, it allowed us to determine the possibility of a reverse scenario: viz. whether, given their normal initial contact with lexical entries, they could fill gaps even for sentences which they often fail ultimately to understand.

Our assessment of gap-filling and the range of possibilities just outlined, turned on a cross-modal lexical priming (CMLP) paradigm (Swinney, Onifer, Prather, & Hirshkowitz, 1979). Subjects listened to a sentence over earphones (delivered uninterruptedly and at a normal speaking rate) and at one point, while listening to the sentence, were required to make a lexical decision for a visually presented letter string flashed on a screen in front of them. (To accommodate the right-side weakness of Broca's patients, all subjects "button-pressed" with their left hand when making their decisions.)

What we sought to discover was whether a letter-string probe forming a word related to the moved constituent (the antecedent) was primed at the gap. Such priming would indicate that the moved constituent was reactivated at the gap (thus providing the prime). So for each of our experimental sentences, we recorded lexical decision times either for antecedent-related probes or for letter string probes that were semantically unassociated control words. For the example given earlier, "The man liked the tailor$_i$ with the British accent[1] who[2] $(t)_i$ claimed to know the queen," the probes were "clothes" (the probe for the antecedent, "tailor") and "weight" (the control probe).

As indicated by the superscripts [1] and [2], priming was examined at two points—at the gap indexed by the trace (superscript [2]) and at a pre-gap position (superscript [1]). The latter served as a baseline; it allowed us to distinguish structurally governed reactivation at the gap site

---

[2] Technically, it is the Wh-element ("who") that is hypothesized to have been moved from the subject position of the relative clause. However, since "who" and "tailor" co-refer, "who" inherits the semantics of "tailor."

TABLE 1
Amount of Priming (msec)

Position	Pregap	Gap
Wernicke's patients	44	125*
Broca's patients	−20	−68

Note. Reaction time to control probes minus reaction time to related probes.
*Signficant priming ($p < .03$).

from any residual activation due simply to the earlier appearance of the antecedent ("tailor"). Of course, in each instance, priming was determined by comparing the lexical decision time for the related probe to that for the unrelated probe.

It should be apparent from our description of the task that the lexical decision itself does not require that the subject consciously seek a relation between the visual probe and anything in the orally presented sentence (as is the case, for example, in probe-latency tasks). Rather, at least until the visual letter string is presented, the subject is simply listening and trying to understand the sentence. (We encourage this by randomly asking comprehension questions between trials.) Once the visual probe is presented, all such normalcy ends, of course. But this happens only after the point of theoretical interest concerning sentence processing has passed.

The findings for the aphasic patients on this task are presented in Table 1. As can be seen, the Wernicke's patients reliably filled gaps immediately (as did our neurologically intact subjects who were used to pretest the sentences—see Footnote 1). The Broca's patients did not fill the gaps immediately.[3] It appears, therefore, that the brain areas respectively implicated in Broca's and Wernicke's aphasia have different functional commitments—the former is crucial for the real-time construction of intrasentence dependency relations in a way that the latter is not.

As mentioned earlier, we also carried out a second study (Swinney et al., 1993). This time we used object-relative sentences. Given the Broca's failure to fill gaps for subject-relatives (sentences that they understand), we had little expectation that they would show gap-filling for object-relatives (sentences that they fail to interpret). However, our interest in using object-relatives had to do mostly with Wernicke's patients (who also show less-than-normal comprehension for such sentences). We wanted to broaden the base of our observations of this group's gap-filling

[3] We emphasize that the Broca's patients' failure to show gap-filling cannot be construed as some global failure to prime. In other nonsentence circumstances, when some of the patients were presented with word lists, they did show priming, even if in a temporally protracted manner.

TABLE 2
Amount of Priming (msec)

Position	Pregap	Gap
Wernicke's patients	3	108*
Broca's patients	122	−9

Note. Reaction time to control probes minus reaction time to related probes.
*Signficant priming ($p < .02$).

capacity, particularly because reactivation in subject-relatives might have been affected by the relativizer "who" in that construction and also because movement within subject-relatives has the special property of being "string-vacuous" (e.g., Clements, McCloskey, Maling, & Zaenen, 1983): such movement does not reorder any of the elements of the sequence.

Accordingly, our second study featured object-relative sentences of the type:

"The priest enjoyed the drink$_i$ that the caterer was[1] serving[2] (t)$_i$ to the guests."

We used the same CMLP task as in the first experiment, and again, we checked for priming both at the gap (superscript *2) and at a baseline, pre-gap position (superscript *1). For the example given, "wine" was the probe for "drink" and "boat," the control probe.

As can be seen in Table 2, the Broca's patients again did not show significant priming at either probe site. Still, even though not significant, they did show some advantage for related probes (relative to control probes) at the pre-gap position. In effect, for this group there was no sign of structurally determined reactivation of the antecedent, only a sign of some residual activation—the consequence, likely, of having processed the earlier appearance of the constituent in a slowed-down fashion. As for the Wernicke's patients, they once more showed priming at the gap and only at the gap, and again, this pattern corresponded to that shown by the neurologically intact subjects with whom we pretested the material.

Caplan, in his discussion at the TENNET Conference, questioned the basis of our Broca's–Wernicke's difference in gap-filling. He claimed that the Wernicke's patients we tested had off-line comprehension scores that were superior to those for the Broca's patients, and he suggested that the patient's ability to fill gaps might, therefore, have more to do with their comprehension level than with their syndrome identification. Granting the claim, the argument is sound. However, we do not grant his claim. On our off-line comprehension assessment accompanying each of our gap-filling experiments, neither the Broca's nor the Wernicke's patients showed normal performance for noncanonicial (object-gap) structures. In fact, in the second gap-filling experiment, the patients comprising the Wernicke's group performed at a lower level on the off-line test than did the Broca's. Notwithstanding Caplan's speculation on the matter, our gap-filling data can be interpreted only in terms of a Broca's–Wernicke's contrast.[4]

Syntactic Processing vs. Mapping: A Second Pass

It was earlier forecast that on-line data would show the processing bottleneck in Broca's aphasia to be at the syntactic level and not at a later stage of processing as suggested by the mapping hypothesis. We now return to this topic.

Consider first the data obtained for the subject-relative sentences. Broca's patients show good understanding for subject-relative sentences. In this circumstance, the mapping hypothesis (e.g., Linebarger et al., 1983) stipulates normal syntactic analysis (normal mapping, too). By contrast, as we have framed it, the syntactic hypothesis [in line with various

---

[4] Mauner (this issue) has also raised some questions about our data, and these, too, are empirically unfounded concerns. In particular, she assumes that Broca's patients have slower absolute reaction times than do Wernicke's patients, and in consequence, expresses the concern that our screening procedure (a two-standard deviation cutoff) would be more likely to exclude data from Broca's than from Wernicke's patients. However, as we have pointed out elsewhere (Zurif et al., 1993), our two-standard deviation screen was uniquely determined from each subject's distribution of reaction times and therefore did not disproportionately exclude Broca's responses. For that matter, contrary to Mauner's suppositions, the Broca's response times were not even systematically greater than those for Wernicke's patients. In the experiment employing subject-relative sentences, the average reaction times for the Broca's patients (for all probes in all locations) and for the Wernicke's patients were, respectively, 1113 and 1041 ms, but, with object-relative sentences, the Broca's patients' mean was only 1248 ms, while that for the Wernicke's was 1472 ms. At any rate, what is critical here is the difference between absolute reaction time and relative reaction time. The absolute reaction time numbers that we have just entered—those that concern Mauner—likely reflect psychomotor slowing and are of no direct relevance to our study. What is relevant are the relative reaction times that have allowed us to factor out this effect. It is these relative times based on experimental-control probe differences that have allowed us to chart lexical activation. When we suggest that there is a slowing of lexical activation in Broca's aphasia, what we are referring to is the failure to find a significant priming effect—a significant experimental-control probe difference—under particular temporal constraints as defined by the probe positions in the sentence; absolute response times have no relevance to this issue. Mauner enters other concerns, these being the amount of data excluded by our screening procedures and the frailty of the gap-filling effect even for neurologically intact subjects. With respect to the latter, she cites the work of McKoon, Ratcliff, and Ward (1994). In this connection we urge the reader to consult the paper by Nicol, Fodor, and Swinney (1994) wherein the McKoon et al. claims are very definitely empirically blunted (in all relevant cases there were shown to be methodological problems inherent in the manner in which McKoon et al. attempted to examine the issues). As for the amount of data we excluded, we note that we also collected more for each subject than is usual when testing college students. Still, in the general spirit of Mauner's cautionary note, we, too, emphasize how much there remains to be understood concerning the gap-filling effect (and, indeed, all on-line effects). However, such cautionary notes fail to explain or blunt the relevance of the differences we report.

representational accounts (e.g., Grodzinsky, 1986; Hickok et al., 1993)] predicts a failure of gap-filling and an abnormal reliance on nongrammatical strategies in Broca's aphasia, whatever the construction and however good their understanding is. Clearly, therefore, our subject-relative data are accountable by the syntactic processing hypothesis, and not by the mapping hypothesis.

We think that our data for object-relative sentences also require an explanation along syntactic lines. To make this argument, however, we need first to fix the processing stage at which gap-filling occurs. Some help in this respect is provided by Shapiro and his colleagues (Shapiro, Zurif, & Grimshaw, 1987, 1989; Shapiro & Levine, 1990; Shapiro, Gordon, Hack, & Killackey, 1993). They have shown that Wernicke's patients are insensitive in real-time to the argument-taking properties of verbs. Unlike neurologically intact subjects, the patients are unable to access momentarily all of the possible argument structure configurations within a verb's entry. They are unable, that is, to generate a fully elaborated thematic grid in the normal manner. Accordingly, it seems reasonable to view gap-filling as being syntactically, not thematically, driven—as reflecting processing at a stage prior to the full availability of a verb's argument structure and to thematic mapping. Indeed, the fact that the Wernicke's patients filled gaps in sentences for which they show uncertain comprehension strengthens this possibility. In light of these data, then, the Broca's patients' inability to fill gaps is to be viewed as a syntactic processing failure, and not a mapping failure.[5]

We emphasize, however, that in respect to judging the relative merits of the syntactic and mapping hypotheses, the critical data remain those provided in our first (subject-relative construction) study. For as we have shown in this study, even though the Broca's patients successfully comprehend subject-relatives, their comprehension is still shakily based on an impoverished (abnormal) syntactic analysis.

FUNCTIONAL LOCALIZATION

Most of the papers in this issue—and most aphasia studies generally—are concerned only with evaluating cognitive theory. The goal is usually to determine if distinctions within a linguistic theory are neurologically defensible—if they correspond to deficit patterns following brain damage.

---

[5] Linebarger avoids this possibility in her preconference paper by claiming that Shapiro's data bear on subcategorization rather than on thematic information. Her claim, however, fails on two counts: (1) She invokes the internal structure of a complement rather than the simple fact of its presence or absence; that is, she has the wrong grain size, and (2) she fails to account for an important finding concerning alternating vs. nonalternating datives—constructions that differ with respect to subcategorization, but not with respect to thematic options.

By contrast, our gap-filling work permits not only a connection to linguistic theory but also to functional neuroanatomy.

Our connection to functional neuroanatomy turns on the fact that the syndromes we have examined here—Broca's aphasia and Wernicke's aphasia—are distinguishable both clinically and also roughly with respect to lesion site. To be sure, the brain area associated with Broca's aphasia now seems to have greater extent than initially proposed: Broca's area in the foot of the third frontal convolution is no longer considered to be singularly important, and adjacent and deeper areas have also been implicated (Alexander, Naeser, & Palumbo, 1990; Naeser, Palumbo, Helm-Estabrooks, Stiassny-Eder, & Albert, 1989). Still, the fact remains that the modal lesion site for Broca's area is distinguishable from that for Wernicke's aphasia. For the latter, the greatest involvement is still typically considered to be in the superior temporal gyrus (Wernicke's area). We note also that approximately 80% of Broca's and Wernicke's aphasias appear accountable by the areas defined by these modal sites (M. Albert & H. Goodglass, personal communication, June, 1994). In this sense, then, the real-time processing differences shown for Broca's and Wernicke's patients appear to index different functional commitments for the areas respectively associated with each syndrome.

Wernicke's Aphasia and Functional Localization

Obviously we are only just beginning to characterize the role of the area associated with Wernicke's aphasia. Our data—alongside those reported by Shapiro and his colleagues (e.g., Shapiro et al., 1993)—suggest that with respect to language capacity, this area broadly sustains semantic processes and not those involved in initial parsing and in the formation of dependency relations. However, crucial data are missing even for this rough formulation. In particular, we have yet to determine if Wernicke's patients reactivate only structurally appropriate constituents at gaps. At present, then, we can tentatively conclude only that the brain area implicated in Wernicke's aphasia is not crucially involved in the syntactic business of recognizing and filling gaps immediately in real-time.

Broca's Aphasia and Functional Localization

By contrast, the brain region usually associated with Broca's aphasia does appear to be necessary for the operation of gap-filling. The data reviewed here show that Broca's patients are unable to form dependency relations—whether for object-relative constructions that they have difficulty understanding or even for subject-relative constructions that do not pose difficulty for them.

The consequences of the problem seem relatively straightforward. Since they do not have the processing resources to establish dependency relations normally—to fill the gap at exactly the right time in the processing sequence—they cannot provide the syntactic information necessary for thematic assignment to moved constituents. Presumably, therefore, the Broca's patients rely abnormally on some nongrammatical strategy to achieve thematic mapping for moved constituents (e.g., Grodzinsky, 1986; Hickok, 1992).

We think it reasonable to link these structural limitations in Broca's aphasia to disruptions of automatic lexical activation. We thereby begin to see that the brain region implicated in Broca's aphasia need not be the locus of syntactic representations per se, but rather might be necessary for providing the resources that sustain lexical activation and its syntactic ramifications.

We have proposed in this paper that these resources sustain the normal speed or rate of activation. But in line with Hagoort et al. (1994) and Ostrin and Tyler (1993), the Broca's failure to integrate a moved constituent might well suggest other possibilities concerning the functional commitment of its associated region. For example, several investigators have suggested that it accommodates the memory storage demands that arise during comprehension (e.g., Ostrin & Schwartz, 1986). And certainly, a prima facie case can be made that long distance dependency relations of the sort described here are especially reliant upon some form of working memory capacity. (See Kolk and Weijts in this issue for a discussion on this matter.)

Another possibility is that the broad cortical area implicated in Broca's aphasia sustains multiple functions, including both speed of activation and memory. Yet another possibility is that memory capacity is diminished only because of the increased cost of slower-than-normal activation.

All are variations on the same theme, namely, that syntactic limitations might be rooted to changes in cortically localizable processing resources.

REFERENCES

Alexander, M., Naeser, M. A., & Palumbo, C. L. 1990. Broca's area aphasias: Aphasia after lesions including the frontal operculum. *Neurology,* **40,** 353–362.

Bock, K. 1991. A sketchbook of production problems. (Special issue on sentence processing). *Journal of Psycholinguistic Research,* **20,** 141–160.

Clements, G., McCloskey, J., Maling, J., & Zaenen, A. 1983. String-vacuous rule application. *Linguistic Inquiry,* **14,** 1–17.

Friederici, A., & Kilborn, K. 1989. Temporal constraints on language processing: Syntactic priming in Broca's aphasia. *Journal of Cognitive Neuroscience,* **3,** 262–272.

Goodglass, H., & Menn, L. 1984. Is agrammatism a unitary phenomenon? In M.-L. Kean (Ed.), *Agrammatism.* Orlando, FL: Academic Press.

Grodzinsky, Y. 1984. *Language deficits and linguistic theory.* Unpublished doctoral dissertation, Brandeis University, MA.

Grodzinsky, Y. 1986. Language deficits and the theory of syntax. *Brain and Language,* **27,** 135–159.

Grodzinsky, Y. 1990. *Theoretical perspectives on language deficits.* Cambridge, MA: MIT Press.

Grodzinsky, Y. 1995. A restrictive theory of agrammatic comprehension. *Brain & Language,* **50,** 27–51.

Hagoort, P., Brown, C., & Swaab, T. 1994. *On the nature of lexical–semantic processing impairments in aphasia.* Paper presented to TENNET, Montreal, Quebec.

Hickok, G. 1992. *Agrammatic comprehension, VP-internal subjects, and the trace-deletion hypothesis.* Occasional Paper #45, Center for Cognitive Neuroscience, MIT.

Hickok, G., & Avrutin, S. 1995. Representation, referentiality, and processing in agrammatic comprehension: Two case studies. *Brain & Language,* **50,** 10–26.

Hickok, G., Zurif, E., & Canseco-Gonzalez, E. 1993. Structural description of agrammatic comprehension. *Brain and Language,* **45,** 371–395.

Kean, M.-L. (Ed.) 1984. *Agrammatism.* Orlando, FL: Academic Press.

Kolk, H., van Grunsven, M., & Keyser, A. 1984. Parallelism in agrammatism. In M.-L. Kean (Ed.), *Agrammatism.* Orlando, FL: Academic Press.

Kolk, H., & Weijts, M. (in press). Judgments of semantic anomaly in agrammatic patients. *Brain & Language.*

Linebarger, M. 1995. Agrammatism as evidence about grammar. *Brain & Language,* **50,** 52–91.

Linebarger, M., Schwartz, M., & Saffran, E. 1983. Sensitivity to grammatical structure in so-called agrammatic aphasics. *Cognition,* **13,** 361–393.

Mauner, G., Fromkin, V., & Cornell, T. 1993. Comprehension and acceptability judgments in agrammatism: Disruptions in the syntax of referential dependency. *Brain and Language,* **45,** 340–370.

McKoon, G., Ratcliff, R., & Ward, G. 1994. Testing theories of language processing. An empirical investigation of the on-line lexical decision task. *Journal of Experimental Psychology. Learning, Memory & Cognition,* **20**(5), 1219–1228.

Meyer, D., Schvaneveldt, R., & Ruddy, M. 1975. Loci of contextual effects on visual word recognition. In P. Rabbit & S. Dornic (Eds.), *Attention and performance.* New York: Academic Press. Vol. 5.

Miceli, G., Mazzucchi, A., Menn, L., & Goodglass, H. 1983. Contrasting cases of Italian agrammatic aphasia without comprehension disorder. *Brain and Language,* **19,** 65–97.

Milberg, W., & Blumstein, S. 1981. Lexical decision and aphasia: Evidence for semantic processing. *Brain and Language,* **14,** 371–385.

Milberg, W., Blumstein, S., & Dworetsky, B. 1987. Processing of lexical ambiguities in aphasia. *Brain and Language,* **31,** 138–150.

Naeser, M. A., Palumbo, C., Helm-Estabrooks, N., Stiassny-Eder, D., & Albert, M. L. 1989. Severe nonfluency in aphasia: Role of the medial subcallosal fasciculus and other white matter pathways in recovery of spontaneous speech. *Brain,* **112,** 1–38.

Neely, J. H. 1977. Semantic priming and retrieval from lexical memory: Roles of inhibitionless spreading activation and limited-capacity attention. *Journal of Experimental Psychology: General,* **106,** 226–254.

Nicol, J., Fodor, J. D., & Swinney, D. 1994. Using cross-modal lexical decision tasks to investigate sentence processing. *Journal of Experimental Psychology: Learning, Memory and Cognition,* **20.**

Ostrin, R., & Schwartz, M. 1986. Reconstructuring from a degraded trace: A study of sentence repetition in agrammatism. *Brain and Language,* **28,** 328–345.

Ostrin, R., & Tyler, L. 1993. Automatic access to lexical semantics in aphasia: Evidence from semantic and associative priming. *Brain and Language,* **45,** 147–159.

Prather, P., Zurif, E. B., & Love, T. 1992a. *The time course of lexical access in aphasia.* Paper presented to the Academy of Aphasia, Toronto, Ontario.

Prather, P., Zurif, E. B., Stern, C., & Rosen, J. 1992b. Slowed lexical access in nonfluent aphasia: A case study. *Brain and Language,* **43,** 336–348.

Shapiro, L., Gordon, B., Hack, N., & Killackey, J. 1993. Verb-argument structure processing in complex sentences in Broca's and Wernicke's aphasia. *Brain and Language,*
45, 423–447.

Shapiro, L., & Levine, B. 1990. Verb processing during sentence comprehension in aphasia.
Brain and Language, **38,** 21–47.

Shapiro, L., Zurif, E., & Grimshaw, J. 1987. Sentence processing and the mental representation of verbs. *Cognition,* **27,** 219–246.

Shapiro, L., Zurif, E., & Grimshaw, J. 1989. Verb processing during sentence comprehension: Contextual impenetrability. *Journal of Psycholinguistic Research,* **18,** 223–243.

Shelton, J., & Martin, R. 1992. How semantic is automatic semantic priming? *Journal of
Experimental Psychology: Learning, Memory, and Cognition,* **18,** 1191–1210.

Swinney, D., & Fodor, J. D., Eds. 1989. *Journal of Psycholinguistic Research,* **18**(1).
[Special Issue on Sentence Processing].

Swinney, D., Onifer, W., Prather, P., & Hirshkowitz, M. 1979. Semantic facilitation across
sensory modalities in the processing of individual words and sentences. *Memory and
Cognition,* **7,** 159–165.

Swinney, D., & Osterhout, L. 1990. Inference generation during auditory language comprehension. In A. Graesser & G. Bower (Eds.), *Inferences and text comprehension.* San
Diego: Academic Press.

Swinney, D., Zurif, E. B., & Nicol, J. 1989. The effects of focal brain damage on sentence
processing: An examination of the neurological organization of a mental module. *Journal of Cognitive Neuroscience,* **1,** 25–37.

Swinney, D., Zurif, E., Prather, P., & Love, T. 1993. *The neurological distribution of
processing operations underlying language comprehension.* Unpublished manuscript,
Department of Psychology, University of California, San Diego.

Zurif, E. B., Swinney, D., & Fodor, J. A. 1991. An evaluation of assumptions underlying
the single-patient-only position in neuropsychological research. *Brain and Cognition,*
16, 198–210.

Zurif, E. B., Swinney, D., Prather, P., Solomon, J., & Bushnell, C. 1993. An on-line
analysis of syntactic processing in Broca's and Wernicke's aphasia. *Brain and Language,* **45,** 448–464.

BRAIN AND LANGUAGE **50,** 259–281 (1995)

The Time Course of Syntactic Activation during Language Processing: A Model Based on Neuropsychological and Neurophysiological Data

Angela D. Friederici

Max Planck Institute for Cognitive Neuroscience, Leipzig, Germany

This paper presents a model describing the temporal and neurotopological structure of syntactic processes during comprehension. It postulates three distinct phases of language comprehension, two of which are primarily syntactic in nature. During the first phase the parser assigns the initial syntactic structure on the basis of word category information. These early structural processes are assumed to be subserved by the anterior parts of the left hemisphere, as event-related brain potentials show this area to be maximally activated when phrase structure violations are processed and as circumscribed lesions in this area lead to an impairment of the on-line structural assignment. During the second phase lexical-semantic and verb-argument structure information is processed. This phase is neurophysiologically manifest in a negative component in the event-related brain potential around 400 ms after stimulus onset which is distributed over the left and right temporo-parietal areas when lexical-semantic information is processed and over left anterior areas when verb-argument structure information is processed. During the third phase the parser tries to map the initial syntactic structure onto the available lexical-semantic and verb-argument structure information. In case of an unsuccessful match between the two types of information reanalyses may become necessary. These processes of structural reanalysis are correlated with a centro-parietally distributed late positive component in the event-related brain potential. The different temporal and topographical patterns of the event-related brain potentials as well as some aspects of aphasics' comprehension behavior are taken to support the view that these different processing phases are distinct and that the left anterior cortex, in particular, is responsible for the on-line assignment of syntactic structure. © 1995 Academic Press, Inc.

The work reported here was supported by the Alfried Krupp von Bohlen und Halbach science prize awarded to A.F. and by a grant from the German Research Foundation (DFG FR 519/12-1). I thank Axel Mecklinger for his advice.

Address correspondence and reprint requests to the author at the Max Planck Institute for Cognitive Neuroscience, Inselstraße 22-26, 04103 Leipzig, Germany.

298

INTRODUCTION

The basic mechanism underlying language comprehension is lexical access. Lexical entries by hypothesis hold all relevant information needed to structure the language input and to assign thematic roles. There are two general accounts framing how the language processor exploits syntactic and semantic information carried by lexical elements: the structure-driven and the lexical-driven account. The structure-driven account claims that there are two processing stages, an initial stage during which the parser identifies the structure of the input based on syntactic word category information and a second stage during which thematic role assignment takes place on the basis of structural and lexical information (e.g., Ferreira & Clifton, 1986; Frazier, 1978, 1990; Frazier & Fodor, 1978; Frazier & Rayner, 1982; Rayner, Carlson, & Frazier, 1983). During this initial first-pass parse lexical information other than word category information is irrelevant. The parser is driven by particular phrase structure heuristics rather than by lexical information. One such heuristic is the so-called minimal attachment principle which holds that phrases are initially assigned to the simplest structure defined by the least distant node in the phrase structure tree (Frazier, 1978, 1990). The lexical-driven account, in contrast, holds that initial sentence parsing is guided by lexical information, especially by the argument structure of the verb, i.e., its subcategorization information. In case of multiple argument structures (e.g., *John reads, John reads the book*) preferences as defined by the frequency of use operative in guiding the first parse (Ford, Bresnan, & Kaplan, 1982; Shapiro, Nagel, & Levine, 1992; Trueswell, Tanenhaus, & Kello, 1993).

From the outline of the two positions it is obvious that any empirical support for either position must focus on the temporal structure of the availability of different information types carried by lexical elements and functional elements during sentence processing. There are several ways to gain information about the temporal structure of comprehension processes. One is to conduct reaction time studies sensitive to the issue in focus. A second possibility is to look into language processing systems whose temporal structure deviates from normal subjects in defined and specific ways, such as in subjects with particular neuropsychological deficits. A third way to monitor the temporal structure of language processing is to register the brain activity as sentences are processed in time, as, for example, in event-related brain potential studies.

There is quite an extensive literature using reaction time paradigms in studies with normal subjects, i.e., non-brain-damage subjects (e.g., Altmann, 1989; Frauenfelder & Tyler, 1987), investigating how syntactic and lexical-semantic information is retrieved and used during normal comprehension. This paper will extend this view by focusing on neuropsychological evidence gathered from patients with circumscribed brain lesions in on-line comprehension studies and on neurophysiological evidence from normal subjects in event-related brain potential studies providing neurotopographic as well as temporal information correlated with semantic and syntactic processes during comprehension.

The model under consideration here is close to the structure-driven account holding that there is an initial parse solely based on word category information with lexical-semantic information coming in at a later point in time. In contrast to the original proposal of Frazier (1978), the present view is open to the possibility that preferences for first-pass parses may not necessarily follow the simplest structure, but rather the most frequent one used in the particular language under investigation. Although we are not able to present data of our own laboratory on the latter issue, findings from other groups suggest that this is possible (Altmann, Garnham, & Dennis, 1992; Crain & Steedmann, 1985).

It should be stated clearly that the experiments reported here were not set up to distinguish between the structure-driven and the lexical-driven account, but rather followed a processing view which assumes different processing systems for structural and lexical-semantic information showing different rise-times in normal subjects, different neuropsychological pattern in language breakdown, and different neurophysiological correlates as revealed by measuring subjects' brain activity during sentence processing. The findings from these experiments, however, suggest a view on the time course of language comprehension processes which is compatible with a modified structure-driven parsing account.

THE NEUROPSYCHOLOGICAL DATA

Earlier work (Friederici, 1985) had revealed differential reaction time patterns for the recognition of elements carrying mainly lexical-semantic information, i.e., open-class words and those carrying mainly structural information, i.e., closed-class words, when these were presented in sentence context. Elements of the closed-class were recognized faster than elements of the open class. Moreover, recognition of open-class words, but not of closed-class words, was a function of whether they appeared in sentence pairs in which the first sentence was semantically related to the second one or not. This result was taken to indicate that closed-class words carrying the structural information are accessed fast and independent of the semantic content given by sentential context.

Interestingly, agrammatic Broca patients with lesions in the anterior part of the left hemisphere, but not Wernicke patients with lesions in the posterior part of the left hemisphere, were selectively slowed down in recognizing closed-class words in a similar experiment (Friederici, 1983, 1985). As these patients' behavioral patterns with respect to the open-class elements were similar to normals, we reasoned that access to lexical-semantic information is relatively intact. Thus, these patients seem to provide a good test for the influence of slow-rise time for syntactic information. This view is supported by some studies showing delayed syntactic processes (Friederici & Kilborn, 1989; Haarmann & Kolk, 1994; Zurif, Swinney, Prather, Solomon, & Bushell, 1993) and intact semantic processes (Hagoort, 1993; Ostrin & Tyler, 1993), but not by other studies which found lexical-semantic processes to be slowed down in agrammatics as well (Blumstein, Milberg & Shrier, 1982; Milberg & Blumstein, 1981; Milberg, Blumstein, & Dworetzky, 1987; Prather, Shapiro, Zurif, & Swinney, 1991). However, unlike our own study, these studies had not compared processing of lexical-semantic and syntactic aspects directly. The data of our experiments also showed slowed recognition times for open-class words for agrammatic Broca's aphasics compared to normals; this effect, however, was minor compared to the massive slowing down in recognizing closed-class words. The latter elements were recognized about 250 ms slower by agrammatic Broca's aphasics compared to normal subjects.

Given this major slowing down in recognizing closed-class elements in spoken sentences, we wondered whether agrammatic Broca's aphasics were able to access the structural information encoded in these elements at all. This question was investigated by using a syntactic priming paradigm in which auditorily presented sentence fragments were continued by either a grammatical or an ungrammatical continuation, e.g., *Het meisje wordt geslagen* vs. *Het meisje wordt gereisd/The girl is being hit* vs. *The girl is being traveled* (Friederici & Kilborn, 1989). The grammaticality of the sentences depended on the combination of the auxiliary and the past participle. If agrammatic Broca's aphasics would be able to access the information carried by the auxiliary, although slowly, these patients should show a grammaticality effect in their lexical decision times on the sentence final word, i.e., faster reaction times in the grammatical than in the ungrammatical condition. The observed reaction times indicated that agrammatic Broca's aphasics are able to access and to use the information carried by the closed-class element under investigation; however, their overall lexical decision times for the past participles in sentence context were dramatically slowed down (by about 200–250 ms) compared to a baseline measure in which a lexical decision task had to be performed on past participle forms in isolation. The reverse was true for normal age matched subjects who demonstrated faster reaction times for targets presented in sentence context versus in isolation. This result was taken to support the hypothesis that a major aspect of agrammatic Broca's aphasia is the loss of fast, automatic access and the use of the structural information carried by grammatical elements.

These findings as well as the data of related studies (Prather et al., 1991) suggest that the Broca and/or adjacent areas subserve the fast syntactic procedures necessary to structure the incoming sequence of linguistic elements. These procedures are assumed to be highly automatic and informationally encapsulated in the adult brain, but only emerge in context with given language experience during development (Friederici, 1983, 1988, 1995). The particular and primary function of these established procedures may be defined as to realize fast buildup of phrasal structures including traces of vowed elements.

The outcome of these procedures, in any case, is a syntactic phrase structure providing the basis for thematic role assignment. The building up of a phrase structure, as well as the ability to keep this structure available until thematic role assignment has taken place, may be the heart of the normal comprehension process which derails in Broca's aphasics. This, in turn, would suggest that those cortical areas involved in Broca's aphasia subserve these procedures. The relation between brain areas involved in Broca's aphasia and the building up of phrasal structure has been discussed quite extensively over the last years in the field of aphasia research (Prather et al., 1991; Haarmann & Kolk, 1990; Frazier & Friederici, 1991; see also Grodzinsky 1984, for a linguistic specification of the agrammatic deficit).

The neuropsychological data reported here support the view that the Broca and adjacent areas subserve those syntactic procedures which guarantee normal on-line processing, i.e., the fast and automatic structuring of the incoming linguistic input into syntactic chains or phrases. A delay of these early structuring processes of about 200 to 250 ms seems to have severe consequences for subsequent processes such as on-line thematic role assignment. How can this be? The idea is that the early structuring processes support the comprehension system insofar as the language input does not have to be kept in verbal memory as a list of words, but can be chucked, i.e., parsed into phrases. This allows the system to keep more words which await thematic roles assignment in verbal memory. The assignment of thematic roles defined as the successful match of structural and lexical information may require the availability of quite a sequence of words in the actual verbal memory, as the entire input information must be available again in case no successful match is possible and a reanalysis of the input becomes necessary. The early structuring processes supported by brain systems located in the anterior part of the left hemisphere may thus provide the basis for an efficient verbal memory keeping information in the form of structured phrases rather than word lists (Friederici & Frazier, 1992).[1]

---

[1] Note that the assumption predicts poor memory performance of agrammatic subjects for structured sequences or elements herein, but not for function words when presented in isolation as proposed by Nicol and Rapscak (1994). What they showed is indeed agrammat-

So far, the present view is based solely on findings from studies with brain-damaged subjects. There is, however, a debate with respect to whether it is valid to generalize from lesion studies to the normal functioning of the brain.

THE EVENT-RELATED BRAIN POTENTIAL DATA

One possibility to investigate the temporal and neurotopological parameters of language processes in the normal brain is to register subjects' brain activity while reading or listening to sentences. A noninvasive registration of brain activity during cognitive processes is the electrophysiological measure of event-related brain potentials. The event-related brain potential (ERP) is the electrical activity of the brain time-locked to the presentation of a stimulus. Its temporal resolution is in the domain of milliseconds and its topographic resolution depends upon the amount of electrodes used for registration. Components of the ERP have been shown to be sensitive in polarity, amplitude, and latency to a variety of sensory and cognitive processes including those underlying language comprehension (Donchin & Coles, 1988; Hillyard & Picton, 1987; Kutas & van Petten, 1988; van Petten & Kutas, 1991).

LEXICALLY BOUND PROCESSES

The meanwhile classical experiment by Kutas and Hillyard (1983) demonstrated a specific waveform in the event-related brain potential measured during sentence reading correlated with the processing of semantic anomalies. This waveform had a negative polarity and peaked 400 ms after the onset of the critical word showing a wide distribution over the posterior areas of both hemispheres. The amplitude of this negativity was a reverse function of the semantic adequacy or fit of the target to the preceding context.

In the same experiment Kutas and Hillyard (1983) had also included sentences containing syntactic errors of subject–verb agreement, but did not find any reliable ERP correlate for this type of error. The absence of an ERP correlate for syntactic processes in this experiment could be due to several reasons. First, it could be due to the fact that agreement markers in English are not very prominent and, therefore, hard to detect. Second, a listener being exposed to language which is only weakly in-

---

ics' poor memory performance for closed-class elements when presented in sentences. They fail to show these subjects performance on word lists consisting of or containing function words. The data of Friederici and Frazier (1992) show that agrammatics' comprehension performance decreases when memory load of the task increases, despite the fact these patients show not particularly poor performance for function word memory versus content word memory when presented in lists.

flected such as English may not have developed a strong sensitivity to inflectional elements. Third, the fact that the stimulus material in this experiment was presented in a word-by-word presentation mode with pauses of 400 and 500 ms between each word may have blurred fast and automatic syntactic processes. We assumed that we might be able to observe an ERP correlate for fast syntactic processes when investigating more salient violations than those used by Kutas and Hillyard (1983) in a highly inflected language such as German in a rapid serial visual presentation mode with pauses of 100 to 200 ms between each word.

In a first experiment we evaluated a quite salient type of syntactic violation, namely, subcategorization violations, e.g., *Der Präsident wurde gefallen/The president is being fallen* (Rösler, Friederici, Pütz, & Hahne, 1993). This type of violation had been proven to show reliable effects in reaction time studies conducted with normal and aphasic subjects (Friederici & Kilborn, 1989). In order to be able to compare waveforms elicited by this type of violation to the known N400 component as a correlate of semantic processes, we also included sentences containing semantic anomalies, i.e., violations of selectional restriction information, e.g., *Der Präsident wurde gewürzt/The president is being spiced*. Sentences of these types together with correct sentences were presented visually in a word-by-word fashion with a 100-ms presentation time for each word and a 100-ms pause for the three words making up the context for the sentence final target word which was presented for 200 ms. Subjects were required to perform a delayed lexical decision task on the last word of the sentence. Brain activity was recorded from six electrodes [Fz, Pz, "Broca left" (Bl), "Wernicke left" (Wl), and the homologous areas of the right hemisphere, i.e., "Broca right" (Br) and "Wernicke right" (Wr)]. ERPs were averaged over 13 subjects in the semantic violation condition and over 15 subjects in the syntactic violation condition.

For the semantic violation we observed a N400 waveform, broadly distributed over the left and the right hemisphere. For the syntactic violation we found a negativity in the same temporal domain, but with a different topography. In contrast to the N400, the negativity elicited by the subcategorization violation had a left anterior distribution with maxima over the left anterior (Bl) and the frontal electrode (Fz).

We interpreted these data with respect to their temporal as well as to their topographic characteristics. The *temporal domain* around 400 ms was taken to reflect the time window at which the full information of a lexical entry is available, i.e., aspects of meaning, for example, selectional restriction information, as well as syntactic aspects, such as subcategorization information. The different *topography* was taken to indicate the respective brain systems involved in processing semantic versus syntactic aspects encoded in the lexical entry with syntactic processes, in particular being subserved by the anterior parts of the left hemisphere.

A similar left anterior negative component around 400 ms was recently observed independently in different laboratories to correlate with aspects of syntactic processes (e.g., Münte, Heinze, & Mangun, 1993; see Kluender and Kutas, 1993, for an overview.[2]

The observed ERP pattern for the subcategorization violation may be valid only for syntactic processes requiring the full access to the lexical entry. Other syntactic processes responsible for different aspects of syntactic parsing may, however, correlate with electrophysiological components different in polarity, amplitude, and timing. These are, for example, processes discussed in models of sentence comprehension assuming different stages of syntactic processing. The structure-driven model by Frazier (1978) assumes two stages: an initial stage, during which the parser builds a phrasal structure solely on the basis of word category information, and a second stage, during which thematic role assignment takes place integrating lexical-semantic and syntactic information (Frazier, 1978, 1987). This position has found its support in some studies (e.g., Frazier & Rayner, 1982; Mitchell, 1987; Rayner, Garrod, & Perfetti, 1992), while other studies rather suggest an approach allowing for preceding sentential and lexical information to influence the initial parse (e.g., Altmann et al., 1992; Shapiro et al., 1993). From the available empirical data it is not clear under which circumstances and at which point in time the reader or listener might consult lexical frame information to guide phrase structure assignment. In theory, the lexical-driven account would predict that full lexical information is available before or at the time when structure is assigned, whereas the structure-driven account would predict the first-pass parsing stage to be based primarily on word category information, with lexical and discourse information coming in only later.

Early Syntactic Processes

A next ERP experiment was carried out focusing on those early syntactic parsing processes which are assumed to be based on word category information (Friederici, Pfeifer, & Hahne, 1993). In this experiment we used an auditory presentation mode presenting the stimulus material as running speech. We reasoned that in this mode we might be able to detect fast and automatic processes which guarantee the early structuring of incoming linguistic information. Previous studies which set out to evaluate syntactic processes during comprehension by event-related brain potentials had mostly used a word-by-word visual presentation mode with

---

[2] Kluender and Kutas (1993) interpret this left anterior negativity around 400 ms to be correlated with working memory involved in gap-filling operations. This interpretation may not hold for the present data, as the stimulus material used did not require an extensive load on working memory.

pauses between each word of 300, 500, or 700 ms long (Kutas & Hillyard, 1983; Münte et al., 1993; Osterhout & Holcomb, 1992). This presentation mode may have covered those early syntactic processes assumed by structure-driven comprehension models.

In our study we included correct sentences and sentences containing violations of three different types. A semantic violation condition, similar to the one used in the previous experiment, i.e., a selectional restriction violation (e.g., *Die Wolke wurde begraben/The cloud is being buried*) was included, in order to see whether we could replicate the N400 effect in the running speech mode (see also Holcomb & Neville, 1990, 1991). In addition, we included sentences containing a morphological error (e.g., *Das Parkett wurde bohnere/The parquet is being polish*) and most importantly sentences containing a phrase structure violation (e.g., *Der Freund wurde im besucht/The friend is being in the visited*). In this latter type of sentences the last word of the sentence violates the syntactically required word category. The preposition indicates a prepositional phrase requiring a noun phrase consisting of either an article and a noun or a pronoun. In this experiment subjects heard the preposition together with the article, which in German is marked for case and in this example glutinated with the preposition, e.g., (*in dem → im/in the*). This prepositional form certainly requires the next word to be a noun. In the incorrect version, subjects, however, heard an inflected verbform (past participle) instead representing an obvious violation of the structure initiated by the preposition. All sentences were presented in random order. After each sentence subjects heard a probe word and had to decide whether this had occurred in the previous sentence. Brain potentials elicited by sentence final words (recorded from seven electrodes (Fz, Cz, Pz, Bl, Wl, Br, Wr) are displayed in Fig. 1.

The results from 16 subjects displayed different patterns of brain potentials as a function of the sentence types. For the semantic condition we observed a N400 waveform previously found in other studies (Kutas & Hillyard, 1989, 1983). For the morphological condition we also observed a negativity around 400 ms, peaking slightly earlier and being somewhat less pronounced at left and right posterior sites (Wl, Wr) than that observed for the semantic condition, but otherwise similar to the semantic N400 in its distribution. This negativity was followed by a posteriorly distributed positivity. For the phrase structure violation we observed an early negativity at the frontal electrodes peaking around 200 ms being only significantly larger than for the correct condition at the left anterior electrode (Bl). A similar early left anterior negativity was reported in correlation with phrase structure violations in a rapid serial visual presentation experiment (Neville, Nicol, Barss, Forster, & Garrett, 1991) and a left anterior negativity with a somewhat later peak was found to correlate with verbal memory functions involved in long-distance syntactic

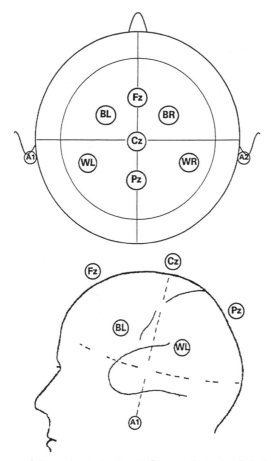

FIG. 1. Placement of the scalp electrodes. Reference electrodes linked mastoids A1 + A2.

operations such as gap-filling (Kluender & Kutas, 1993). This left anterior negative component contrasts to another component identified to correlate with syntactic processes (e.g., Neville et al., 1991; Osterhout & Holcomb, 1992; Hagoort, Brown, & Groothusen, 1993) which will be discussed below.

The different patterns in the distribution and the time-course of the waveforms for the different types of linguistic violations in this experiment suggest that different brain systems are involved in the processes dealing with lexical-semantic information as opposed to local phrasal information and that these are activated at different points in time. The anterior parts of the left hemisphere seem to particularly support those early syntactic processes responsible for structure building and maintenance as assumed by structure-driven models. These processes seem to precede processes requiring full lexical information.

Before drawing firm conclusions on the nature of the early left anterior negativity, we felt that a further investigation concentrating on the processing of phrase structure violations was necessary (Friederici, Hahne, & Mecklinger, submitted). This study's goal was twofold. First, it was designed to allow for a higher topographic resolution using a total of 25 electrodes. Second, it was planned to allow a direct comparison of syntactic processes involved in parsing connected speech. Moreover, in contrast to the experiment discussed above, we investigated not only the processing of phrase structure violations, but also the processing of phrase structure preferences.

The stimulus material used in this study consisted of sentences containing a violation of an obligatory phrase structure induced by an incorrect word category (1) or a violation of a preferred phrase structure induced by a nonpreferred word category (3) or represented the correct counterparts, (2) and (4).

(1) *Das Metall wurde zur veredelt von einem Goldschmied den man auszeichnete.*
   The metal was to the refined by a goldsmith who was honored. (literal translation)

(2) *Das Metall wurde veredelt von einem Goldschmied den man auszeichnete.*
   The metal was refined by the goldsmith who was honored.

(3) *Das Metall wurde Veredelung von einem Goldschmied den man auszeichnete.*
   The metal was refinement by a goldsmith who was honored.

(4) *Das Metall wurde zur Veredelung gebracht von einem Goldschmied den man auszeichnete.*
   The metal was to the refinement given by a goldsmith who was honored. (literal translation)

The critical word (*veredelt/refined*) in the obligatory phrase structure violation condition (1) created a mismatch between the obligatory phrasal context (noun-context) and the actual target (verb). In the preferred phrase structure violation condition (3), the critical word (*Veredelung/refinement*) created a mismatch between the preferred phrase structure (verb-context) and the actual target (noun). The nonpreferred structure, however, can take a noun after the word *wurde,* as this word has two readings, (a) an auxiliary reading, i.e., *wurde/is being,* and (b) a main verb reading, i.e., *wurde/became.* The latter reading allows the sentence to be continued with a noun (e.g., *Das Gesetz wurde Standard/The law became standard*). Thus, the actual sentence *Das Gesetz wurde Veredelung/The law is being/became refinement* could either be viewed to contain a syntactic violation when considered the preferred reading of *wurde,* namely, the auxiliary reading, or as a lexical error when considering the nonpreferred reading of *wurde,* namely, the main verb reading. Sentences were constructed in a way that would allow us to determine the word category uniqueness point between the noun and the verb reading. The vowel in the syllable prior to the disambiguating suffix was defined as the uniqueness point in order to stay free of the possible influence of coarticulation effects that the suffix might have on the consonant immediately preceding it.

Results from 17 subjects listening to 40 sentences with violations of obligatory phrase structure and their correct counterparts are displayed in Fig. 2a and to 40 sentences with violations of the preferred structure and their correct counterparts are displayed in Fig. 2b. The waveforms are elicited by the critical words in each of the conditions.

Similar to the previous experiment violations of obligatory phrase structure elicited a left anterior negativity peaking about 270 ms after the defined word category uniqueness point. The early negative peak was followed by a sustained negativity most pronounced over the left anterior electrodes. Around 600 ms after the word category uniqueness point we observed a positivity widely distributed over the posterior electrodes of both hemispheres (T_5, P_3, O_1, O_2, P_4, T_6 and Wl, Po, Wr). For the violation of the preferred phrase structure we also found a negativity most prominent over left anterior electrode sites which, however, started somewhat later than for the obligatory phrase structure violation condition. In this condition the negativity was also followed by a centro-parietal positivity.

The data of the phrase structure violation condition of this experiment replicate the early left anterior syntactic negativity observed in the earlier study. This early negativity is correlated with local phrase structure violations induced by word category errors. The negativity observed in the phrase structure preference condition started only around 400 ms after the word category uniqueness point, suggesting that this negativity reflects processes different from those eliciting the early left anterior negativity. Under this condition the parser may keep the preferred and the nonpreferred structure active until lexical access of the critical element is completed. Differently in the phrase structure violation condition, in which ungrammaticality can be flagged on the basis of word category information alone, ungrammaticality in the phrase structure preference condition can be flagged only once lexical access is completed. Thus, the left anterior negativity around 400 ms may well be correlated with syntactic processes based on lexical information other than word category information (see also Rösler et al., 1993, for a similar temporal and topographic component correlated with the processing of subcategorization information).

Given the two different latencies of the left anterior negativity observed in correlation with the processing of two different aspects of syntactic information encoded in a verb's lexical entry, one could assume a temporally (hierarchically) ordered access to these different aspects of syntactic information, with syntactic word category information being available earlier (Friederici Pfeifer et al., 1993; Friederici et al., submitted) than argument structure information (Rösler et al., 1993).

Late Syntactic Processes

Other groups investigating syntactic processes during language comprehension using ERP as the dependent variable found yet another component related to syntactic processes, that is a positivity around 600 ms and later widely distributed over the posterior parts of both hemispheres (Osterhout & Holcomb, 1992; Osterhout, Holcomb, & Swinney, 1995; Hagoort, Brown, & Groothusen, 1993). This positivity was observed for the processing of sentences which either lead subjects up to a garden-path (Osterhout, Holcomb, & Swinney, 1995) or an incorrect structure (Osterhout & Holcomb, 1992; Hagoort et al., 1993). Garden-path sentences allow for more than one syntactic structure up to a certain point. Mostly one of these structures can be viewed as highly preferred. At some critical point in the sentence, it becomes clear which of the different structures is the valid one. In case a nonpreferred structure turns out to be valid, reanalysis of the initially preferred structure becomes necessary. As similar positivities were also observed for sentences containing syntactic anomalies indicating at some point in the sentence that the structural analysis carried out was incorrect (Osterhout & Holcomb, 1992; Hagoort et al., 1993), this positive component may be correlated with the necessity for syntactic reanalysis,[3] rather than with the initial build up of a syntactic chain.

In a next study we investigated these processes of syntactic reanalysis further. We focused on the processes of syntactic ambiguity resolution using event-related brain potentials as the dependent variable (Mecklinger, Schriefers, Steinhauer, & Friederici, in press). The stimulus material consisted of relative clause sentences which were structurally ambiguous up to the last word in the clause (5).

(5) *Das ist die Managerin, die die Arbeiterinnen gesehen [hat/haben].*
   This is the manager who the workers seen [has/have]. [literal translation]).

The last word in the clause, i.e., the auxiliary, determined whether the clause had to be read as a subject relative clause or an object relative clause. In addition to this factor, we varied the factor of semantic bias either using a "neutral" verb (e.g., *sehen/to see*) or a semantically biasing verb (e.g., *entlassen/to fire,* assuming that it is more plausible that manager fire workers than workers manager).

---

[3] The distribution of this late positivity is similar to that of the so-called P300 which has been correlated with a general (non-language-specific) context updating process (Donchin, 1981). It is discussed whether the observed positivity in relation to processes of reanalysis is language specific or not (Osterhout & Holcomb, 1992).

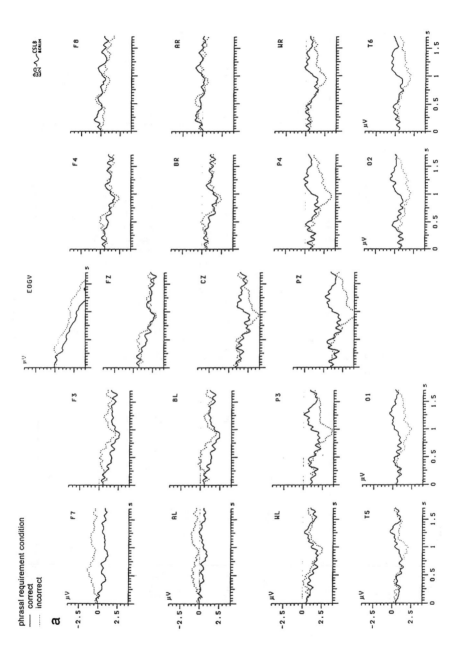

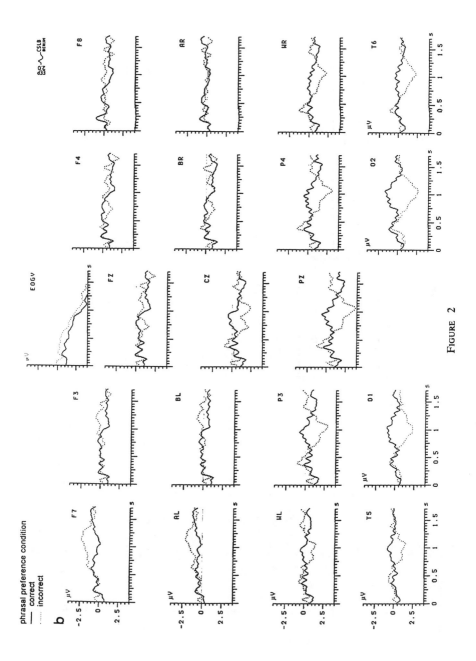

FIGURE 2

Thus, in this experiment only syntactically correct subject and object relative clause sentences were presented. They were displayed visually in a word-by-word fashion. Sentences containing the biasing verb were constructed such that the semantic bias always supported the ultimate reading of the sentence, i.e., the bias never ran against the ultimate reading of the sentence. After each sentence subjects had to answer a question concerning the agent and the patient of the sentence just read. As the subjects' behavioral performance on this task had a bimodal distribution, they were subgrouped into a fast comprehension group with short answering latencies and a slow comprehension group with long answering latencies. The fast comprehension group showed particularly interesting results. The ERPs for the reading of the past participle of the main verb (e.g., *gesehen/seen* vs. *entlassen/fired*) differed in their amplitude around 400 ms post onset. The "neutral" verb elicited a larger negativity than the semantically "biasing" verb. The distribution of this negativity resembled that of a classical N400 and was taken to reflect lexical-semantic integration processes which are easier in case of "biasing" verbs than in case of "neutral" verbs.[4]

For the disambiguating auxiliary we observed a positivity peaking 345 ms post onset with a larger amplitude in the object relative clause sentences than in the subject relative clause sentences (Fig. 3). Note that this effect was observed independent of the semantic bias of the preceding main verb.[5]

This positivity's distributional pattern was similar to that found in other studies investigating the processing of garden-path sentences and syntactic anomalies (Osterhout & Holcomb, 1992; Osterhout et al., 1995; Hagoort et al., 1993). The positivity observed in the latter studies, however, differed from that observed in the former study in its latency. While the

---

[4] We also observed a syntactically induced N400 amplitude difference. In the condition with semantically biased verbs, the N400 amplitude was larger when they biased an objective reading than when they biased a subject relative reading. To interpret this result, it is important to recall that the two relative clause types differed only with respect to the order of the two nouns preceding the past participle. An explanation for this N400 effect might be that readers initially assume the syntactic structure of a subject relative clause. When the past participle is encountered in the subject relative condition, the chosen syntactic preference and semantic information are consistent resulting in less effort to integrate the past participle's semantic information. In contrast, in the object relative condition, the initially preferred syntactic structure does not match the semantic information carried by the past participle. In this case the past participle receives less priming from the preceding context resulting in more effort to integrate the past participle.

[5] This independence of semantic and syntactic aspects during sentence processing is furthermore supported by a reaction time study with similar material (Schriefers, Friederici, & Kühn, in press) in which we found a main effect of semantic bias for the processing of the main verb and a main effect of clause type for the processing of the auxiliary, but no interaction of the factor verb bias and clause type for the auxiliary reading times.

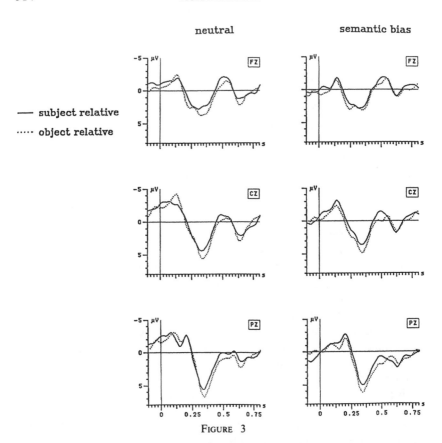

FIGURE 3

positivities in the latter studies was found at 600 ms and later, the positivity in the former peaked at 345 ms. The difference in latency may reflect the complexity of processing necessary for the revision of the initially preferred reading. The structure-driven model (Frazier, 1978) would predict that during the initial parse only one structure is built up, i.e., in case of structural ambiguities the least complex one. Furthermore, this may lead to a situation in which the parser has considered the incorrect structure and will have to reanalyze the initially considered structure. For the sentences used in the studies by Osterhout and co-workers (1992, 1993, 1995), the parser has to revise the hierarchical structural tree in order to achieve a correct structural representation. This, however, is not the case for the subject and object relative clause sentences used by Mecklinger, Schriefers, Steinhauer, and Friederici (in press). In case of an incorrect reading of the critical German relative clause the parser only has to reindex the subject noun phrase and the object noun phrase to the relative pronoun, while the hierarchical structure of the sentence remains the same. The process of hierarchical restructuring is more complex than the process of reindexation, and this may be reflected in the differential latencies observed for the positivity under the different processing conditions in the studies discussed above. The shorter latency seems to be correlated with processes of reindexation, and the longer latency with processes of structural reanalyses requiring a complete restructuring of the hierarchical tree.

The data reported by Mecklinger, Schriefers, Steinhauer, and Friederici (in press) were taken to support a comprehension model in which syntactic processes are independent of lexical-semantic processes. Only such a model would predict the syntactic effect to be uninfluenced of the semantic bias of the preceding verb with respect to the thematic role assignment. The ERP results strongly support a structure-driven account (Frazier, 1978) according to which the parser considers only one, namely, the least complex structure in case of syntactic ambiguity, such as the subject–object relative clause ambiguity tested. The data indicate that subjects primarily considered the subject relative clause reading, even when the lexical-semantic information biased an object relative clause reading.

A SYNTACTIC PROCESSING MODEL BASED ON NEUROCOGNITIVE DATA

When reviewing the event-related brain potential data with respect to language comprehension, we are left with four different language-related ERP components manifest in three different time windows: first, an early negativity around 200 ms at the left anterior sites associated with the processing of local phrase structure information; second, two negativities with different distributions around 400 ms, (a) the N400 elicited by semantic anomalies widely distributed over the posterior areas and (b) a more localized negativity in the same time window with left anterior maxima associated with the processing of lexically bound syntactic information, such as subcategorization information; and third, a late positivity which is widely distributed centrally and over the posterior parts of both hemispheres and which seems to correlate with processes of structural reanalysis.[6]

A review of the neuropsychological findings suggests that those anterior parts of the left hemisphere, usually lesioned in Broca's aphasia, subserve the fast and early structuring processes necessary to build up

---

[6] Note that a left anterior negativity around 400 ms has also been found to correlate with the processing of filler-gap dependencies. Whether the left anterior negativities observed at different time windows are variants of one component or two different components cannot be univocally decided by the data at hand and must await further confirmation.

syntactic structure including traces of moved elements on-line. The alteration of lexical processes often coincides with lesions in the posterior parts of the left hemisphere. The selective breakdown of processes of syntactic reanalysis has not been identified so far. However, it may be interesting to note that patients with lesions in the posterior part of the left hemisphere are far worse in judging a sentence's grammaticality than those with lesions in the anterior parts of the left hemisphere (Huber, Cholewa, Wilbertz, & Friederici, 1990; Linebarger, Schwartz, & Saffran, 1983).

The combined findings from neuropsychological and electrophysiological studies may suggest the following temporal and neurotopographically specified language comprehension model with three phases, two of which are primarily syntactic in nature. A first syntactic processing phase reflected by the early left anterior negativity correlates with a first-pass parse defined as the assignment of the initial phrase structure including traces of moved elements. A second phase reflected by negativities around 400 ms seems to represent the phase during which full lexical access is completed and during which lexically bound semantic (meaning and selectional restrictions) and syntactic information (subcategorization information) is processed to achieve the thematic role assignment. The differential scalp distribution of these two negative components around 400 ms suggests that the processing of the subcategorization information, in particular, is subserved by the anterior parts of the left hemisphere, whereas the processing of lexical-semantic is subserved by brain systems distributed over both hemispheres.[7] The third phase reflected by the broadly distributed late positivity appears to be related to processes of structural reanalysis which may become necessary when the initially build syntactic structure cannot be successfully mapped onto the semantic information and verb argument information provided by the lexical elements.

However, in the view of the finding that structure building processes are correlated with activities in the left anterior cortex, one might expect these cortical areas to be involved in processes of syntactic reanalysis as well. In the absence of such an ERP pattern one might be inclined to take the data reported here and in the literature to support the modified structure-driven view according to which in case of structural ambiguity

---

[7] The finding that word category information is processed prior to all other types of information carried by a lexical element requires a specific assumption about the organization of the lexical entry or its access to it. Under a structural view we would have to assume a lexical entry with a hierarchical structure in which word category information is at the top of the hierarchy and therefore available first. Under an activation view we would have to assume that word category information reaches the critical threshold for activation more easily and therefore earlier than other types of information.

the parser activates both structures, not, however, without giving a clear preference to one of them (Hickok, 1993). Depending on heuristics which are either guided by structural simplicity, as proposed by Frazier (1978), by language-specific frequencies for particular structures (e.g., subject versus object relative clauses in English, German, and Italian), or even by individual preferences (Shapiro et al., 1993), structural preferences may be set during the first-pass parse. Thus, when the need for the recovery of the nonpreferred structure is detected, this structure may be made available by raising the amount of activation for the initially nonpreferred structure. This assumption would be compatible with a computational model proposed by Kempen and Vosse (1989).

The finding, however, that the latency of the late positivity has been found to be related to the type of reanalysis required, i.e., reindexation versus hierarchical restructuring, could be taken to challenge this latter assumption. If both structures of an ambiguous sentence are active, one might expect the activation of the nonpreferred structure to be equally fast and easily retrievable, independent of whether the nonpreferred structure differs from the preferred one minimally or maximally. The observed difference in the latency of the late positivity in the different studies rather seems to suggest that these processes of reanalysis are not independent of the degree of structural similarity between the initially preferred and the nonpreferred structure.

The combined findings discussed here suggest that on-line structuring processes are subserved by brain systems located in the anterior part of the left hemisphere, whereas processes of structural reanalysis seem to involve different brain systems. The former processes may be instantiated as highly automatic procedures working on the given linguistic input and outputting structured sequences. The latter processes which take place only when structural and semantic information cannot be matched successfully on-line may require the involvement of different processing components. Further research investigating this issue may help to resolve the open questions concerning the processes of reanalysis during language comprehension.

For the time being we may take the available data to suggest a parser with two subcomponents, a first subcomponent responsible for the early structuring of the input seemingly working in a highly time-dependent procedural manner and a second subcomponent responsible for syntactic integration and reanalysis consulting grammatical knowledge which may be represented in a less time-dependent form. With such an architecture the human syntactic processing system would (a) be fast in assigning structure to the incoming information and would (b) be most flexible in selecting the valid structure for adequate thematic role assignment and the ultimate interpretation.

REFERENCES

Altmann, G. T. M. 1989. Parsing and interpretation: An introduction. *Language and Cognitive Processes*, **4**, S11–S121.

Altmann, G. T. M., Garnham, A., & Dennis, Y. 1992. Avoiding the garden-path: Eye movements in context. *Journal of Memory and Language*, **31**, 685–712.

Blumstein, S. E., Milberg, W., & Shrier, R. 1982. Semantic processing in aphasia: Evidence from an auditory lexical decision task. *Brain and Language*, **17**, 301–315.

Crain, S., & Steedmann, M. 1985. On not being led up the garden-path: The use of context by the psychological parser. In D. Dowty, L. Kartunnen, & H. Zwicky (Eds.), Natural language parsing. Cambridge: Cambridge University Press.

Donchin, E., & Coles, M. G. H. 1988. Is the P300 component a manifestation of context updating? *Behavioral and Brain Science*, **11**, 357–374.

Ferreira, F., & Clifton, C. 1986. The independence of syntactic processing. *Journal of Memory and Language*, **25**, 348–368.

Ford, M., Bresnan, J. W., & Kaplan, R. M. 1982. A competence-based theory of syntactic closure. In J. W. Bresnan (Ed.), *The mental pre-presentation of grammatical relations*. Cambridge, MA: MIT Press.

Frauenfelder, U. H., & Tyler, L. K. 1987. The process of spoken word recognition: An introduction. *Cognition*, **25**, 1–20.

Frazier, L. 1978. On comprehending sentences: Syntactic parsing strategies. Doctoral dissertation, University of Connecticut.

Frazier, L. 1987. Sentence processing: A tutorial review. In M. Coltheart (Ed.), *Attention and performance XII*. Hillsdale, NJ: Erlbaum. Pp. 559–586.

Frazier, L. 1990. Exploring the architecture of the language-processing system: In G. T. M. Altmann (Ed.), *Cognitive models of speech processing*. Cambridge, MA: MIT Press. Pp. 409–433.

Frazier, L., & Fodor, J. D. 1978. The sausage machine: A new two-stage parsing model. *Cognition*, **6**, 291–325.

Frazier, L., & Friederici, A. D. 1991. On deriving the properties of agrammatic comprehension. *Brain and Language*, **40**, 51–66.

Frazier, L., & Rayner, K. 1982. Making and correcting errors during sentence comprehension: Eye movements in the analysis of structurally ambiguous sentences. *Cognitive Psychology*, **14**, 178–210.

Friederici, A. D. 1983. Aphasics' perception of words in sentential context: Some real-time processing evidence. *Neuropsychologia*, **21**, 351–358.

Friederici, A. D. 1985. Levels of processing and vocabulary types: Evidence from on-line comprehension in normals and agrammatics. *Cognition*, **19**, 133–166.

Friederici, A. D. 1988. Autonomy and automaticity: Accessing function words during sentence comprehension. In G. Denes, C. Semenza, P. Bisiacchi, & E. Adreewsky (Eds.), *Perspective in Neuropsychology*. Hillsdale, NJ: Lawrence Erlbaum. Pp. 115–133.

Friederici, A. D. 1995. The temporal structure of language processes: Developmental and neuropsychological aspects. In B. M. Velichkovsky & D. M. Rumbaugh (Eds.), *Biological and cultural aspects of language development*. Princeton: Princeton University Press.

Friederici, A. D., & Frazier, L. 1992. Thematic analysis in agrammatic comprehension: Syntactic structures and task demands. *Brain and Language*, **42**, 1–29.

Friederici, A. D., & Kilborn, K. 1989. Temporal constraints on language processing: Syntactic priming in Broca's aphasia. *Journal of Cognitive Neuroscience*, **1**, 262–272.

Friederici, A. D., Pfeifer, E., & Hahne, A. 1993. Event-related brain potentials during natural speech processing: Effects of semantic, morphological and syntactic violations. *Cognitive Brain Research*, **1**, 183–192.

Friederici, A. D., Hahne, A., & Mecklinger, A. The temporal structure of syntactic parsing: Event-related potentials during speech perception and word-by-word reading. Submitted for publication.

Grodzinsky, Y. 1984. The syntactic characterization of agrammatism. *Cognition,* **16,** 99–120.

Haarmann, H. J., & Kolk, H. H. J. 1990. A computer model of the temporal course of agrammatic sentence understanding: The effects of variation in severity and sentence complexity. *Cognitive Science,* **15,** 49–87.

Haarmann, H. J., & Kolk, H. H. J. 1994. On-line sensitivity to subject–verb agreement violations in Broca's aphasics: The role of syntactic complexity and time. *Brain and Language,* **46,** 493–516.

Hagoort, P. 1993. Impairments of lexical-semantic processing in aphasia: Evidence from the processing of lexical ambiguities. *Brain and Language,* **45,** 189–232.

Hagoort, P., Brown, C., & Groothusen, J. 1993. The syntactic positive shift as an ERP-measure of syntactic processing. *Language and Cognitive Processes,* **8,** 439–483.

Hickok, G. 1993. Parallel parsing: Evidence from reactivation in garden-path sentences. *Journal of Psycholinguistic Research,* **22,** 239–250.

Hillyard, S. A., & Picton, T. W. 1987. Electrophysiology of cognition. In V. B. Mountcastle, F. Plum, & S. R. Geiger (Eds.), *Handbook of Physiology, Higher Functions of the Brain.* Bethesda: American Physiological Society. Vol. 5, Part 2. Pp. 519–584.

Holcomb, P. J., & Neville, H. 1990. Auditory and visual semantic priming in lexical decision: A comparison using event-related brain potentials. *Language and Cognitive Processes,* **5,** 281–312.

Holcomb, P. J., & Neville, H. 1991. Natural speech processing: An analysis using event-related brain potentials. *Psychobiology,* **19,** 286–300.

Huber, W., Cholewa, J., Wilbertz, A., & Friederici, A. D. 1990. *What the eyes reveal about grammaticality judgments in aphasia.* 28th Annual Meeting of the Academy of Aphasia, Baltimore, MD.

Kempen, G., & Vosse, Th. 1989. Incremental syntactic tree formation in human sentence processing: A cognitive architecture based on activation decay and simulated annealing. *Connection Science,* **1,** 273–290.

Kluender, R., & Kutas, M. 1993. Bridging the gap: Evidence from ERP's on the processing of unbounded dependencies. *Journal of Cognitive Neuroscience,* **2,** 196–214.

Kutas, M., & Hillyard, St. A. 1983. Event-related brain potentials to grammatical errors and semantic anomalies. *Memory and Cognition,* **11,** 539–550.

Kutas, M., & van Petten, C. 1988. Event-related potential studies of language. In P. K. Ackles, J. R. Jennings, & M. G. H. Coles (Eds.), *Advances in psychophysiology.* Greenwich: JAI Press. Vol. 3.

Kutas, M., & Hillyard, St. A. 1989. An electrophysiological probe of incidental semantic association. *Journal of Cognitive Neuroscience,* **1,** 38–49.

Kutas, M., & Hillyard, St. A. 1993. Event-related brain potentials to grammatical errors and semantic anomalies. *Memory and Cognition,* **11,** 539–550.

Linebarger, M. C., Schwartz, M., & Saffran, E. M. 1983. Sensitivity to grammatical structure in so-called agrammatic aphasia. *Cognition,* **13,** 361–392.

Martin, R. C. 1987. Articulatory and phonological deficits in short-term memory and their relation to syntactic processing. *Brain and Language,* **32,** 159–192.

Mecklinger, A., Schriefers, H., Steinhauer, C., & Friederici, A. D. Processing relative clauses varying on syntactic and semantic dimensions: An analysis with event-related potentials. *Memory and Cognition,* in press.

Milberg, W., & Blumstein, S. E. 1981. Lexical decision and aphasia: Evidence for semantic processing. *Brain and Language,* **14,** 371–385.

Milberg, W., Blumstein, S. E., & Dworetzky, B. 1987. Processing lexical ambiguities. *Brain and Language,* **31,** 138–150.

Mitchell, D. C. 1987. Lexical guidance in human parsing: Locus and processing characteristics. In M. Coltheart (Ed.), *Attention and performance XII*. Hillsdale, NJ: Erlbaum.

Münte, T. F., Heinze, H.-J., & Mangun, G. R. 1993. Dissociation of brain activity related to syntactic and semantic aspects of language. *Journal of Cognitive Neuroscience, 5*, 335–344.

Neville, H. J., Nicol, J., Barss, A., Forster, K., & Garrett, M. 1991. Syntactically based sentence processing classes: Evidence from event-related brain potentials. *Journal of Cognitive Neuroscience, 3*, 155–170.

Nicol, J., & Rapscak, B. 1994. *The closed class account revisited: Impaired memory for function words in Broca's aphasia*. Paper presented at TENNET V, Montreal, Canada, May 1994.

Osterhout, L., & Holcomb, P. J. 1992. Event-related brain potentials elicited by syntactic anomaly. *Journal of Memory and Language, 31*, 785–804.

Osterhout, L., & Holcomb, P. J. 1993. Event-related potentials and syntactic anomaly: Evidence of anomaly detection during the perception of continuous speech. *Language and Cognitive Processes, 8*, 413–437.

Osterhout, L., Holcomb, P. J., & Swinney, D. A. 1995. Brain potentials elicited by garden-path sentences. Evidence of the application of verb information during parsing. *Journal of Experimental Psychology: Learning, Memory and Cognition*.

Ostrin, R. K., & Tyler, L. K. 1993. Automatic access to lexical-semantic in aphasia: Evidence from semantic and associative priming. *Brain and Language, 45*, 147–159.

Prather, P., Shapiro, L., Zurif, E., & Swinney, D. 1991. Real-time examination of lexical processing in aphasics. *Journal of Psycholinguistic Research, 20*, 271–281.

Rayner, K., Carlson, M., & Frazier, L. 1983. The interaction of syntax and semantics during sentence processing: Eye movement in the analysis of semantically biased sentences. *Journal of Verbal Learning and Verbal Behavior, 22*, 358–374.

Rayner, K., Garrod, S., & Perfetti, C. A. 1992. Discourse influences during parsing are delayed. *Cognition, 45*, 109–139.

Rösler, F., Friederici, A. D., Pütz, P., & Hahne, A. 1993. Event-related brain potentials while encountering semantic and syntactic constraint violations. *Journal of Cognitive Neuroscience, 5*, 345–362.

Schriefers, H., Friederici, A. D., & Kühn, K. The processing of local ambiguous relative clauses in German. *Journal of Memory and Language*, in press.

Shapiro, L. P., Nagel, H. N., & Levine, B. A. 1993. Preferences for a verb's complements and their use in sentence processing. *Journal of Memory and Language, 32*, 96–114.

Trueswell, J. C., Tanenhaus, M. K., & Kello, C. 1993. Verb-specific constraints in sentence processing: Separating effects of lexical preference from garden-paths. Unpublished manuscript. University of Rochester, Rochester, NY.

van Petten, C., & Kutas, M. 1991. Influences of semantic and syntactic context on open and closed class words. *Memory and Cognition, 19*, 95–112.

Zurif, E., Swinney, D., Prather, P., Solomon, J., & Bushell, C. 1993. An on-line analysis of syntactic processing in Broca's and Wernicke's aphasia. *Brain and Language, 45*, 448–464.

BRAIN AND LANGUAGE **50,** 282–303 (1993)

A Time-Based Approach to Agrammatic Production

HERMAN KOLK

Nijmegen Institute for Cognition and Information, Nijmegen, The Netherlands

A time-based approach to agrammatic speech is presented. The paper consists of three parts. In the first part, the literature which deals with agrammatic comprehension as a problem of disrupted timing, that is, as a slow-down of syntactic computation and/or a rapid decay of the results of syntactic processing, is reviewed. In a second part, the hypothesis that similar timing problems cause difficulties in production as well is discussed. Two possible ways in which this can happen are described. First, slow down or rapid decay can lead to desynchronization within the process of syntactic tree formation. Second, a slow down of syntactic processing can cause asynchrony between the production of a syntactic slot and the retrieval of the proper grammatical morpheme from the mental lexicon. This hypothesis predicts that morphemes which are dependent on a relatively complex part of the syntactic tree will elicit relatively many errors. Results from the literature which seem to confirm this prediction are discussed. In the third part of the paper, the possible ways in which a patient can adapt to the reduced temporal window that would result from a timing deficit are discussed. Message simplification will reduce the size of the required temporal window and will therefore have a beneficial effect on the error rate. Restart of the computational process will profit from previously reached activation levels so that synchrony is easier to reach and error rate is reduced. Empirical work which appears to support these hypotheses is reviewed. © 1995 Academic Press, Inc.

DESYNCHRONIZATION AS A POSSIBLE SOURCE OF AGRAMMATIC COMPREHENSION

Language comprehension and production are exceedingly complex tasks in which numerous pieces of information have to be juggled within fractions of seconds. All parts have to fall in the right place at the right time. The disruption of this temporal fine-tuning could well be the deficit responsible for the difficulties aphasics have in expressive and receptive language tasks. This has been the claim of a number of authors in the so-called chronogenetic tradition in aphasiology (see Kolk & van Grunsven, 1985, for references). As early as 1885, Grashey proposed that lack

Address correspondence and reprint requests to the author at NICI KUN, P.O.Box 9104, 6500 HE Nijmegen, The Netherlands. E-mail: kolk@nici.kun.nl.

of synchrony between the representations of word meaning and word form can lead to word-finding difficulties. He reported on a patient with severe naming difficulties. This patient was very impaired in naming objects presented to him by means of pictures. But he had another problem as well. If the patient was given a picture and the picture was taken away and immediately replaced by the correct picture and one or more other pictures, he was unable to identify the correct one. Grashey suggested that the pictorial representation was subject to very rapid decay and that, as a consequence, activation of the word form had too little time to develop, hence the word-finding difficulties (Grashey, 1885). The great Carl Wernicke commented very favorably upon this hypothesis stating that ". . . I would not hesitate to suggest that it may be considered the most significant contribution in the development of the doctrine of aphasia during the past decade. In his work Grashey pursues an entirely new and very fruitful notion by postulating the temporal factor as an important consideration in the formation of the spoken word, which can be likewise applied to reading and writing" (Wernicke, 1885).

Not only semantic information but also word-form (phonological) information itself could be subject to pathological decay. Just recently, Martin, Dell, Saffran, and Schwartz (1994) simulated the speech errors of a jargon aphasic by means of Dell's (1986) interactive spreading activation model of language production. By assuming a high decay rate in the semantic–lexical–phonological network, they were able to simulate various qualitative error patterns in the speech of this patient, not only as they varied over tasks (naming versus repetition), but also as they varied over time (spontaneous recovery). In a follow-up study, Schwartz, Dell, Martin, and Saffran (1994) investigated the naming errors of 17 fluent aphasics. They found that patients fell into three groups. For one group, the error pattern could be simulated by means of a fast decay, just as with the jargon aphasic described above. For another group, however, a different change in the temporal parameters was necessary. The behavior of this subgroup could only be simulated by assuming a slow activation of word–form information within the network. Still another group seemed to have both kinds of temporal disruption. So the behavior of these 17 patients could be accounted for by either a fast decay or a slow activation, or a combination of both.

In 1985, Kolk and van Grunsven (1985; Kolk, van Grunsven, & Keyser, 1985) proposed a general framework for the explanation of agrammatic sentence processing as a timing disorder. In this framework, it is assumed that every element needed to build a sentence representation has some activation that determines the availability of that element. It takes some time for elements to reach a critical level of activation and after a peak level, the activation is subject to decay. A third assumption is that activations of elements are typically interdependent. This means that the activity of one element is required for the activation of another element. For instance, information about the subject of the sentence must be active in order for the right form of the verb to become activated. Between these two types of information, there must therefore be computational simultaneity or synchrony. When the parameters, determining the various activation levels, are changed, this delicate simultaneity can be jeopardized, leading to a premature disintegration of sentence structures. Two changes to the normal situation were suggested. In the "slow activation" case, it takes longer for an element to reach its critical level of activation and occasionally, this level is reached too late. "Fast decay" makes elements unavailable when they fall below their critical level too soon to be combined with other elements in the sentence representation.

Haarmann and Kolk (1991a) have constructed a computational model to investigate these possibilities. This model, SYNCHRON, simulates the temporal course of the building up of a hierarchical phrase-structure representation. The nodes, needed to construct a syntactic tree, take some time to reach their "memory time phase," that is, to become available to interact with other nodes. Furthermore, this memory time is limited; if it is exceeded, elements disappear from memory. A particular syntactic category, say a VP, can be retrieved only if all immediate daughter categories (e.g., V, NP, PP) are available. The model successfully reproduces the agrammatic performance profile over reversible active, locative, and passive sentences at two different levels of severity (reported by Kolk & van Grunsven, 1985). It does so both by slowing down computation and by limiting memory time; the fit with the empirical data is equally good in the two cases. The type of elements affected by the temporal deficit do make a difference, however. When function word nodes are affected, the required pattern does not emerge. It appears only when phrasal category nodes are impaired.

The SYNCHRON model has a number of clear advantages over most existing hypotheses on agrammatic comprehension (see Kolk & Weijts, in press, for a discussion of these other hypotheses). First of all, it accounts for the finding that sentences with a more complex constituent structure pose more problems than sentences with a simpler structure, not only in comprehension (cf. Caplan & Hildebrandt, 1988; Kolk & Weijts, in press) but also in the detection of ungrammaticality (Haarmann & Kolk, 1994). Second, it can explain that agrammatic comprehension is a phenomenon that varies in degree. That is, even though for instance passives are generally harder to understand than actives, the absolute level of performance can vary. Thus, one finds patients who perform at chance on both actives and passives and other patients who are above-chance on both actives and passives (Kolk & van Grunsven, 1985; Mitchum, Haendiges, & Berndt, 1993). Third, the model produces a complexity × severity interaction, a trend of which was present in the Kolk

and van Grunsven data and, more convincingly, in Caplan and Hildebrandt's (1988) findings. Finally, SYNCHRON can, at least in principle,
give an account for the well-known dissociation between agrammatic
comprehension and grammaticality judgment (Linebarger, Schwartz, &
Saffran, 1983). To do so, it must be assumed that comprehension, entail-
ing both role assignment and the selection of the correct picture or the
acting-out of the proper event, requires a longer availability of the syntactic representation than grammaticality judgment and is therefore more
easily disrupted by rapid decay or slow activation of syntactic information.

In its present form, SYNCHRON also has a number of clear limitations. First of all, there is no stage of role assignment. Adding this process
to the model would make it possible to see whether in fact desynchronization within the parser would leave grammaticality judgments relatively
unimpaired. Second, there is no chain formation. Chain formation would
put additional constraints on synchronization, because the trace and the
moved argument, including their coindexations, must be simultaneously
available for correct role assignment. If SYNCHRON would be provided
with this facility, it would be possible to investigate how much the movement factor contributes to the performance deterioration, independent
from constituent structure complexity. Finally, SYNCHRON's precise
assumptions regarding the synchrony requirement may need revision.
Haarmann and Kolk (1991a) demonstrate that the predictions SYN-
CHRON makes with respect to sentence types other than actives, locatives, and passives are far from optimal. These predictions could be improved, the authors argue, by requiring *all* daughter nodes to be available
for a particular mother category to be retrieved, rather than only the
immediate daughter nodes (see Cornell, 1995, for a computational model
of agrammatic comprehension, which can be regarded as an extension of
SYNCHRON).

There are various kinds of empirical evidence to support the claim
that desynchronization of language processing contributes to agrammatic
sentence comprehension. Swinney and Zurif (1995) discuss data to show
that at least some agrammatics suffer from a slowing down of lexical
activation and, as a consequence, are not able to reactivate moved arguments at the point in time that such reactivation is needed: at trace positions. Friederici (1995) reviews a number of studies she conducted which
led her to conclude that agrammatics are slowed down in the first-pass
assignment of syntactic structure to the incoming sentence. Furthermore,
she presents ERP data which suggest a very early activity (around 300
ms) over the frontal areas of the left hemisphere, an activity she thinks
reflects this early assignment process. Hagoort (1990) reports two studies
which are suggestive of a processing slow down. In both experiments,
ambiguous words were presented in a sentence context. Research with
normals has shown that both meanings of an ambiguous word are active

for a short period of time and then the contextually inappropriate meaning is quickly suppressed (cf. Onifer & Swinney, 1991). Hagoort found evidence that Broca's are slowed down in this respect: they do suppress the inappropriate meaning but only at a relatively late point in time (750 ms). This was true not only when the appropriate meaning of the ambiguous word was biased by the meaning of the sentence but also when it was biased by the syntactic context. The first effect—disambiguation slowed down by the sentence meaning—has very recently been replicated in an ERP study. At an interstimulus interval of 100 ms, Broca's aphasics showed an N400 effect of semantic priming in response to both meanings of the ambiguous noun. Only at 1250 ms was the N400 effect selective for the appropriate meaning (Hagoort, 1994). Haarmann and Kolk (1991b) tested 12 agrammatics in a syntactic priming paradigm in which they varied grammaticality and SOA between context sentence and target word (SOAs of 300, 800, and 1200 ms were employed). Only at 1200 ms was a significant priming effect obtained. In a subsequent word monitoring study, again grammaticality was varied as well as interstimulus interval between the point at which the sentence became ungrammatical and the target word (Haarmann & Kolk, 1994). This time, there was no evidence for slow activation, even though to a large extent the same group of patients was used. However, there was evidence for rapid decay, as the effect of ungrammaticality had disappeared after an ISI of 750 ms, although the elderly controls still showed a significant effect. Why there is this difference between the syntactic priming task and the word monitoring task is unclear. Taken together, the evidence for a slow activation or fast decay looks promising although the issue is far from settled.[1]

A TIME-BASED APPROACH TO (PAR)AGRAMMATIC PRODUCTION

In view of the progress that has been made with the timing approach to agrammatic comprehension, it seems reasonable to explore the possibilities of this approach to agrammatic sentence production. A few years ago, one of my doctoral students, Mart van de Kerkhof, and I designed a first-time-based model (Kolk, 1987) of agrammatic sentence production. In this model, we employed the Kempen and Hoenkamp (1987) Incremental Procedural Grammar, an algorithm which generates grammatical sentences in Dutch. It does so in an "incremental" fashion; that is, as soon as a particular part of the syntactic tree is ready, the corresponding part of the sentence is produced (see also Levelt, 1989, for an extensive de-

---

[1] Tyler, Ostrin, Cooke, and Moss (1995) have recently demonstrated by means of a word-monitoring paradigm, that at least some agrammatic patients can retrieve some types of grammatical information quite rapidly. Tyler et al., however, did not manipulate SOA or ISI. Therefore, there could still be slow activation in some patients and/or for some types of information. There also could be fast decay.

scription and discussion of the IPG model). Similarly to what was later done by Haarmann and Kolk (1991a), we assumed that for correct production of the sentence, synchrony between the various parts of the syntactic tree was necessary. We were able to show that with both rapid decay and slow activation, the required synchrony often failed to materialize, so that a grammatical sentence could not be produced. The number of failures was dependent upon (a) the complexity of the sentence and (b) the activation and decay rates. No attempt was made to actually generate sentences on the basis of disintegrated syntactic representations.

In addition to problems with complex sentences, agrammatics have difficulty producing the correct grammatical morphology. In the well-known classification of Goodglass and Kaplan (1972), these two symptoms are represented by means of different rating scales. It has been proposed that we are dealing here with two separate and dissociable deficits, a syntactic and a morphological one (cf. Berndt, 1987; Saffran, Berndt, & Schwartz, 1989). Although the syntactic and the morphological component could indeed be independently damaged in some individual cases, this does not exclude the possibility that a purely syntactic deficit has consequences for the production of grammatical morphology. In particular, if one thinks of syntactic and lexical processes to be partially autonomous production routines, morphological errors could arise as a result of an asynchrony between these two lines of processing. This is a possibility I will elaborate below.

What precisely do I mean by "morphological" errors? In our previous work we have demonstrated that there are, at least in Dutch and German, large differences in type of output between "spontaneous speech" (that is, free conversation) and elicited speech (various kinds of picture description and cloze tasks). Our research has demonstrated that in free conversations, patients typically produce *agrammatic* speech: output that—according to Kleist's original definition of agrammatism (1916)—lacks much of the required grammatical morphology but contains relatively few erroneously produced morphemes. Elicited speech is typically more *paragrammatic:* it contains a high number of wrongly selected morphemes and relatively few omissions (Heeschen, 1985; Kolk et al., 1985; Haarmann & Kolk, 1992; Kolk & Heeschen, 1992; Hofstede & Kolk, 1994). Our theory of this task effect (see the above references) holds that elicited speech largely reflects the underlying deficit, but that the agrammatic character of spontaneous speech is primarily due to the way in which the patients adapt themselves to this underlying deficit. I will first discuss our views on the deficit and explain how a timing disorder can lead to paragrammatic speech. I will then describe how patients can adapt to such a deficit in a way that leads to agrammatic output.

There are relatively few models of paragrammatic speech. One important processing account of paragrammatism is given by Butterworth and Howard (1987). The paragrammatic output they tried to explain was produced by a group of jargon aphasics. Butterworth and Howard assume that, in this group at least, the sentence production system itself is intact. There is no selective loss of a particular component but rather an impairment of the processes controlling the operation of the various components. These control operations involve the transfer of information between system components, the initiation and termination of component processes, and the checking of the output of components. An omission of a word, for instance, could be due to a failure in initiation of lexical selection or a loss in the transfer from lexical selection to phonology assembly. As to why these control processes are impaired, Butterworth and Howard refer to Freud (1890), who thought there was a transient attentional disturbance leading to a failure of inhibition. Given the assumption of such a global impairment, affecting all components of the sentence production system to some extent, one would expect close similarity between normal speech errors and aphasic paragrammatisms and this is indeed what their data suggest.

My theory is similar to that proposed by Butterworth and Howard, in that I assume no change in the overall structure of the sentence production system but only in the mode of processing. Instead of a transient attentional deficit that can affect any set of components, I propose a slowing down of the syntactic component that affects not only the computation of structure but also the selection of the proper grammatical morphology. How could slowing down have such an effect? In most psycholinguistic theories (cf. Levelt, 1989), sentence production is seen to involve the generation of syntactic frames, with categorized slots (e.g., Det, Adj, N). The slots are filled with morphemes, retrieved from the mental lexicon. Garrett (1975, 1980) has argued, on the basis of speech error data, that there is a fundamental distinction between closed-class elements (function words and inflections) on the one hand and open-class elements (content words) on the other. Whereas open-class words are generated by lexical processes and have to be inserted into the syntactic frame, closed-class items would be generated by the syntactic process itself: they are part of the frame and need no independent retrieval. Stemberger (1984, 1985), however, has shown that one can interpret the critical speech error data in a different way, without making the assumption that closed-class elements and syntactic frame are accessed within a single operation.[2] Furthermore, if the closed-class vocabulary would be

---

[2] Stemberger relates the different behaviors of open- and closed-class elements primarily to frequency differences between the two sets of elements. Evidence for the important role of frequency has been obtained by Stemberger and MacWhinney (1986) and by Dell (1990). Another argument against Garrett's hypothesis is Bock's (1989) finding that "syntactic

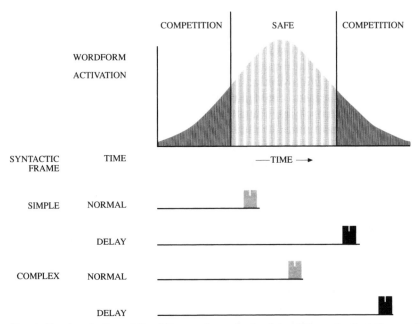

FIG. 1. Synchronization of the delivery of a syntactic slot and the activation of a word form. (Top) The growth and decay of activation of the word form is depicted. The dark gray areas indicate that at the beginning and at the end of the activation period, when the amount of activation is relatively small, competition with other lexical candidates is relatively high, and the chance to select the wrong word form is equally high. In the light gray area, competition is low and there is a low chance to make errors. (Bottom) Time at which the syntactic slot is delivered is indicated with simple and complex sentences and with normal and delayed rate of syntactic processing. Optimal syntacto-lexical integration is obtained when the slot is delivered in synchrony with the "safe" period of lexical activation.

generated by the syntax, there is no possibility to get an asynchrony between syntax and lexicon with respect to these items and we have no way to account for paragrammatic errors within our general framework. In the theory I am going to propose, therefore, not only content but also function morphemes are represented in the syntactic representation by means of a categorized slot and both types of morphology have to be integrated with their syntactic slots. This integration requires synchrony and a processing delay can disrupt this synchrony.

In Fig. 1, I have given a pictorial sketch of the theory. The activation curve at the top represents the lexical activation process of one particular item, as it develops over time. With current models of spreading activa-

---

persistence,'' i.e., the tendency to repeat a particular phrase structure across successive sentences, was equally strong when the closed-class members of these phrase structures were different or the same.

tion (e.g., Dell, 1986), I assume that both at the beginning and at the end of the activation period, when the amount of activation is relatively low, competition from alternative lexical candidates is relatively high. At these two periods, the selection process is error prone. The middle period, on the other hand, is relatively "safe." In Fig. 1, the safe and the unsafe regions are indicated by different shades of gray.

The lower part of Fig. 1 represents the syntactic process, in particular the point in time at which this process delivers a syntactic slot for integration with a lexical filler. Two assumptions are reflected. First of all, in agrammatics the process of slot delivery is slower than in normals. Second, in both normals and aphasics, a slot that is part of a complex syntactic structure is produced at a later point in time than a slot in a simpler structure. The latter assumption follows from our general line of reasoning, also evident in the SYNCHRON model, that a more complex structure requires more computational steps and therefore more time to be computed.

As can be derived from Fig. 1, the theory predicts that complex structures will elicit more morphological errors than simple structures. I will follow the Kempen and Hoenkamp (1987) model discussed above in assuming that for a particular morpheme to be produced, it is *not* necessary that a syntactic tree for a full sentence be available. Production of morphology is possible, as soon as a *minimally required* syntactic representation has been made available. For the production of plural inflections of nouns, for instance, the minimally required structure is the NP. For lexical prepositions to be produced, a PP would have to be available. Of course, what will count as a minimally required structure will change from language to language.

In three studies evidence in support of this prediction has been obtained. The first study was conducted by Goodglass and Berko (1960). These authors presented 21 unclassified aphasics with a sentence completion task. In this task, they elicited 10 different grammatical morphemes. Of particular interest is the contrast they observed between the plural, verb, and possessive inflections, because the same phonological forms are involved in each case ($-s$, $-z$, or $-z$). First of all, they found the plural inflection to elicit significantly fewer errors than the verb inflection. This is what one would expect, assuming that for the production of a plural inflection, only an NP has to be available, whereas an S-node is required for a verb inflection to be produced. Goodglass and Berko also found the possessive inflection (e.g., "the horse's blanket") to be significantly harder than both the plural and the verb inflections. That possessive inflections are harder than plurals is to be understood, given the fact that possessives require the availability of a compoud NP. Why the possessives are harder than the verb inflections is less obvious, since the two critical structures are of comparable complexity (a compound

NP, consisting of two NPs on the one hand, and an S, consisting of an NP and a VP). Perhaps possessives have a lower frequency. If this is the case, it could be argued that the structure takes more time to develop and as a consequence leads more readily to errors in lexical selection.

A second relevant finding was reported by Friederici (1982). She elicited prepositions in a cloze task. Prepositions that could occur in different functional roles were employed. Thus, the German preposition *auf* can occur not only as a lexical preposition (*Peter steht auf dem Stuhl—Peter stands on the chair*) but also as a subcategorized preposition (*Peter hofft auf dem Sommer—Peter hopes for the summer*). With her group of Broca's aphasics, Friederici found that subcategorized prepositions were much harder to produce than the lexical ones. With respect to our hypothesis, this result makes sense, since for the production of the subcategorized preposition, the integrity of a complex VP seems to be required (a VP with an embedded PP), whereas the lexical preposition can be produced solely on the basis of a PP being available.

In a recent study, Haarmann and Kolk (1992) compared various types of grammatical morphology in a cloze task.[3] It is important to realize that, unlike in the previous two studies, the phonological form of the grammatical morpheme was not kept constant, so variation in the properties of these morphemes, such as frequency and the number of morphological options in a given category, could have played a role (Menn & Obler, 1991). Three types of inflectional morphology were studied. (a) The plural-noun inflection; here the minimally required structure is the NP. (b) The inflection of adjectives in attributive position; here the minimally required structure is a complex NP, in which the head noun is modified by an adjective. (c) The inflection of verbs in present or past tense; here the minimally required structure is the S. There is a clear order of structural complexity of these three structures: NP < NPadj < S. On this basis, we predict a corresponding order of difficulty for the three types of inflection: Plural inflection < adjectival inflection < verb inflection. This was indeed the result obtained by Haarmann and Kolk.

Besides inflectional morphology, three types of function words were tested. (a) Determiners (articles and possessive pronouns); these elements require the availability of an NP. (b) Lexical prepositions (locative, directional, or instrumental); for these elements, minimally a PP must be

---

[3] The Haarmann and Kolk study was set up primarily to investigate the difference between Broca's and Wernicke's. For this reason, the various sets of morphemes tested were not as homogeneous as one would want. This was particularly true for the category "pronouns," which we will therefore not consider. Furthermore, the category "adjective inflections" contained a few items in which the comparative and superlative inflections were elicited, and in the category "prepositions," 4/12 items were not lexical prepositions. Leaving these elements out, however, did not change the overall order of difficulty reported by Haarmann and Kolk.

available. (c) Auxiliaries; for these elements, the required structure is the S (the task asked for the production of an inflected auxiliary). Again, the structural complexity is clearly ordered: NP < PP < S. So the predicted order of difficulty is determiners < prepositions < auxiliaries. Haarmann and Kolk observed this order of difficulty in their task.

Taken together, these data seem to indicate that structural complexity at least partially determines the number of errors made in the production of morphology. Of course, I have only loosely defined what "minimally required" complexity is; whether the complexity order that I have presented is the right one remains to be seen. Furthermore, the role of other factors such as frequency and number of morphological options still has to be worked out.

So far, I have assumed that paragrammatisms were brought about by syntactic delay. However, the general scheme, depicted in Fig. 1, allows for another possibility. Selection of the wrong lexical alternative would also take place if the syntactic slot would be delivered in synchrony with the early phase of lexical selection (the dark area in the left part of the activation curve). If lexical activation would be delayed, integration with the syntactic slot would be attempted too early and errors of selection could arise. This is the kind of paragrammatism one could expect from a patient with a lexical deficit. Obvious candidates, of course, would be Wernicke's aphasics, who show paragrammatism in their spontaneous speech and are also sometimes claimed to have a lexical impairment (cf. Berndt & Caramazza, 1980). This hypothesis would predict that for Wernicke's aphasics, there should be a *reversed* complexity effect: since complex structures are produced more slowly, their slots would become available later, at a point in time where there is relatively little response competition and integration with the correct morpheme will succeed more often (see Fig. 1). Haarmann and Kolk (1992), however, have given their cloze task also to a group of Wernicke aphasics. Contrary to the prediction of the lexical hypothesis, the Wernicke group shows the same order of difficulty as the Broca group. Given these data then, the most parsimonious hypothesis is that the Wernicke group also suffers from a slowdown in the syntactic part of their production system.

ADAPTING TO A REDUCED TEMPORAL WINDOW IN PRODUCTION

According to the argument given above, a syntactic slow down will lead to desynchronization, both within the process of syntactic encoding and in integrating syntactic slots with lexical fillers. Such asynchronies will also occur in normals, but only under more extreme circumstances, that is, with very complex syntactic structures. The difference between aphasics and normals could be described as one in size of the temporal window available for syntactic computation and syntacto-lexical integration. This makes it understandable why aphasics make more grammatical errors than normals, but not qualitatively different ones, as was shown by Butterworth and Howard (1987). What it does not explain, however, is why the normals make as few errors as they do. Since the syntactic system, given its recursive nature, is in itself capable of producing a structure of any given complexity, why is there not a continuous overload, leading to a constant flow of speech errors? This argument, of course, is equally valid if one believes that the capacity limitation common to aphasics and normal speakers is not of a temporal nature but rather one characterized in terms of parsing-work space, as has been assumed by Caplan and Hildebrandt (1988).

The answer to this question must be that somehow the sentence production system as a whole is adapted to its limited capacity. In terms of current models (e.g., Garrett, 1975; Levelt, 1989), such adaptation could occur at the message level, the level at which the "what-is-to-be-said" is represented in conceptual terms. Complexity at this level leads to structurally complex sentence forms. If these message level representations are fine-tuned to the capacity of the syntactic system, a situation of continuous overload is prevented. All this fine-tuning, of course, would be the effect of a long learning process and would therefore, in the adult speakers at least, be highly automatized.

Now back to the aphasic speakers. If they suffer from a reduction in the size of their temporal window, the fine-tuning between message level and syntactic process is disrupted and the patients are confronted with continuous overload. There is little reason to suppose that the pressure towards fine-tuning that was assumed in the normal speakers would no longer be present in the aphasic. This means that there will be a tendency for simpler message level structures to be selected up to a point at which the system is no longer overloaded and relatively error-free output is possible. However, such selection can no longer occur automatically, as it does in the normal speaker. Readaptation will start as a controlled process that can gradually become automatic again. If it succeeds, it will have a double effect. Not only will it eliminate errors due to overload, it will also create simpler sentence forms. This is basically the hypothesis that my colleagues and I have been defending over the last 10 years. Agrammatic spontaneous speech results from message simplification and message simplification is the adaptive reaction from the aphasic speaker to capacity overload.

The hypothesis that agrammatic speech results from message simplification was first proposed by Isserlin (1922). "It is not damage to sentence finding so much as damage to sentence creation that lies at the root of the grammatical disturbance in aphasia. There is not a derailment of ordinary speech: the telegram style is laid down, a priori; and we must assume that there is a schema of telegram thought that anticipates the creation of telegram speech'' [English translation, p. 336].

Isserlin obviously limited his message simplification hypothesis to telegraphic speech: the output pattern characterized by a tendency to omit grammatical morphology. I will have more to say about telegraphic speech below. First, I will discuss another property of speech produced by Broca's aphasics, to which the hypothesis can be extended. This is the symptom of simple but complete sentence form, known as "reduced variety of grammatical form" (Goodglass & Kaplan, 1972) or "structural simplicity" (Berndt, 1987; Saffran et al., 1989). Its most important features are paucity of phrasal elaboration and relative absence of sentence embedding. Research by Saffran et al. (1989) has shown that both features are reliably present in nonfluent speakers, classified as Broca's aphasics. Hofstede (1992) looked at sentence embedding in a group of 16 Dutch-speaking Broca's aphasics and found that the aphasics produced significantly fewer embedded sentences than the controls (6% vs. 22% for the controls). However, there is considerable variation between patients: one patient scored just below the control level (21%) whereas 5 patients produced 0% embedded sentences. In the theory we have proposed (cf. Kolk et al., 1985; Kolk & van Grunsven, 1985; Kolk, 1987; Kolk & Heeschen, 1990), structural simplicity results from message simplification on the part of the aphasic speaker in an attempt to prevent computational overload. In Kolk et al. (1985), a model is sketched which demonstrates how simplified messages lead to structurally simple sentences.

Besides structural simplicity, we have telegraphic speech: the so-often described pattern of output that, at least for languages like English, German, and Dutch, is characterized by a tendency to omit grammatical morphology. Hofstede and Kolk (1994) have made an attempt to quantify this phenomenon in their recent study with a group of 16 Broca's and three German speaking aphasics. Both for prepositions and determiners an average omission rate of 49% for the Broca's was observed, with a range from 5% to 97%. The normal controls omitted about 4% of these morphemes, significantly less than the Broca's. It is important to observe the gradual variation between patients in the amount of telegraphic speech: from 4% up to 97%, almost every decile contains one or more patients. Contrary to what is implicitly assumed in the bulk of the agrammatism literature, agrammatic speech is *not* an all-or-none phenomenon but varies in degree. Following Isserlin, we have proposed that telegraphic speech results from message simplification, though a more austere form of it than underlies structurally simple speech. In the message-simplification model referred to above, we have indicated how this could occur.

Most of our research has been devoted to the question of whether telegraphic speech in Broca's aphasics is indeed due to adaptation. We have provided two types of evidence to suggest an affirmative answer. The first type of evidence is that the constructions used in telegraphic speech are part of the normal repertoire. The second kind of evidence is that it seems possible for at least a number of telegraphic speakers to shift to a different, more paragrammatic type of output.

Let us first discuss the argument that telegraphic speech is normal. Isserlin's hypothesis is that by means of message simplification, aphasics select sentence forms that their impaired processing system is still able to handle. This implies that these sentence forms are a subset of the normal repertoire. My colleague Claus Heeschen and I have proposed that this subset is the set of elliptical constructions normal speakers use under particular circumstances (1992). We have made a list of eight properties of normal ellipsis in German and Dutch and have shown that these properties are significantly more characteristic of the spontaneous speech of German speaking Broca's aphasics than of Wernicke's aphasics. The properties are the following.

(A) Normal ellipsis allows for the omission of function words. Accordingly, Broca patients showed an omission rate of 56%, and Wernicke patients omitted only 13% of their function words.

(B) Normal ellipsis does not allow for the omission of bound morphology. Therefore, if a normal speaker wants to be very short, he can say "two tables here" instead of "I want you to put two tables here." But he is not allowed to say "*two table_ here." Here the theory makes a nontrivial prediction. Counter to the standard view that agrammatic speech consists of "omission of free and bound grammatical morphology," it is predicted that agrammatics do not omit this bound morphology. The prediction was confirmed, not only for the German-speaking but also for a group of Dutch speaking Broca patients studied by Kolk and Heeschen. It was again confirmed by Hofstede and Kolk (1994) for a different group of Dutch agrammatics. The group of Wernicke patients also showed a near absence of inflection omission. The impression that Broca's omit inflections probably derives from the fact that in English, the infinitive of the verb has the same form as the verb stem and as we will show, Broca patients do overuse infinitives, also in German and Dutch.

(C) Normal ellipsis does not allow for morphological substitutions. Although elliptical speech is deplete of "errors" of omission, substitution errors would make the utterance ungrammatical, just as is the case for full sentences. Taking free and bound morphemes together, Kolk and Heeschen found a 3% substitution rate for the German speaking Broca's and one of 13% for the Wernicke's. The Dutch agrammatics made 1% substitutions. Hofstede and Kolk (1994) observed a similarly low substitution rate in their Dutch agrammatics.

(D) Normal ellipsis allows for the use of nonfinite verb forms (e.g., "Me leaving showbusiness? Never!"). If agrammatics overuse ellipsis, we predict a higher incidence of infinitive use—without accompanying auxiliary—for Broca's than for Wernicke's. Kolk and Heeschen observed percentages of 53 and 9, respectively.

(E) Normal ellipsis allows for main verb omission. So besides "buying flowers for Sally," we have "flowers for Sally" as a regular form of ellipsis. Overuse of ellipsis would therefore lead to a high omission rate for main verbs. The percentages found by Kolk and Heeschen were 41 and 9, for Broca and Wernicke patients, respectively.

(F) Normal ellipsis allows for omission of the grammatical subject (see the examples in the previous paragraph). The percentages for the two groups of German speaking patients were 50 and 18, respectively.

(G) Normal ellipsis prescribes the word order of the subordinate (S-O-V) rather than that of the main clause (S-V-O). S-O-V word order was observed in 41% with Broca's and in 10% with Wernicke's.

(H) Normal ellipsis prescribes, at least in German, a strong adjective inflection. So a normal speaker can say "Der blaue Engel" (the blue angel). He is allowed to omit the article, but then he has to inflect the adjective differently (e.g., "Blauer Engel"). The German-speaking agrammatics had this strong inflection with 74% of their adjectives, and Wernicke's had it in 34%.

Another strategy to demonstrate the normality of agrammatic speech has been followed by Hofstede (1992). Instead of looking at the relative frequency with which elliptical features are present in agrammatic speech, he selected telegraphic utterances from both agrammatic and normal speech and compared the two sets of constructions. A "telegraphic utterance" was defined as any utterance in which finiteness was omitted. Finiteness was considered to be omitted whenever (a) the main verb was omitted or (b) a nonfinite form of the main verb was used, without there being an additional auxiliary. This criterion was chosen because finiteness omission appears to represent the clearest break with the full sentence. It turned out to be a good choice: most of the omissions Hofstede observed in the speech samples he studied were covered by this criterion (92% of the agrammatic omissions and 83% of the normal omissions). Three samples of speech were obtained: (a) Speech obtained in conversations with normal adults, matched in age and education with the aphasics. During these conversations, an attempt was made to create an informal atmosphere, which we know stimulates the production of elliptical speech. (b) Speech produced by municipal officials talking to foreigners, the so-called "foreigner talk." (c) Speech obtained from Broca's aphasics during free conversations.

The normal telegraphic utterances were categorized first. The most frequent category was labeled "isolated predicates" (91%). The following subtypes were observed.

(1) Nonfinite verbs, e.g., "in China geboren" (born in China).
(2) Noun phrases, e.g., "mooi huis" (beautiful house).
(3) Prepositional phrases, e.g., "naar een feestje" (to a party).
(4) Adjectives, e.g., "heel normaal" (very normal).
(5) Adverbials, e.g., "nog een keer" (one more time).
The other main category was called "subject–predicate constructions" (9%). The same five subtypes occur here as in the category "isolated predicates," this time preceded by an NP.
(6) Noun phrases followed by a nonfinite verb , e.g., "ik nooit gezien" (I never seen).
(7) Noun phrases followed by another noun phrase, e.g., "rode wijn tien gulden" (red wine ten guilders).
(8) Noun phrases followed by a prepositional phrase, e.g., "zoon twee dagen in bed" (son in bed for two days).
(9) Noun phrases followed by an adjective, e.g., "mensen in Spanje vriendelijk" (people in Spain friendly).
(10) Noun phrases followed by an adverb, e.g., "mijn vrouw terug" (my wife back).
The samples of foreigner talk showed the same 10 categories of telegraphic expressions. Furthermore, more or less the same relative frequencies were observed in the two samples: isolated predicates by far outnumbered the subject–predicate connections and within the first category, isolated NPs were the most frequent, followed by the isolated nonfinite verbs; the other categories had about the same (low) frequency.
The interesting question, of course, was what do the aphasic utterances look like? As it turned out, all categories of expressions present in the two normal samples were also present in the aphasic samples and vice versa. Furthermore, as was the case with foreigner talk, the relative frequencies of the two main categories and of the two most frequent subcategories (1 and 2 in the above list) were the same. The main difference between the aphasic and the normal samples concerned the complexity of the telegraphic constructions. The aphasic showed less phrasal elaboration (e.g., adding a determiner or an adjective to a noun) than was present in the normal conversations, although the amount of elaboration of foreigner talk was less than in the aphasic speech. Furthermore, the aphasics produced fewer grammatical objects (direct, indirect, or prepositional object) with the nonfinite verbs (e.g., "op Jan wachten"—waiting for John).
It is interesting to note that Saffran et al. (1989) describes a subcategory of agrammatic utterances they call "topic-comment structures." The five examples they present (Saffran et al., 1989, p. 471) correspond exactly with our subcategories 6 to 10: "dancing Cinderella and prince" (6); "Cinderella washerwoman" (7); "Cinderella in the house" (8); "Cinderella very pretty" (9); "party over" (10). Isolated predicates were observed as well; they were put into the class of "Other utterance catego-

ries, NP, VP, etc.'' Unfortunately, no examples or frequencies of occurrence were provided.

I think it is no exaggeration to say that, as far as structural similarity is concerned, the evidence for the ellipsis hypothesis is pretty strong. Let us now turn to the other type of evidence, that at least some agrammatics can shift from agrammatic to more paragrammatic speech. We have assumed that agrammatic speech results form message simplification and that this simplification is under control of the subject. This implies that a patient should be able to at least partially refrain from message simplification. This will result in more overload for the grammatical system, synchrony will be harder to achieve, and more errors of substitution will occur. On the other hand, the omission rate for function words will go down (omissions of inflections are true errors and will therefore show a rise).

Heeschen (1985) asked a group of German-speaking Broca and Wernicke patients to describe a picture to an experimenter who could not see the picture. He observed that, in comparison to spontaneous speech, Broca's produced fewer errors of omission and more of substitution. The Wernicke patients showed no such effect. In terms of omissions and substitutions of grammatical morphology, the output patterns of the two groups were indistinguishable. Kolk and Heeschen (1992) analyzed a larger data set from Heeschen's original study and came to the same conclusion. Hofstede and Kolk (1994) demonstrated with a large group of Dutch-speaking agrammatics that, at least in a number of patients, one can obtain a shift toward paragrammatism simply by giving the patients pictures to describe, without hiding the pictures from the experimenter. Hiding the pictures gave an additional effect for a number of patients. Bastiaanse (1994) described a case of a Dutch-speaking agrammatic woman, who—in the middle of an interview—demonstrated a complete change in type of output. Whereas in the beginning her sentences were complete but with many morphological as well as constructional errors, later on she shifted to a classical form of telegraphic speech. A final demonstration comes from Kolk and Hofstede (1994). In a case study of an agrammatic patient, they compared spontaneous speech to a condition in which the patient simply was *requested* to "talk in complete sentences." Each time the patient produced a telegraphic utterance, he was reminded of the instruction. A dramatic decrease in omission rate resulted from this manipulation, accompanied by a significant rise of the percent of substitutions.

Two recent studies (Goodglass, Christiansen & Gallagher, 1993; Hesketh & Bishop, in press) appear to indicate that there is only a limited shift toward paragrammatism in English-speaking agrammatics. On the one hand, it could be that a language-specific factor is responsible for this finding, having to do with the existence and form of an elliptical register in English. On the other hand, there are a number of important procedural differences between the two studies and ours, having to do with baseline, elicitation procedure, response parameters, and the like (see Kolk & Heeschen, in press, where the Hesketh and Bishop study is discussed in detail). The question whether substantial shifts toward paragrammatism can also be obtained with English-speaking agrammatics is therefore still unanswered.

It does appear, therefore, that at least some patients can make a shift from agrammatic to a more paragrammatic type of output, as predicted by our theory.

Let us now return for a moment to the Kolk and Hofstede (1994) study, where it was shown that a shift from agrammatism to paragrammatism could be produced "upon request." In this study, we also looked at speech rate and number of word repetitions. We observed that the shift to more complete utterance forms was accompanied by (a) a sharp reduction in speech rate and (b) a large increase in number of word repetitions. How do we account for these changes?

In 1985, Marianne van Grunsven and I proposed that besides simplification of sentence form, there is another way a patient could react to the newly acquired capacity limitation (see also Kolk & Heeschen, 1990, where this point is elaborated in more detail). Instead of trying to prevent premature disintegration of sentence representation by means of message simplification, a patient could try to repair the disintegrated representation. We called these two reactions *preventive adaptation* and *corrective adaptation*, respectively. Whereas preventive adaptation leads to structural simplicity and telegraphic speech, corrective adaptation leads to the symptom of nonfluency, one of the hallmarks of the syndrome of Broca's aphasia. Increased nonfluency is what we observe in Kolk and Hofstede's (1994) patient, when he gives up telegraphic style. Because the patient tries to produce more complex utterance forms, he finds himself more often in a situation of capacity overload. As a consequence, more errors occur at what Levelt (1989) calls the level of "inner speech" (also referred to as the "phonetic plan"). The patient can allow these errors to come out and produce paragrammatic errors. He can also, by means of "covert repairing" (Levelt, 1989) edit these errors out and produce relatively error-free speech. This will take time, hence the nonfluencies.

How does this covert repairing take place? In the normal speaker, one could conceive of this repair process as involving a sequence of steps: (a) error identification; (b) computation of the correct element; (c) replacement of the erroneous for the correct element. If this were to be the case, it is hard to see how an aphasic patient with a severely limited capacity would be able to do any repairing at all. I do not think, however, that all this processing is necessary. After step (a), the normal speaker can simply *restart* the production of the sentence, or part of the sentence. Since the likelihood of making a speech error is very low, it is highly unlikely that he will make two errors in a row. Restarting therefore automatically leads to repairing. In the aphasic speaker, however, the situation is different. Here the likelihood of making errors is high and, other things being equal, it will remain high, even if a second attempt is made. How then can restarting lead to improvement?

For an answer to this question, it is necessary to consider again the nature of the capacity limitation we have proposed. Suppose the critical limitation would consist in a reduction of the size of a syntactic buffer, as has been suggested by Caplan and Hildebrandt (1988). If a particular construction would be too complex for this small buffer, restarting would have no benefit whatsoever: a structure that does not fit into the buffer will never fit. When the limitation is a temporal one, however, the situation is different. The basic difficulty that results from a timing deficit, as I have defined it, is that a particular representational element decays before other elements, with which it has to be in synchrony, are activated. Now restarting does offer an advantage. After decay, the element may still have a relatively high level of activation, because of the fact that it has just been activated. Reactivation can occur from this level, rather than from the rest level, and the critical element will reach the threshold sooner. In this way, restarting leads to faster processing and to improved performance.

We can conclude therefore that there is evidence for both preventive and corrective adaptation. Is it possible for a patient *not* to adapt, by neither simplifying nor restarting the sentence? In such a case, we would expect fast and complex speech, full of errors. The speech of Wernicke patients is like this and consequently, my colleague Claus Heeschen and I have proposed that the difference between Broca's and Wernicke's, as far as sentence production is concerned, is a difference in adaptation, not in type of grammatical impairment. Evidence that both groups of patients have the same production deficit comes from two studies, already described above. Kolk and Heeschen (1992) have shown that in the constrained picture description task, overall omission and substitution rates are the same for the two groups. Haarmann and Kolk (1992) gave a cloze task to the two groups. They compared the error profiles over seven types of grammatical morphemes and found no significant difference. The same was true for the profile of response rates, as well as for the average rates overall. So the hypothesis that there is a common production deficit in the two groups receives some support.

Suppose for the moment that the two groups do have the same impairment; then another question arises: why do the Wernicke's aphasics not adapt? This is a tough question that we have not yet been able to answer satisfactorily. We have considered the possibility that Wernicke's aphasics are less aware of or less concerned about their errors and therefore do not bother to avoid them (Heeschen, 1985). This led us to expect that the behavior of the two groups in the cloze task would be very different. The Broca's would be expected to be slow and accurate, the Wernicke's to be fast and sloppy in their performance. What we found, however, was that both groups were equally slow and equally accurate (Haarmann & Kolk, 1992). The fact that the two groups were equally slow was remarkable, because in their free conversations, the Wernicke patients spoke three times faster than the Broca patients. An alternative explanation that we suggested in Kolk and Heeschen (1992) is that, as a side effect of their brain damage, Wernicke's suffer from a press of speech and have therefore little time to notice their errors. But this leaves another question unanswered: why is no press of speech observable in the cloze task?

CONCLUSION

It will be clear from the above that the timing approach to agrammatism, both in production and comprehension, has its problems and open ends. However, I believe it also has a number of virtues. (a) It gives an explicit description of the capacity limitation underlying agrammatic behavior. (b) It suggests a model for the genesis of paragrammatic errors. (c) It also suggests a model for the genesis of agrammatic errors. The strategies that are assumed to underlie these errors make sense within the time-based approach as a whole. They are not postulated in an ad hoc fashion. (d) Finally, an integrated account is given of an aspect of agrammatic speech that is often considered to be less interesting: nonfluency.

REFERENCES

Bastiaanse, R. 1994. Broca's aphasia: A syntactic and/or a morphological disorder? A case study. *Brain and Language*, **48**, 1–32.

Berndt, R. S. 1987. Symptom co-occurrence and dissociation in the interpretation of agrammatism. In M. Coltheart, G. Sartori, & R. Job (Eds.), *The cognitive neuropsychology of language*. New Jersey: Lawrence Erlbaum Associates.

Berndt, R., & Caramazza, A. 1980. A redefinition of the syndrome of Broca's aphasia. *Applied Psycholinguistics*, **1**, 245–299.

Bock, J. K. Closed-class immanence in sentence production. *Cognition*, **31**, 163–186.

Butterworth, B., & Howard, D. 1987. Paragrammatism. *Cognition*, **26**, 1–37.

Caplan, D., & Hildebrandt, N. 1988. *Disorders of syntactic comprehension*. Cambridge, MA: MIT Press.

Cornell, T. L. 1995. On the relation between representational and processing models of asyntactic comprehension. *Brain and Language*, **50**, 304–324.

Dell, G. S. 1986. A spreading-activation theory of retrieval in sentence production. *Psychological Review*, **93**, 283–321.

Dell, G. S. 1990. Effects of frequency and vocabulary type on phonological speech errors. *Language and Cognitive Processes*, **5**, 313–349.

Freud, S. 1890. *On aphasia.* Translated by E. Stengel, 1951. London: Imago.

Friederici, A. 1982. Syntactic and semantic processes in aphasic deficits: The availability of prepositions. *Brain and Language,* **15,** 249–258.

Friederici, A. D. 1995. The time course of syntactic activation during language processing: A model based on neuropsychological and neurophysiological data. *Brain and Language,* **50,** 259–281.

Garrett, M. F. 1975. The analysis of sentence production. In G. H. Bower (Ed.), *The psychology of learning and motivation.* New York: Academic Press. Vol. 9.

Garrett, M. F. 1980. Levels of processing in sentence production. In B. Butterworth (Ed.), *Language production.* London: Academic Pres. Vol. 1.

Goodglass, H., & Berko, J. 1960. Agrammatism and inflectional morphology in English. *Journal of Speech and Hearing Research,* **3,** 257–267.

Goodglass, H., Christiansen, J. A., & Gallagher, R. 1993. Comparison of morphology and syntax in free narrative and structured tests: Fluent vs. nonfluent aphasics. *Cortex,* **29,** 377–407.

Goodglass, H., & Kaplan, E. 1972. *The assessment of aphasia and related disorders.* Philadelphia: Lea & Febiger.

Grashey. 1885. Über Aphasie und ihre Beziehungen zur Wahrnemung. *Arch. für Psychiatrie und Nervankrankheiten,* **16,** 654–688. [Translated by R. de Bleser in *Cognitive Neuropsychology,* 1989, **6.**]

Haarmann, H. J., & Kolk, H. H. J. 1991a. A computer model of the temporal course of agrammatic sentence understanding: The effects of variation in severity and sentence complexity. *Cognitive Science,* **15,** 49–87.

Haarmann, H. J., & Kolk, H. H. J. 1991b. Syntactic priming in Broca's aphasics: Evidence for slow activation. *Aphasiology,* **5,** 49–87.

Haarmann, H. J., & Kolk, H. H. J. 1992. The production of grammatical morphology in Broca's and Wernicke's aphasics: Speed and accuracy factors. *Cortex,* **28,** 97–112.

Haarmann, H. J., & Kolk, H. H. J. 1994. On-sensitivity to subject–verb agreement violations in Broca's aphasics': The role of syntactic complexity and time. *Brain and Language,* **46,** 493–516.

Hagoort, P. 1990. *Tracking the time course of language understanding in aphasia.* Dissertation, University of Nijmegen.

Hagoort, P. 1994. *Agrammatic aphasia as an interface between the cognitive and the neural architecture of language.* Paper presented at the 1st European Summer Institute of Cognitive Neuroscience. Nijmegen, June.

Heeschen, C. 1985. Agrammatism versus paragrammatism: A fictitious opposition. In M.-L. Kean (Ed.), *Agrammatism.* New York: Academic Press.

Hesketh, A., & Bishop, D. V. M. Agrammatism and adaptation theory. *Aphasiology,* in press.

Hofstede, B. T. M., & Kolk, H. H. J. 1994. The effects of task variation on the production of grammatical morphology in Broca's aphasia: A multiple case study. *Brain and Language,* **46,** 278–328.

Hofstede, B. M. T. 1992. *Agrammatic speech in Broca's aphasia: Strategic choice for the elliptical register.* Dissertation University of Nijmegen. [Available as NICI Technical Report 92-07.]

Isserlin, M. 1922. Uber Agrammatismus. *Zeitschrift für die gesamte Neurologie und Psychiatrie,* **75,** 332–416. [English translation by H. Droller, D. Howard, & R. Campbell in *Cognitive Neuropsychology,* 1985, **1,** 308–345.]

Kempen, G., & Hoenkamp, E. 1987. An incremental procedural grammar for sentence formulation. *Cognitive Science,* **11,** 201–258.

Kleist, K. 1916. Uber Leitungsaphasie und grammatische Störungen. *Monatschrift für Psychiatrie und Neurologie,* **40,** 119–199.

Kolk, H. H. J. 1987. A theory of grammatical impairment in aphasia. In G. Kempen (Ed.),

Natural language generation; new results in artificial intelligence, psychology and linguistics. Dordrecht: Martinus Nijhoff.

Kolk, H. H. J., & van Grunsven, M. F. 1985. Agrammatism as a variable phenomenon. *Cognitive Neuropsychology,* **2,** 347–384.

Kolk, H. H. J., van Grunsven, M. F., & Keyser, A. 1985. On parallelism between production and comprehension in agrammatism. In M.-L. Kean (Ed.), *Agrammatism.* New York: Academic Press.

Kolk, H. H. J., & Heeschen, C. 1990. Adaptation symptoms and impairment symptoms in Broca's aphasia. *Aphasiology,* **4,** 221–231.

Kolk, H. H. J., & Heeschen, C. 1992. Agrammatism, paragrammatism and the management of language. *Language and Cognitive Processes,* **7,** 82–129.

Kolk, H. H. J., & Heeschen, C. The malleability of agrammatic symptoms: A reply to Hesketh and Bishop. *Aphasiology,* in press.

Kolk, H. H. J., & Weijts, M. Judgments of semantic anomaly in agrammatic patients. Argument movement, syntactic complexity and the use of heuristics. *Brain and Language,* in press.

Kolk, H. H. J., & Hofstede, B. M. T. 1994. The choice for ellipsis: A case study of stylistic shifts in an agrammatic speaker. *Brain and Language,* **47,** 507–509.

Levelt, W. J. M. 1989. *Speaking: From intention to articulation.* Cambridge, MA: MIT Press.

Linebarger, M., Schwartz, M. F., & Saffran, E. M. 1983. Sensitivity to grammatical structure in so-called agrammatic aphasics. *Cognition,* **13,** 361–392.

Martin, N., Dell, G. S., Saffran, E., & Schwartz, M. F. 1994. Origins of paraphasias in deep dysphasia: Testing the consequences of a decay impairment to an interactive spreading activation model of lexical retrieval. *Brain and Language,* **47,** 609–660.

Menn, L., & Obler, L. K., Eds. 1990. *Agrammatic Aphasia. A cross-language narrative sourcebook.* Amsterdam: John Benjamin.

Mitchum, Ch.C., Haendiges, A. N., & Berndt, R. S. 1993. *Patterns of sentence comprehension in "agrammatism."* Paper presented at the Annual Meeting of the Academy of Aphasia, Tucson, Arizona, October 24–26.

Onifer, W., & Swinney, D. 1991. Accessing lexical ambiguities during sentence comprehension: Effects of frequency of meaning and contextual bias. *Memory & Cognition,* **9,** 225–236.

Saffran, E. M., Berndt, R. S., & Schwartz, M. F. 1989. The quantitative analysis of agrammatic production: Procedure and data. *Brain and Language,* **37,** 440–479.

Schwartz, M. F., Dell, G. S., Martin, N., & Saffran, E. M. 1994. Normal and aphasic naming in an interactive spreading activation model. *Brain and Language,* **47,** 391–394. [Abstract]

Stemberger, J. P. 1984. Structural errors in normal and agrammatic speech. *Cognitive Neuropsychology,* **1,** 281–313.

Stemberger, J. P. 1985. An interactive model of language production. M. A. Ellis (Ed.), *Progress in the psychology of language, Vol. 1.* London: Erlbaum.

Stemberger, J. P., & MacWhinney, B. 1986. Frequency and the lexical storage of regularly inflected forms. *Memory and Cognition,* **14,** 17–26.

Swinney, D., & Zurif, E. 1995. Syntactic processing in aphasia. *Brain and Language,* **50,** 225–239.

Tyler, L. K., Ostrin, R. K., Cooke, M., & Moss, H. E. 1995. Automatic access of lexical information in Broca's aphasics: Against the automaticity hypothesis. *Brain and Language,* **48,** 131–162.

Wernicke, C. 1885. Einige neuere Arbeiten über Aphasie. *Fortschritte der Medizin,* **3,** 463–482. [English translation in G. H. Eggert, 1977, *Wernicke's works on aphasia. A sourcebook and review.* The Hague: Mouton. Pp. 175–205. Also translated by R. de Bleser in *Cognitive Neuropsychology,* 1989, **6,** 547–569.

BRAIN AND LANGUAGE **50**, 304–324 (1995)

On the Relation between Representational and Processing Models of Asyntactic Comprehension

Thomas L. Cornell

University of Tübingen, Tübingen, Germany

Most accounts of asyntactic comprehension fall along a spectrum from pure representational accounts to pure processing accounts. The double dependency hypothesis of Mauner, Fromkin, and Cornell (1993) is an example of the former, while the SYNCHRON model of Haarman and Kolk (1991; see also Kolk, this volume) is an example of the latter. This paper attempts to demonstrate some of the ways that these two approaches interact. We introduce GENCHRON, a computer model based on Haarman and Kolk's SYNCHRON. GENCHRON is a parser subject to the kinds of processing deficits examined in Haarman and Kolk (1991). We present a simple grammar which leads GENCHRON to produce the kinds of semantic representations which Mauner, Fromkin, and Cornell (1993) propose for asyntactic comprehenders. © 1995 Academic Press, Inc.

BACKGROUND

Most accounts of asyntactic comprehension fall along a spectrum from pure representational accounts, in which the details of the parser are largely irrelevant but properties of the grammar are very important, to pure processing accounts, in which the details of the grammar are largely irrelevant but properties of the parser are very important. The double dependency hypothesis of Mauner, Fromkin, and Cornell (1993) is an example of the former, while the SYNCHRON model of Haarman and Kolk (1991; see also Kolk, 1995) is an example of the latter. This paper attempts to demonstrate some of the ways in which these two approaches interact. We introduce GENCHRON, a computer model based on Haarman and Kolk's SYNCHRON. GENCHRON is a parser subject to the kinds of timing-based processing deficits explored in Haarman and Kolk (1991), which can output the semantic interpretations of the fragments

Address correspondence and reprint requests to the author at Seminar für Sprachwissenschaft, Kleine Wilhelmstrasse 113, 72074 Tübingen Germany. e-mail: cornell@sfs.nphil.uni-tuebingen.de.

343

which it is able to parse, even when it cannot assign a complete syntactic analysis to its input. We present a simple constraint-based phrase structure grammar from which GENCHRON produces the kinds of semantic representations which Mauner et al. (1993) argue underlie asyntactic comprehension (and see also Hickok, Zurif, & Canseco-Gonzalez, 1993).

The Computational Simultaneity Condition

The parsing model that Haarman and Kolk propose has several important features. First, it is strictly bottom-up, i.e., nonpredictive. Second, it is parallel. Words come in at a steady rate, independent of the parser's task-load, and they are processed immediately. Third, grammatical constituents are resource-consumers, and their allowed resource consumption is strictly limited. In particular, it takes time before they become available to the parser, and they subsequently persist in the parser's working memory for a limited period of time. Finally, the construction of new constituents from old is governed by the *computational simultaneity condition*.

> *Computational Simultaneity Condition*
> Construct a superordinate constituent node only if there is a point in time at which all of its subordinate constituent nodes are simultaneously available in memory.

There are thus three temporal parameters which are important in the life of a constituent: the time at which the parser begins its construction (i.e., the point at which the simultaneous presence of all its daughter constituents is verified), the point at which it becomes available to other parsing tasks, and the point at which it dies away from working memory and is no longer available to the parser. Following Haarman and Kolk (1991) we can hypothesize that the kind of brain damage we see in agrammatism affects the brain's computations by either (a) slowing down the rate at which new elements are constructed or (b) increasing the rate at which they decay.

The parsing rule can then be expressed, semiformally, as follows.

> *Parsing Rule*
> If there is a rule of the grammar $A \rightarrow B_1, \ldots, B_n$ and there are available in working memory n adjacent constituents labeled B_1 through B_n, then construct a new constituent labeled A, with daughters labeled B_1 through B_n, and set the time at which its construction begins to the earliest point in time at which the B_i are simultaneously available.

Constraint-Based Phrase-Structure Grammars

We will not be able to make use of the kind of simple context free grammar that Haarman and Kolk (1991) use in their simulations. We will need to associate features (such as case, θ role, index) and other sorts of information with constituents, and we will need special computational tools to manipulate them. A context free grammar rule is a rule of the form

$$A \rightarrow B_1, \ldots, B_n,$$

where A denotes a single category label drawn from the list of nonterminal categories (like NP, IP, V0), and the B_i each denote a category drawn from either the nonterminal or terminal vocabularies (the latter consisting of words or morphemes).

A *constraint-based* grammar (Shieber, 1992) adds expressive power along two dimensions. First, categories can now have features associated with them, so we can speak not only of a constituent of category NP, but also of the referential index of that constituent, or its case or θ role or even its semantic interpretation. Second, we can place constraints on these features, where for our purposes we will take constraints to be simple formulas in a predicate-calculus-like language. So, for example, we might have a rule like

S → NP VP,
    agreement(NP) = agreement(VP),
    case(NP) = nominative,
    apply(semantics(VP), semantics(NP), semantics(S)).

The equality constraints in this (somewhat unrealistic) example enforce subject–verb agreement and the assignment of case to the NP; the predicate *apply* is meant to hold just in case the third argument (*semantics*(S)) is the result of applying the semantics of the VP (assumed to be a function of some sort) to the semantics of the NP (assumed here to be its argument).

Note that the rule combines both syntactic and semantic constraints. No claim is being made here about modularity; only that all syntactic constituents have semantic interpretations which are a function of the interpretations of their subconstituents (the principle of semantic *compositionality*). The information associated with a particular constituent can be strictly divided between syntactic information (case and agreement features, here) and semantic information. In general, syntactic constraints will involve only syntactic or semantic information, not both.

We can now extend the computational simultaneity condition straightforwardly so that it handles our new type of grammar.

> *Extended Computational Simultaneity Condition*
> Construct a superordinate constituent node, *and solve its associated constraints,* only if there is a point in time at which all of its subordinate constituent nodes are simultaneously available in memory.

These added grammatical constraints will give us the computational devices we need to construct movement-chains and logical forms in accordance with the theory underlying Mauner et al. (1993).

Because we take semantics to be compositional, and we wish to see what constraints on semantic interpretation may survive parse-breakdown, we must be very careful to say not only what it means to pass the simultaneity condition (it means that the superordinate node gets built) but also what it means to fail the simultaneity condition. Haarman and Kolk (1991) merely equate parse failure (i.e., the failure of any one rule due to the simultaneity condition) with comprehension failure, inducing guessing behavior on experimental tasks. This means that whenever the deficit has an effect on processing, comprehension is a matter of guesswork. The Mauner et al. (1993) approach (and also Hickok's approach) holds that the deficit affects all processing (of relevant structures). The syntactic parser never sends complete information to the semantic interpreter; sometimes the incomplete information delivered by the syntax is enough to drive the semantics to a single conclusion, and other times it is insufficient to force the semantics one way or another. Therefore, to simulate the operation of this theory we must be able to represent partial syntactic structures, and in particular we must say what representation the parser returns if a particular constituent cannot be built due to a failure of synchronization.

In this paper the simplest possible assumption is made. The output of the parser will be a list of all of those trees which it was able to construct successfully. So, for example, if there is a rule like $S \rightarrow$ NP VP and the NP and the VP are constructed successfully, but the NP has faded from memory before the VP arrives (or vice-versa—it can happen!), then the semantics will be delivered just the sequence of logical forms associated with the NP and the VP. If, for example, the NP itself was never constructed due to a failure of a rule like NP $\rightarrow$ Det N S', but the VP was still constructed successfully, then the semantic interpreter will behave as if it received the sequence Det, N, S', VP. We will see that this is enough to give us quite detailed information about how the semantic interpretation will turn out.

The simulations discussed here were run using the GENCHRON system currently under development at the University of Arizona. The core of the system is a parser, whose operation is dependent on (1) a grammar file and (2) a parameter file. The parameter file allows the user to control the rate at which nodes become active in memory and with which they decay away for arbitrary classes of categories, with pretty much arbitrary probability distributions. However, for the purposes of this exercise, the stochastic aspects of the system were not used. All the files making up the GENCHRON system are Prolog programs and were run under SICStus Prolog on a Sun SPARCstation/330 in the University of Arizona Psycholinguistics Lab.

The Syntax

We begin by discussing the grammar file. Before anything else, note that the grammar about to be described was constructed solely with an eye toward assigning particular structures to sentences of the sort often used in comprehension experiments. No attempt has been made to rule out ungrammatical structures. So, for example, this grammar allows for a parse of the relative clause *who is chasing the boy* as having *who* in subject position. Ruling out such examples requires adding more constraints to the grammar, but does not significantly alter the rules and constraints we will employ, so I have chosen simply to let the grammar overgenerate, ignoring the ill-formed structures it assigns.

The grammar I have constructed for this exercise, which I will henceforth refer to as MFCG1, is a standard X-Bar theoretic grammar. There are six basic categories: *V(erb)*, *N(oun)*, *P(reposition)*, *I(nflection)*, *C(omplementizer)*, and *D(eterminer)*. Each category "projects" syntactic constituents at three "bar levels," e.g., V0, V1, and VP, where V0 is the lowest and VP is the highest. Thus for each basic category we have at least the following pair of rules (where *Specifier* is a phrasal category—YP, for some Y—and *Complements* is a sequence of phrasal categories):

(R1) *XP → Specifier X1*
(R2) *X1 → X0 Complements*

In addition, we allow for the adjunction of modifiers to the basic structures given by rules R1 and R2, as in R3, below.

(R3) *XP → XP Modifier*

This is sufficient to allow for modification of NPs by relative clauses and VPs by prepositional phrases, which are the only instances of modification that we will take an interest in here.

Following Koopman and Sportiche (1988) and many others, and in accordance with the theory underlying Mauner et al. (1993), let us adopt the VP-internal subject hypothesis, according to which a verb assigns all of its θ roles within the VP. Following Stowell (1981), let us implement θ role assignment as the coindexation of an argument category (always DP—"Determiner Phrase"—in these examples) with a position in a predicate's θ grid. (In these examples predicates will always be projections of verbs.) So minimally, we will need to associate our DPs with indices and our V0s and V1s with θ grids. In addition, it will be convenient to indicate whether the argument DP has received an *internal* or *external* θ role. The rules expanding V1 constituents then become

V1 → V0 DP,
theta_assign(index(DP), grid(V0), grid(V1)),
role(DP) = internal.

$$V1 \rightarrow V0$$
$$grid(V1) = grid(V0),$$

and the VP rule becomes

$$VP \rightarrow DP \ V1$$
$$theta\_assign(index(DP), \ grid(V1), \ grid(VP)),$$
$$grid(VP) = [\ ],$$
$$role(DP) = external.$$

The constraint-language predicate *theta_assign* is defined as a relation between an index and two θ grids which holds just in case the index is equated with the first available slot in the first grid, with the remaining, unbound grid positions returned as the second grid. Thus, for example, if the index of the DP were *i* and the θ grid of a V0 were [*Int, Obl, Ext*] then *theta_assign*(*i*, [*Int, Obl, Ext*], *G*) would be true just in case *Int* was set equal to *i* and *G* was set equal to [*Obl, Ext*].

Besides receiving a θ role, every DP must in addition be assigned an abstract case. In the MFCG1 grammar, subjects receive nominative case from I1, direct objects receive accusative case from V0, and prepositional objects receive oblique case from P0. Note that not all V0 can assign accusative case. In particular, neither intransitive verbs nor passive participles license the assignment of accusative case. Therefore DPs receiving internal θ roles from passive participles must receive case elsewhere, and DPs receiving external θ roles must always find their cases elsewhere. In GB theory this provides the essential repellent force which induces syntactic movement, or chain-formation.

A simple way to implement this is to supply verbs with "case grids" analogous to θ grids. Case assignment is then analogous to θ role assignment. In particular, if the grid is empty, then the verb cannot assign case. We thus expand the V1 rule for transitive verbs as follows:

$$V1 \rightarrow V0 \ DP,$$
$$theta\_assign(index(DP), \ grid(V0), \ grid(V1)),$$
$$role(DP) = internal,$$
$$case\_assign(case\text{-}grid(V0), \ case(DP)).$$

The constraint-language predicate *case_assign* marks the direct object with whatever is in the verb's case-grid (invariably *accusative* in these examples) or, if there is nothing in the case-grid, leaves the DP unmarked.

Chain Formation in MFCG1

We will handle chain formation using the constraint-language predicate *chain_link* which takes three arguments: a chain-link and two link buffers. It holds true if the first buffer differs from the second only in that it contains the given link. Informally, the second buffer equals the first minus the link. Note that this predicate can be used computationally either to remove a link from the first buffer, yielding the second, or to add a link to the second buffer, yielding the first. We will also allow the first argument to be *nil* (represented as [ ], the empty list), in which case the two link buffers must be identical: the second equals the first minus zero, as it were.

In this grammar, we will always allow DP to dominate a trace— wherever a DP may occur, a trace may occur. When a DP node dominates a trace, then a chain-link crosses the DP boundary, and so the chain-link-buffer associated with the DP must be nonempty—in fact it must contain just the link which extends into the DP. (For the moment we represent chain links as triples containing the crucial information that must be shared along the chain: index, case and θ role. Later we will add semantic interpretations to this list.)

$DP \rightarrow$ [ ],
   $link(DP) = \langle index(DP), case(DP), role(DP) \rangle.$

If on the other hand the DP is lexicalized, then we will stipulate that the value of *link(DP)* be [ ]. In either case, the following rule template will work (where X and Y can be any categories). It states that the links-buffer of the mother node X must contain an antecedent for any traces domi-nated by DP, which is removed to yield the set of links crossing into the sister node Y. If the DP dominates no traces (it is lexical) then the chain links passing into constituent X must all pass into constituent Y as well.

$X \rightarrow DP\ Y$ (order irrelevant)
   $chain\_link(link(DP), links(X), links(Y)).$

We can always identify a trace because it dominates no lexical material. Furthermore, because DPs must always be associated with (a) a θ role, (b) a case and (c) some sort of semantic content, we can always identify a DP which must be the antecedent of one or more traces. For example, the specifier of IP position is (in MFCG1) always case-marked, but never θ-marked. Thus any DP appearing in surface subject position will have to be the antecedent of a chain-link which provides it with a θ role (but not a case!). The specifier of CP position (the position of relative pronouns, in MFCG1) is neither case-marked nor θ-marked, so its occupant, if there is one, will have to be the antecedent of a chain in order to acquire a case and a θ role. We can handle antecedents with the following template (where L is just a local variable aiding readability).

$X \rightarrow DP\ Y$ (order irrelevant)
   $L = \langle index(DP), case(DP), role(DP) \rangle,$
   $chain\_link(L, links(Y), links(X)).$

Here the call to *chain_link* takes L, which is instantiated to a chain-link symbol containing the essential information about the DP, and adds it to the links buffer associated with the mother node X to yield the links buffer associated with the sister node Y.

Note that a DP can find itself at both the bottom of one chain link and the top of another. For example, in the question *Who is chasing the girl?* the subject position is occupied by the trace of the interrogative pronoun *who*, which is itself the antecedent of the trace in the external argument position in VP: *who$_i$ t$_i$ is t$_i'$ chasing the girl*. The following rule combines the effects of both templates.

$IP \rightarrow DP\ I1$,
  $L = \langle index(DP), case(DP), role(DP) \rangle$,
  $chain\_link(link(DP), links(IP), X)$,
  $chain\_link(L, links(I1), X)$.

If the subject DP is a trace, then the first *chain_link* constraint will trigger the removal of a chain-link from the buffer associated with IP, leaving the results in a temporary variable X. (Otherwise, X equals *links(IP)*.) The second *chain_link* constraint then adds the link L to X to yield the buffer associated with I1. In the example of *Who is chasing the girl?*, the buffer associated with IP contains only the link added by *who*.

	$links(IP) = [\langle index(who), \ldots \rangle]$
first call to *chain_link:*	$link(DP) = \langle index(who), \ldots \rangle$,
	$X = [\ ]$
second call to *chain_link:*	$links(I1) = [L]$ (i.e., X plus L)

Passive in MFCG1

The theory of passive employed in Mauner et al. (1993) is implemented here in two rules: the rule expanding VP to the external argument position and V1 and a rule adjoining the *by*-PP to VP. In accordance with the underlying syntactic theory, we in fact do nothing to the VP $\rightarrow$ DP V1 rule. All of the work is done by the VP $\rightarrow$ VP PP rule, and in the construction of the PP itself.

First note that we treat the preposition *by* as little more than a case marker and not as a predicate with independent semantic content. Therefore the features of the *by*-PP are essentially those of its DP argument, plus the fact that the preposition marks the phrase as being in the oblique case.

The *by*-PP is an adjunct in this theory, and not an argument; therefore it is not in a θ-marked position. It must receive a θ role by being linked to a θ-marked position. In fact, the *by*-phrase can be linked only to the external argument position. While no theory of syntax known to us proposes that the *by*-phrase is *moved* from an underlying external argument position, nonetheless the link established between the oblique case marked *by*-phrase and the external θ position is formally very similar to the link between the external argument position and the nominative case marked surface subject; indeed, we use exactly the same tools and techniques to deal with this link. (In the following rule, subscripts are used solely to distinguish the two instances of the VP category.)

$VP_0 \rightarrow VP_1\ PP$

$\ldots,$

$X = \langle index(PP),\ case(PP),\ role(PP) \rangle,$

$chain\_link(link(PP),\ links(VP_0),\ LL),$

$chain\_link(X,\ links(VP_1),\ LL),$

$\ldots,$

Note that this grammar allows extraction from the *by*-phrase, as in *Who is the girl being chased by?*, but we will not do anything with *by*-phrase extraction here.

Semantic Interpretation

The logical forms which the MFCG1 grammar assigns are based on the following theory. First, verbs are interpreted as predicates, with as many places as they assign θ roles. Thus a transitive verb like *chase* is interpreted as a two place predicate $chase(X,\ Y)$, where we interpret the first argument as the chaser and the second as the chase-ee, the quarry. Nominal expressions (DPs) are interpreted in general as "valence reducers." In particular we will follow work in generalized quantifier theory and treat DP interpretations as functions from n-place predicates to $(n - 1)$ place predicates. Sentences denote propositions, or zero-place predicates.

We represent the meaning of a DP such as *the bear* as a restricted quantifier, to be read as something like "the x such that x is a bear" and written as $the(X,\ bear)$. We write the application of this function to a predicate like $yawned(X)$ as

$the(X,\ bear)(yawned(X)).$

This expression is meant to evaluate to the zero-place predicate interpretation "true" just in case there is a unique salient individual of type *bear* who is a member of the set of individuals that yawned. Where two or more DPs are present in a sentence the meaning may depend on which one takes scope over the other. However, for the purposes of this paper we have no particular interest in quantifier scope, that is, in the order in which quantifiers apply to a predicate, and so we will skirt the issue using the following representation for propositions:

$\{every(X,\ student),\ some(Y,\ book)\}\ (read(X,\ Y)).$

The use of the set braces is to indicate that we do not care what order the two functions denoted by *every student* and *some book* apply in. We just care which argument position of the predicate denoted by *read* each one binds, as indicated by the shared variable names. Let us refer to the predicate *read(X, Y)* as the *nuclear predicate* or just *nucleus;* we will refer to the set of DP denotations as the *prefix* of the expression.

The only aspect of semantics which we are interested in here is what we might term "thematic semantics": the semantics of "who verbed whom." This is what the standard comprehension tasks usually test. Since scope, temporal semantics, propositional attitudes, and, in general, all semantic contributions from outside the DP and VP fall outside our investigation, I will assume that the semantics of the clause is essentially the semantics of the VP; that is, DPs are interpreted in their base positions. This means that the interpretation of a V1 constituent is the same no matter whether the direct object is lexicalized or a trace. This very much simplifies the task of writing a usuable grammar. Accordingly, we augment the VP and V1 rules along the following lines.

> *VP → DP V1*
> . . . ,
> *chain_link(link(DP), links(VP), links(V1)),*
> *q_rule(lf(V1), lf(DP), lf(VP)).*

The constraint-language predicate *q_rule* adds the logical form assigned to the DP to the prefix of the logical form associated with the V1 to yield the logical form associated with the VP. So, for example, *q_rule* (*yawned(Y), the(X, bear), Z*) will be true if *Z* is set equal to {*the(X, bear)*}(*yawned(X)*).

Note that, since the external argument position is never case-marked, it always contains a trace, so that we cannot actually determine the value of the quantifier that this DP denotes by inspecting the DP constituent itself—it is empty. However, in MFCG1 logical forms are transmitted along chains, so solving the *chain_link* constraint will connect that trace to its antecedent, which provides the logical form to be associated with the external argument, either by itself or by inheritance via higher chain-links. This move actually makes no difference to the results of the simulation reported here; we could get the same outcomes if we applied the logical forms of the DPs *in situ,* but it would make the grammar harder to write and harder to understand.

Finally, note that the interpretation of a *Wh*-operator like the relative pronoun is different from the interpretation of a standard DP. The function which relative *who* denotes (which I will write *wh(X)*) just maps *n*-place predicates to *n*-place predicates, but with the side effect of binding the relevant argument position in the nucleus predicate to the variable associated with the "head" of the relative clause.

The sorts of relative clauses discussed in the literature are *restrictive modifiers.* So while the expression *bear* just denotes the set of bears, the expression *bear who the tiger chased* denotes the intersection of the set of bears with the set of things that the relevant tiger chased to yield a set containing just those things which are both bears and chased by that tiger. This expression could then function as an argument of, e.g., *every*, just as well as *bear* could. We have already determined that the meaning of *who the boy chased* will be represented as $\{wh(X), the(Y, boy)\}$ $(chase(X, Y))$, according to the rules sketched so far. We will then denote *girl who the boy chased* as

$(girl)$ & $(\{wh(X), the(Y, boy)\}(chase(X, Y)))$

and *the girl who the boy chased* as

$the(X, ((girl)$ & $(\{wh(X), the(Y, boy)\}(chase(X, Y)))))$.

For the purposes of this paper we will most be concerned with the representation of just the relative clause, so the representation should not often become this cumbersome.

The relation between syntax and semantics, that is, the mechanics of semantic interpretation, is handled fairly straightforwardly. Variables in the semantic representations correspond exactly to indices in the syntactic representation. Therefore we will simply identify them: the syntactic expression $[_{DP}the\ boy]_I$ becomes the semantic expression $the(I, boy)$. Furthermore, as mentioned above, we follow Stowell (1981) in treating θ role assignment as coindexation. The verb's θ grid will just be represented as a list of variables, each corresponding to a grid position. Thus a verb like *chase* would have a θ grid like $[Int, Ext]$, and θ assignment to a DP like $[_{DP}the\ boy]_I$ (say in direct object, i.e., internal argument position) is just a matter of asserting $Int = I$. Then, in the lexical entry for *chasing*, if we write the θ grid as $[Int, Ext]$, we must write the logical form as $chase(Ext, Int)$. In that case, binding the grid position to the DP index I will have the immediate effect of binding the predicate argument position in the logical form to the same variable bound by the quantifier *the* in the DP's logical form. This is an instance of a general approach to θ grids as essentially mediating between syntactic information and variables in a predicate's conceptual structure.

Premises:	$index(DP) = I,$	$lf(DP) = the(I, bear)$
	$grid(V0) = [Int, Ext],$	$lf(V0) = chase(Ext, Int)$
θ-assignment:	$Int = I$	
Conclusion:	$lf(V0) = chase(Ext, I)$	
(Equivalently:	$lf(DP) = the(Int, bear).)$	

The key connections between syntax and semantics are thus established in the lexicon, and then the syntax (theta theory, in particular) drives the composition of more complex logical forms from simpler ones.

To see better how the syntax and the semantics are connected it is helpful to examine a "pure" version of the index-deletion model explored in Mauner et al. (1993). Currently, chain links contain the following information, given a particular DP α:

$\langle index(\alpha), case(\alpha), role(\alpha), lf(\alpha)\rangle$.

Given, following Mauner et al. (1993), that chain-link formation does not entail coindexation, we can implement this deficit simply by removing the first element from every chain-link. We can do this most easily by altering the grammar file so that all chain-links are just triples

$\langle case(\alpha), role(\alpha), lf(\alpha)\rangle$.

As expected, running GENCHRON with this altered grammar file and setting the timing parameters so that the computational simultaneity constraint is never violated give us exactly the logical forms in Mauner et al. (1993). So, for example, given as input *The boy is chasing the girl*, the parser returns an IP with the logical form

$\{the(A, boy), the(B, girl)\}(chase(C, B))$.

That is, in effect, the girl is known to be the individual being chased, and it is known that the boy is doing something, and it is known that someone is doing the chasing. There is, of course, only one way to read this logical form so that it is a zero-place predicate, i.e., a proposition, i.e., the proper denotation of a sentence, and that is by insisting that $A = C$.

This result is due to the fact that the DP-trace in external argument position has index C, and it is the lower end of a link of the form

$\langle nominative, external, the(A, boy)\rangle$

whose logical form component comes from the antecedent in IP-specifier (i.e., surface subject) position, whose index is A. However, since that information is not conveyed to the trace in VP-specifier (i.e., external argument) position, there is no way for the syntax to constrain the linking of the quantified-variable/subject-index A with the predicate-variable/external-argument index C.

When both θ positions contain traces, as in the passive sentence *The boy is chased by the girl*, GENCHRON returns the logical form

$\{the(A, girl), the(B, boy)\}(chase(C, D))$.

As per Mauner et al. (1993), this logical form has two distinct (well-typed) interpretations, which differ depending on whether we decide that $A = C$ and (therefore) $B = D$—the correct interpretation—or that $A = D$ and $B = C$ (the role-reversed interpretation). The logical form of the *by*-PP is *the(A, girl)*, and its index is A, but only the logical form gets passed to the external argument trace position, which therefore has logical form *the(A, girl)* but index C, and, since it is the index of the θ position which matters to the θ role assignment process, it is the "unbound" index C which marks the external argument position of the predicate *chase*.

THE SIMULATION

The foregoing demonstration shows only that the phrase structure grammar I am using in this exercise is faithful to the syntactic and semantic theory underlying Mauner et al. (1993). It does what it does because it was designed specifically to behave this way. The question that we are really interested in here is whether or not, and under what conditions, these same effects can be derived in a less direct manner consonant with the processing theory underlying Haarman and Kolk (1991). Recall that their hypothesis is that the actual process of phrase-structure tree-building breaks down.

Given that the results of the Haarman–Kolk deficit model are much more drastic than the results of the Mauner–Fromkin–Cornell deficit model, we would expect it to be easy to disrupt the flow of information through the phrase-structure tree. In fact, it is quite tricky to find a set of parameters which yield the correct complexity hierarchy—when we do cause the hard constructions to break apart in the right way, we find that the easy constructions are just as badly fragmented. So far I have found only one parameter setting that works, but this is not to say that there are not more, or that subtle changes in the grammar may not provide more.

SYNCHRON, and its descendant GENCHRON, provide two parameters of the processor which may be varied to give a particular deficit model. First, the user must specify the length of time which it takes to construct an element (called "retrieval time" in Haarman & Kolk, 1991). Lengthening this time period increases the likelihood that earlier arriving constituents will have faded from working memory by the time the later arriving constituents are finally constructed. Let us refer to deficit models which lengthen the retrieval time parameter as *retrieval time models*. Second, the user may vary the length of time a completed constituent remains available in working memory. Shortening this time period increases the likelihood that earlier arriving constituents will have faded from memory before later arriving constituents are made available. We will refer to this class of deficit models as *memory time models*.

One further dimension which the user can control is in the construction of a type system which allows one to vary retrieval time and memory time parameters according to the type of particular constituents. With GENCHRON the user can specify a complete type hierarchy dividing the universe of constituents in many different ways. In the experiments reported here, however, I have followed closely the open-class/closed-class distinction which has been so important in the study of agrammatism.

Open-Class/Lexical: {VP, V1, V0, NP, N1, N0}
Closed-Class/Functional: {DP, D1, D0, IP, I1, I0, CP, C1, C0, PP, P1, P0}

Note that we are here hewing closer to the psychologist's typology of categories, according to which the prepositional categories PP, P1, and P0 belong with the closed class, rather than the linguist's typology, according to which the prepositional categories belong with the lexical categories. Of course, the only preposition we use here is *by,* and it appears only in passive constructions, where it is clearly an uninterpreted case marker. It is not at all clear that we would want to treat locative prepositions in this way, since in locative constructions, for example, they provide the nuclear predicate of the whole sentence, and even as modifiers they clearly provide significant semantic constraint.

Haarman and Kolk's SYNCHRON was constructed to get the pattern of results reported in Schwartz, Saffran, and Marin (1980) and replicated in Kolk and van Grunsven (1985), which involves active, passive, and locative sentences. We are here interested in active and passive sentences and relative clauses and will have little more to say about locative sentences.

I have so far been unable to find any retrieval time model that will work, that is, that yields (fragmented but) unambiguous logical forms for active sentences and subject relative clauses, and ambiguous logical forms for passive sentences and object relative clauses. I have been able to find one memory time model that does work, however, which I will present here.

Open-class items persist for:	6 clock cycles.
Closed-class items persist for:	3 clock cycles.
Retrieval time for all items:	1 clock cycle.

Given the MFCG1 grammar discussed above, and these parameters, GENCHRON returns the tree fragments in Figs. 1–4 for the sentences and relative clauses in (1–4), below.

(1) *The boy is chasing the girl.*
(2) *The boy is chased by the girl.*
(3) *. . . who is chasing the boy . . .*
(4) *. . . who the boy is chasing . . .*

In the figures, the time interval during which each constituent is available is given next to the category label of that constituent. Features and other data structures associated with each constituent are indicated in brackets below the category label. Since DPs are always parsed completely and correctly, I have sacrified their internal details for readability.

In processing the active sentence *The boy is chasing the girl* the deepest failure point is in the attempt to combine the external argument DP with the V1 using the VP → DP V1 rule. The DP containing the subject-trace is available from Time 4 to Time 10, but the V1 does not become available until Time 11. Therefore the VP node is never built. Since the

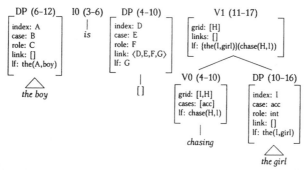

FIG. 1. Fragments returned by GENCHRON attempting to parse the active sentence *The boy is chasing the girl.*

VP cannot be constructed, no node dominating VP can be constructed. Therefore the link associated with the external argument trace in VP-specifier position is never identified with the link associated with the surface subject in IP-specifier position. The syntax thus delivers the following two fragments to the semantics.

the(A, boy), {the(I, girl)}(chase (H,I))

The first fragment is a function from *n*-place predicates to $(n - 1)$-place predicates, and the second is a 1-place predicate. The only way to get a zero-place predicate (the proper type for a sentence interpretation) is to apply the first fragment to the second, yielding in effect

{the(A, boy), the(I, girl)}(chase A, I)).

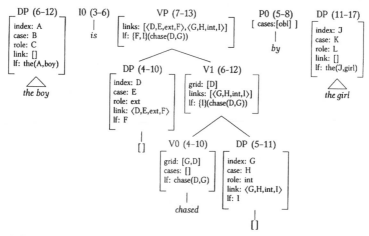

FIG. 2. Fragments returned by GENCHRON attempting to parse the passive sentence *The boy is chased by the girl.*

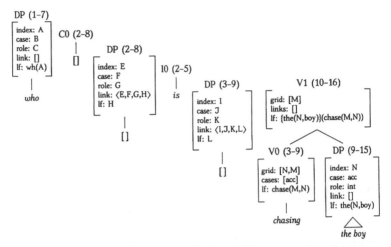

FIG. 3. Fragments returned by GENCHRON attempting to parse the subject-extracted relative clause *who is chasing the boy.*

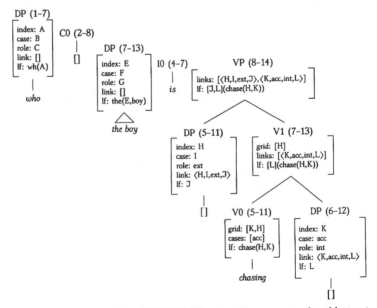

FIG. 4. Fragments returned by GENCHRON attempting to parse the object-extracted relative clause *who the boy is chasing.*

In the passive sentence *The boy is chased by the girl* (see Fig. 2) the VP is parsed completely, chiefly because it takes much less time to process traces in the highly parallel parsing model inherited from Haarman and Kolk (1991). The time taken to process a constituent depends heavily on the length of the string it dominates, and a DP dominating a trace dominates very little. However, since the VP contains only traces, it yields a highly underspecified logical form.

Our decision to throw prepositional categories in with the closed-class/functional group becomes crucial at this point. Because *by* fades away so fast, the *by*-PP cannot be built, and therefore no connection is established between the intended agent DP *the girl* and the predicate denoted by the VP. The semantic processor is provided with the following sequence of three fragmentary logical forms.

$$the(A, boy), \{F, I\}(chase(D,G)), the(J, girl)$$

The "higher-order" variables F and I stand for functions; their presence is to some degree a side effect of the implementation of the grammar. We can think of $\{F, I\}(chase(D, G))$ as denoting a zero-place predicate, whose consequences cannot be determined until we decide whether, e.g., $F = the(A, boy)$ or $F = the(J, girl)$. Alternatively we can think of it as no different from the 2-place predicate $chase(D, G)$. In any case there are two possible interpretations, depending on whether we decide that $A = D$ or $A = G$.

The processing of the relative clauses (see Figs. 3 and 4) yields strongly analogous results. Once again, processing never gets beyond the V1 or VP nodes, and everything else in the sentence is disconnected.

Several slight variations of the parameter file were tried. It turns out not to matter, for example, whether we treat all functor categories (e.g., DP, D1, and D0) or just the head-level preterminal categories (D0, in this case) as affected by the deficit. Nor does it matter whether traces are affected or not. It only matters that the closed-class head categories D0, I0, C0, and P0 are affected. This makes a certain kind of sense given the way these categories work in the grammar. The closed-class items are the glue that connects phrases to other phrases. Every open-class phrase is encased in one or more closed-class shells, which determine whether it will fit into the structure. Although they have very little inherent semantic content in and of themselves—in particular as we restrict our attention to thematic semantics—nonetheless they are essential to the semantics because and to the extent that they are essential to the syntax and the syntax is essential to the semantics. This gives a certain very concrete interpretation to the old observation that agrammatics' comprehension breaks down just where it depends on syntax.

DISCUSSION

The computational exercise described in this paper was conceived with very limited intentions, and from it we are entitled to derive only very limited conclusions. The fact that GENCHRON, together with the grammar MFCG1, produces the right kinds of semantic outputs for the four constructions of interest is not yet a proof that a processing account along the lines of Haarman and Kolk (1991) is the correct one for accounting for asyntactic comprehension. For one thing, the extreme fragmentation of the parse tree required to break it in just the right places means that there is no way the model presented here could make grammaticality judgments at the level of accuracy found in Linebarger, Schwartz, and Saffran (1983) or Shankweiler, Crain, Gorrell, and Tuller (1989), for example. What it can provide, however, is an indication of how processing and representational models of a deficit can inform each other and lead to advances in understanding the computational foundations of processing breakdown and, hence, of processing in general.

So, for example, I believe this GENCHRON experiment is a step forward from SYNCHRON largely because the grammar is an improvement over the grammar of Haarman and Kolk (1991), although it remains manifestly inadequate in very many details. Because of the more expressive formalism I have employed here, it is possible to actually record the impact of even the most mangled parse on the downstream process of semantic interpretation.

In Haarman and Kolk (1991) all that was required to force the simulation to guess at a correct response was (global) parse failure. There is no indication in that paper that the *location* of the parse failure was taken into account. If this is true, then, for example, the parser may fail on a sentence like *The boy who the girl is chasing is tall* because the main clause predicate fades away before the subject becomes available. Nonetheless it may have succeeded in parsing the relative clause *who the girl is chasing,* which is the part of the sentence whose comprehension is really being tested in the standard picture-pointing tasks, especially. Theories like those of Mauner et al. (1993) or Hickok et al. (1993) are based on taking account of the parser's local successes in spite of its global failures. Therefore it is essential that an appropriate complexity hierarchy and specific timing deficit (e.g., the Memory Time model discussed here) conspire to break the phrase structure tree in just the right locations.

Immediately, however, we see the problem we will have in deriving correct grammaticality judgments from such a model. If we have to break the tree completely, and thwart the propagation of all information from node to node, then we cannot hope to use that information in making grammaticality judgments. To take a single example, in the structures given in this paper the subject DP is never connected to the I0 node with which it must agree. Therefore there is no way this parser could reject a sentence like *The boy are chasing the girl, even if we added constraints to the grammar imposing subject-verb agreement.

One fairly obvious remedy would be to appeal to the generally accepted claim that grammaticality judgment is a strictly easier task than picture pointing or act-out tasks (see, e.g., Kolk, 1995, and the discussion of the trade-off hypothesis in Linebarger et al., 1983; Kolk & Weijts, 1995; Linebarger, 1995). Accordingly we could claim that the degree to which memory time decreases or retrieval time increases is dependent on the nature of the task being attempted. It would be a trivial matter to alter GENCHRON or SYNCHRON along these lines, but it should be clear that such a solution is purely stipulative, based on an empirical fact (relative task complexity) and not on a theory with that fact among its consequences. (Although note that Kolk (this volume) does attempt to extend the timing-based theory of the deficit to capture this complexity distinction.) Worse, it is empirically insufficient. We are not faced with a situation in which comprehension is asyntactic but grammaticality judgment is uniformly good. There are constructions which are typically very hard to judge correctly, such as agreement between a reflexive pronoun and its antecedent. As noted in Mauner et al. (1993), the generalization that these constructions involve coindexation (e.g., Schwartz, Linebarger, & Saffran, 1985) can be extended to a detailed account of comprehension failure, which I have tried to illustrate computationally here. Any lessening of the syntactic damage due to timing problems, to the extent that it repairs the damage to phrase structure trees, should also allow again for the free passage of indices along their branches.

The challenge to a processing account of asyntactic comprehension is thus clear. The complexity metric one derives must be such as to highlight index-mediated grammatical dependencies (at least) for special attention. A node-counting metric based solely on tree geometry and not on the content of grammatical relations—like the *antecedent* or *specifier* or *governor* relations—will most likely fail the grammaticality judgment test.

The question we should ask is how far away from such a model we are with simulations like SYNCHRON, and now GENCHRON. With this in mind let me propose the following as the logical next step. The version of GENCHRON used in these simulations is subject to the extended simultaneity condition; it waits until all subtrees have been parsed and then attempts to solve all of the constraints at once. In line with a great deal of work on logic grammars (Pereira & Warren, 1980; Pereira & Shieber, 1987; Dahl & Abramson, 1989), we can essentially do away with the formal distinction between the rewrite rule and its associated constraints. We can think of the task of parsing a VP, given a rule like VP → DP V1 together with its associated constraints, as composed of subtasks, one of which is the task of parsing a DP and another of which is a *theta_assign* task, and so on.

With some significant modifications, we should still be able to speak of computational simultaneity in this framework. Suppose that we generalize the idea that constituents take time to build, and decay away over time, to cover constraints as well. Every constraint represents a computational task, whose accomplishment may depend on the accomplishment of other tasks. Therefore, for example, the accomplishment of the *vp* task rests on the accomplishment of the *dp*, *v1*, *theta_assign*, *chain_link* and *q_rule* tasks. In addition, each task, on completion, supplies information to the task that called it. Accordingly we can offer the following generalized simultaneity condition.

> *Generalized Simultaneity Condition*
> The output of a particular task only becomes available when and if the output of all of its subtasks is available at some point in time. At that point in time the superordinate task begins to make its output available.

Now we can distinguish types of tasks just as we distinguished types of category (closed-class heads vs. everything else, in the current case). We could, for example, make the categorical predicates like *vp* and *dp* fast with respect to lexical predicates like *theta_assign*, so as to simulate the division of parsing labor into a fast first-pass parse with subsequent use of argument-structure information (see, e.g., Friederici, this volume; Linebarger, this volume; but cf. Shapiro & Nagel, 1995). And, of course, we can isolate predicates that manipulate indices and chain-links.

This approach does more than just expose coindexation to the kind of stipulative deficit illustrated in grammar MFCG2. Just as the difficulty in establishing a VP constituent in SYNCHRON—or GENCHRON with MFCG1—depends on the subconstituents of that VP, so too the difficulty of establishing a coindexation between two constituents should depend on the subtasks involved. And of course, what subtasks are involved depends in large part on the theory of chain formation and anaphoric dependencies inherited from syntactic theory. And so we close on a recapitulation of the theme of this study, that the investigation of processing deficits need not be, and perhaps cannot be, independent of the investigation of representational deficits.

REFERENCES

Dahl, V., & Abramson, H. 1989. *Logic grammars*. New York: Springer-Verlag.

Friederici, A. 1995. The time course of syntactic activation during language processing: A model based on neuropsychological and neurophysiological data. *Brain and Language*, **50**, 259–281.

Haarman, H., & Kolk, H. 1991. A computer model of the temporal course of agrammatic sentence understanding: The effects of variation in severity and sentence complexity. *Cognitive Science*, **15**, 49–87.

Hickok, G., Zurif, E. B., & Canseco-Gonzales, E. 1993. Structural description of agrammatic comprehension. *Brain and Language, 45,* 371–395.

Kolk, H. 1995. A time-based approach to agrammatic production. *Brain and Language,* **50,** 282–303.

Kolk, H., & van Grunsven, M. 1985. Agrammatism as a variable phenomenon. *Cognitive Neuropsychology,* **2,** 347–384.

Kolk, H., & Weijts, M. 1995. Judgments of semantic anomaly in agrammatic patients: Syntactic complexity and word-order heuristics. *Brain and Language,* in press.

Koopman, H., & Sportiche, D. 1988. Subjects. Unpublished manuscript, UCLA.

Linebarger, M. 1995. Agrammatism as evidence about grammar. *Brain and Language,* **50,** 52–91.

Linebarger, M., Schwartz, M., & Saffran, E. 1983. Sensitivity to grammatical structure in so-called agrammatic aphasics. *Cognition,* **13,** 361–393.

Mauner, G., Fromkin, V., & Cornell, T. 1993. Comprehension and acceptability judgments in agrammatism: Disruption in the syntax of referential dependency. *Brain and Language,* **45,** 340–370.

Pereira, F., & Warren, D. 1980. Definite clause grammars for natural language analysis. *Artificial Intelligence,* **13,** 231–278.

Pereira, F., & Shieber, S. 1987. *Prolog and natural language analysis.* Chicago: Chicago University Press.

Schwartz, M., Saffran, E., & Marin, O. 1980. The word-order problem in agrammatism: I. Comprehension. *Brain and Language,* **10,** 249–262.

Schwartz, M., Linebarger, M., & Saffran, E. 1985. The status of the syntactic deficit theory of agrammatism. In M.-L. Kean (Ed.), *Agrammatism.* Orlando: Academic Press.

Shankweiler, D., Crain, S., Gorell, P., & Tuller, B. 1989. Reception of language in Broca's aphasia. *Language & Cognitive Processes,* **4,** 1–33.

Shapiro, L., & Nagel, N. 1995. Lexical properties, prosody, and syntax: Implications for normal and disordered language. *Brain and Language,* **50,** 240–257.

Shieber, S. M. 1992. *Constraint-based grammar formalisms: Parsing and type inference for natural and computer languages.* Cambridge, MA: MIT Press.

Stowell, T. 1981. *Origins of phrase structure.* Unpublished Ph.D. dissertation, MIT.

BRAIN AND LANGUAGE **50,** 325–338 (1995)

Issues Arising in Contemporary Studies of Disorders of Syntactic Processing in Sentence Comprehension in Agrammatic Patients

David Caplan

Neuropsychology Laboratory, Massachusetts General Hospital

This paper reviews recent studies of sentence comprehension in agrammatic patients. The conclusion is reached that more detailed study of individual patients is necessary to support hypotheses that have been presented concerning the deficit in these patients and that the rationale for studying comprehension in this group of patients is not well developed. A set of suggested criteria is presented for patient analysis in this field. © 1995 Academic Press, Inc.

My goal in this paper is to raise a number of general points regarding theories of sentence comprehension by agrammatic patients. My comments focus on the adequacy of the empirical support for these theories.

Since the publication of Caramazza and Zurif's (1976) seminal paper on disorders of syntactic processing in sentence comprehension in agrammatic aphasics, accounts of the deficits in syntactic comprehension that are attributed to agrammatic patients have been phrased in extremely detailed terms. These analyses have been closely linked to models of syntactic structure and language processing that have been developed in linguistics and in psycholinguistic research, leading to research into these disorders that utilizes a highly articulated framework and that has a powerful deductive component. The integration of research into disorders of syntactic processing in sentence comprehension in agrammatic aphasics with linguistic theory and psycholinguistic models thus constitutes a great advance over previous work that described these disorders in less precise terms.

However, in my view, despite these accomplishments, research in this area suffers from a number of serious limitations. Essentially, although disorders of syntactic processing in sentence comprehension in agram-

This work was partially supported by a grant from NIDCD (DC00942). Address correspondence and reprint requests to the author at the Neuropsychology Laboratory, Vincent Burnham 827, Fruit Street, Boston, MA 02114.

matic aphasics have been linked to linguistic theory and psycholinguistic models, the data that support these links are very weak. I shall discuss the problems with the literature under three headings: (1) inadequacies in experimental methods; (2) overly narrow interpretation of patients' deficits; and (3) inappropriate patient grouping. The first of these problem areas is not specifically due to researchers focusing on agrammatic patients—these are simply problems that weaken the database. Problems in the second area partially stem from the focus on agrammatism, and those in the third area are a direct consequence of assumptions that researchers make about sentence comprehension in agrammatism.

1. INADEQUACIES IN METHODS

There are problems with the methods used in many papers in the literature on agrammatic comprehension. It is not my intention to review these problems here in detail, but to indicate their existence and to illustrate them with a few examples.

One problem deals with inadequacies in the construction of materials. For instance, Grodzinsky (1988, 1990) proposed that agrammatic patients tend to omit prepositions that are not governed and to retain those that are. Grodzinsky (1988) had subjects do a grammaticality judgment task in which the independent variable of interest was whether a prepositional phrase was governed or ungoverned. Grodzinsky reported that performance was worse on two sentence types that contained governed prepositions—active sentences with prepositions subcategorized by the verb and lexical passives—than on the sentence type that contained ungoverned prepositions—syntactic passives. However, the syntactic passives were classifiable into acceptable and unacceptable sets purely on the basis of the preposition that was present. All the acceptable syntactic passives had PPs beginning with *by* and 9 of 10 unacceptable syntactic passives had PPs beginning with *on*. Subjects in this experiment could have simply been classifying all sentences with PPs with *by* as grammatical and all sentences with PPs with *on* as ungrammatical; the results may have nothing to do with whether the subjects could construct certain types of phrase markers and with whether they retained ungoverned PPs.

A second problem regards inadequate matching of lesioned controls and experimental (i.e., agrammatic) subjects. For instance, Zurif, Swinney, Prather, Solomon, and Bushell (1993) reported that four agrammatic patients did not show cross-modal lexical priming for the antecedents of traces in subject position in relative clauses, while four Wernicke's aphasics did. However, inspection of the off-line performance of the patients indicates that the Wernicke's aphasics were not as impaired as the Broca's aphasics. It is not surprising to find that aphasic patients with more severe syntactic comprehension problems on off-line tasks are more matic aphasics have been linked to linguistic theory and psycholinguistic models, the data that support these links are very weak. I shall discuss the problems with the literature under three headings: (1) inadequacies in experimental methods; (2) overly narrow interpretation of patients' deficits; and (3) inappropriate patient grouping. The first of these problem areas is not specifically due to researchers focusing on agrammatic patients—these are simply problems that weaken the database. Problems in the second area partially stem from the focus on agrammatism, and those in the third area are a direct consequence of assumptions that researchers make about sentence comprehension in agrammatism.

1. INADEQUACIES IN METHODS

There are problems with the methods used in many papers in the literature on agrammatic comprehension. It is not my intention to review these problems here in detail, but to indicate their existence and to illustrate them with a few examples.

One problem deals with inadequacies in the construction of materials. For instance, Grodzinsky (1988, 1990) proposed that agrammatic patients tend to omit prepositions that are not governed and to retain those that are. Grodzinsky (1988) had subjects do a grammaticality judgment task in which the independent variable of interest was whether a prepositional phrase was governed or ungoverned. Grodzinsky reported that performance was worse on two sentence types that contained governed prepositions—active sentences with prepositions subcategorized by the verb and lexical passives—than on the sentence type that contained ungoverned prepositions—syntactic passives. However, the syntactic passives were classifiable into acceptable and unacceptable sets purely on the basis of the preposition that was present. All the acceptable syntactic passives had PPs beginning with *by* and 9 of 10 unacceptable syntactic passives had PPs beginning with *on*. Subjects in this experiment could have simply been classifying all sentences with PPs with *by* as grammatical and all sentences with PPs with *on* as ungrammatical; the results may have nothing to do with whether the subjects could construct certain types of phrase markers and with whether they retained ungoverned PPs.

A second problem regards inadequate matching of lesioned controls and experimental (i.e., agrammatic) subjects. For instance, Zurif, Swinney, Prather, Solomon, and Bushell (1993) reported that four agrammatic patients did not show cross-modal lexical priming for the antecedents of traces in subject position in relative clauses, while four Wernicke's aphasics did. However, inspection of the off-line performance of the patients indicates that the Wernicke's aphasics were not as impaired as the Broca's aphasics. It is not surprising to find that aphasic patients with more severe syntactic comprehension problems on off-line tasks are more formed the basis for Grodzinsky's original theory was tested for his/her comprehension of sentences containing PRO, pronouns, and/or reflexives. Grodzinsky's more recent study of the comprehension of pronouns in agrammatic patients (Grodzinsky, Wexler, Chien, Marakovits, & Solomon, 1993) does not test PRO. To my knowledge, there is not a single study in the literature in which an individual patient has been shown to have a disturbance in off-line comprehension that is restricted to the co-indexation of traces and that spares all other referentially dependent NPs. The patient K.G. studied by Hildebrandt, Caplan, and Evans (1987) comes closest to this profile, but K.G. had difficulty with PRO under some circumstances; moreover, K.G. was not agrammatic—a point to which I shall return below. If agrammatic patients have trouble with all these referentially dependent NPs, the theory that their deficits are specific to traces is incorrect.

To take another example, Linebarger (this volume) cites data indicating that agrammatic patients can make correct grammaticality judgments about sentences which as *When/*who did the teacher smile*, *Which records are you going to give to Louise/*Which are you going to give records to Louise*, and *Bill dropped a plate that (*the stove) was too hot*. She claims that this indicates that these patients "must associate a fronted Wh-element with the "hole" of the same category in the phrase structure." But these judgments could be made without patients' being able to associate fillers with gaps. The discrimination between *When did the teacher smile* and *Who did the teacher smile* can be made if a subject can classify *who* as an NP and *when* as an adverbial and if he or she accepts sentences as grammatical if the number of NPs equals the number of arguments of the verb. A similar process can lead to correct discrimination of *Which records are you going to give to Louise* vs. *Which are you going to give records to Louise*. The case of *Bill dropped a plate that the stove was too hot* is more complex. Depending upon how the copula is treated with respect to the assignment of the thematic roles, simply determining whether the number of NPs equals the number of verb arguments could lead to this sentence being accepted. But it is not necessary that subjects relate fillers and gaps for this sentence to be rejected. If subjects classify *that* as a determiner, they could reject this sentence because two determiners precede a noun (*that the plate*). If subjects take *that* as a complementizer, they could reject the sentence because *drop* does not allow a sentential complement—a lexically listed item of information. If subjects take *that* as a relative pronoun, they are again in a situation in which there are more NPs than verb arguments. If patients made their judgments in these sentences in any of these ways, the conclusion Linebarger draws—that these patients relate a fronted Wh-word to a gap—is too strong. In this case, the subsequent claim that patients postulate gaps but fail to interpret them correctly semantically is not supported by these data.

To make a final example, consider the intriguing dissociation reported by Hickok and Avrutin (this volume) between the performance of two patients on sentences such as *Who was pushed by the woman*, which was interpreted extremely well, and *Which man was pushed by the woman*, which was interpreted at chance. The authors attribute the dissociation to differences in the patients' abilities to coindex elements in government chains and binding chains. However, the visual processing associated with matching the expression *which man* to an item may be greater than that associated with matching the expression *who* to an item in a picture.

What is needed in all these studies is a series of control studies that rule out these alternative explanations. However, it has been argued that these controls are unnecessary. Grodzinsky (1990) has claimed that it is legitimate to assume that a patient can accomplish a psycholinguistic function on which he or she has not been tested, because the patient had a normal language processing system before his or her illness. Whatever its philosophical merit, this argument is misplaced on empirical grounds. Given that these patients have cerebral injuries that interfere with language functions, we cannot simply assume that untested functions are normal. Dissociations abound in neuropsychology—a patient whose production of words referring to a man-made object is intact may have an impairment affecting words referring to fruits and vegetables (Hart, Berndt, & Caramazza, 1985), patients may read regularly spelled words but not irregularly spelled words (Coltheart, Masterson, Byng, Prior, & Riddoch, 1983), etc. Specifically in the area of disorders of syntactically mediated sentence comprehension, patients with disturbances affecting co-indexation of traces may or may not have impairments affecting the ability to co-index other referentially dependent NPs, as judged by performance on off-line tests of comprehension (Caplan & Hildebrandt, 1988). For a patient's performance to constitute strong evidence for a particular theory, the integrity or disruption of a psycholinguistic process that figures in that theory cannot be established on the basis of arguments grounded in the philosophy of science, but requires empirical investigation.

There is another justification for the practice of not providing baseline data on patients that is more prevalent in this literature—the claim that we can assume that a patient would perform in a particular way because he or she is agrammatic. This assumption is also unjustified.

An example of such an assumption is the work by Swinney et al. (this volume). These researchers report that four agrammatic aphasic patients failed to show priming in a cross-modal lexical decision task for the antecedents of traces in object position in relative clauses. However, it is not reported whether these patients showed priming for single words in isolation. If not, the absence of priming in the sentence context has no implications for the sentence processing deficits in these patients. Swinney and his colleagues cite the fact that Prather, Zurif, Stern, and Rosen (1992) reported priming in agrammatism as a reason to believe that their patients would do so as well. However, Prather et al.'s results were found in a single patient and cannot be assumed to be true of Swinney et al.'s patients. In this particular case, there is specific evidence that this assumption is not warranted (Milberg & Blumstein, 1981; Milberg, Blumstein, & Dworetzky, 1987).

Overall, the literature on deficits in syntactically mediated sentence comprehension has generated a number of extremely interesting, narrow hypotheses, linked to rich theories of syntactic representations and their processing. However, the empirical support for these theories is weak, in part because inappropriate assumptions have been made about how patients would perform on control tasks.

A final issue about the characterization of deficits is how to interpret coexisting phenomena that can be related to a single aspect of a syntactic theory. For instance, Grodzinsky (this volume) argues that agrammatic patients are sensitive to constraints on X^0 (head) movement, citing the fact that Linebarger, Schwartz, and Saffran (1983) show that their patients could detect violations of constraints on subject-aux inversion and that Lonzi and Luzzatti (1993) found that patients were able to place adverbs correctly around verbs (i.e., adverbial placement was a function of the finiteness of the verb). Let us, for the moment, overlook the fact that these results were obtained in different patients on different tasks and ask how we might interpret the hypothetical finding that a pattern of sensitivity to these two types of structural constraints arose in a single patient in a single task. Would such a finding automatically imply that the patient was sensitive to the constraints on head movement enunciated in Rizzi (1990), as Grodzinsky suggests? Could the patient be sensitive to separate patterns of acceptability that apply to subject-aux inversion and adverbial-verb placement? The same question arises when we are concerned with coexisting deficits. Grodzinsky (1986, 1990) argued that agrammatics' chance performance on passives and object relativized sentences was due to a disturbance related to traces, but how can we know that poor performance on each of these two sentence types was not due to a different functional disturbance?

There may be no unequivocal answer to these questions, but evidence that strengthens the position that a single capacity or deficit is at issue can be adduced. Such evidence would consist of enunciating clear predictions regarding the structures that are and are not affected if the capacity or deficit were stated in terms of a given theory, and the provision of data that a single patient's performance corresponded to those structures on a single task or, better, on each of a set of tasks. It is a major accomplishment of present research that it utilizes linguistic theory to generate descriptions of performances in abstract, theory-internal terms. However, these descriptions need to be treated as hypotheses to be investigated and not as analyses to be accepted simply because they achieve the highest generalization possible within the best available theory.

3. PROBLEMS WITH GROUPING TOGETHER AGRAMMATIC PATIENTS

I have just indicated that patients are not always tested on tasks that are needed to establish the specificity of their deficits, in part because it is assumed that a patient's being agrammatic is sufficient to allow his or her performance to be compared to that of another agrammatic patient. The justification for building a theory of a deficit in syntactic processing on the basis of these comparisons is directly related to validity of considering patients together for studies of sentence comprehension on the basis of their being agrammatic. This is not a legitimate way to proceed, for several important reasons.

The first reason that we should not be developing theories of the syntactic processing deficit in agrammatism is that agrammatism is a disorder affecting sentence production, not comprehension. In the immediate aftermath of Caramazza and Zurif's paper, researchers appreciated that the rationale for selection of agrammatic patients to study syntactic comprehension disorders must be a relationship between deficits found in sentence comprehension and the production disorder found in agrammatic patients (Bradley, Garrett, & Zurif, 1980; Berndt & Caramazza, 1980; Zurif, 1982). However, the theories that attempted to articulate this relationship were never developed to the point that the algorithms or computations that were common to sentence production and comprehension were specified, and they collapsed under the weight of a series of nonreplications of experimental results and of double dissociations between syntactic comprehension disorders and expressive agrammatism (Gordon & Caramazza, 1982, 1983; Berndt, 1987). The absence of a credible basis upon which to relate expressive agrammatism and syntactic comprehension disorders poses a serious problem for theories that maintain that there is a specific syntactic processing deficit in agrammatism. *In principle,* any such a deficit would have to be an unrelated phenomenon, if sentence production and sentence comprehension are separate processes. But then, why study agrammatic patients as a special group? Why not study all patients with certain types of syntactic comprehension disorders?

This question is rendered more pressing because the criteria for identifying agrammatic patients are so poorly defined. The clinical diagnosis of "agrammatism" is made on the basis of a therapist's impressions of the qualitative nature of a patient's speech in a single conversational session that may last as little as a few minutes, which is not recorded, in which no quantitative measurements are made of aspects of speech production, whose inter-observer reliability is unknown, and which reflect performance at a single point in what may be a changing clinical picture. Thus, basic features pertinent to inclusion of individuals in the population under study are unrecorded and largely unknown. More detailed documentation of agrammatic patients' conversational speech (e.g., Saffran, Berndt, & Schwartz, 1989) has rarely been used to select patients in the studies that focus on syntactic comprehension in agrammatic patients. Even such approaches face serious problems with segmentation of utterances and with attributing intent to patients in conversational settings. More constrained tasks such as sentence completion have not been used as the basis for patient selection in the studies under consideration, and it is not clear that patients' performance on them would parallel their spontaneous speech. Regardless of how patients are selected, agrammatic patients differ considerably from one another within and across studies, both with respect to their other speech output disturbances and with respect to the features of their agrammatism (Menn & Obler, 1990; Miceli, Silveri, Romani, & Caramazza, 1989). For all these reasons, it is difficult, if not impossible, for a researcher interested in replicating another's results or in testing a theory to be sure that he or she is selecting a group of patients that are similar in potentially crucial respects to those already tested. This raises the possibility that any nonreplication of results or nonconfirmation of a theory can be dismissed as being due to differences in patient selection and that any apparent replication of results or confirmation of a theory can have occurred in a different patient population than the one originally tested. These issues raise the question of whether it is possible and advisable to select agrammatic patients for study on operational grounds. But the more general question is why we would want to select patients to study comprehension on the basis of their output, even if we could describe that output more clearly, if sentence production and comprehension are unrelated.

One possible answer to this question is that sentence production and comprehension might make use of a single set of syntactic representations, even if they do not utilize the same algorithms. The situation may be similar to that which some researchers maintain is true of the lexicon—there is a single phonological lexicon that is accessed by separate processes for input and output. If this is the justification for selecting agrammatic patients for studies of comprehension, it would be important to determine whether the assumption that sentence production and comprehension share a single set of representations is true. The way to approach this in neuropsychological studies is to find a patient in whom there is evidence that a representation is lost from this set in both comprehension and production. This might not be easy to demonstrate, since the effect of the loss of a representation might be different in these two tasks. However, with well-specified theories of the representations and processes involved, it might be possible to make and test specific predictions about the effects of such a loss. Such theories need to be developed and tested if the idea that loss of shared representations justifies the selection of agrammatic patients to study of sentence comprehension. It should also be noted that this justification would, in any case, apply only to patients with loss of these shared representations (if any such representations and/or patients exist).

A second answer to the question of why we might select agrammatic patients to study comprehension is that, even if sentence production and comprehension are unrelated, choosing agrammatic patients is a way to increase the likelihood of finding "interesting" patients (Zurif et al. 1989). The use of agrammatism as a discovery procedure is a legitimate way to find single cases to study, but it does not license grouping agrammatic patients together a priori in a sentence comprehension study or developing a generalization about agrammatic comprehension on the basis of the performances of different agrammatic patients on different tasks.

There is a variant of the approach to selecting agrammatic patients for studies of syntactic processing in comprehension that consists of selecting patients for study who are both agrammatic and show certain syntactic processing deficits—e.g., who fail to understand reversible passive but not active sentences. Although somewhat different from selecting patients simply because they are agrammatic, this approach is still based upon the notion that there is something special about agrammatic patients' comprehension: syntactic comprehension problems in patients who are not agrammatic are assumed to be different from these problems in patients who are agrammatic.

At the present state of knowledge, however, there is no reason to believe that this assumption is correct. The now-classic finding of impaired sentence-picture matching for semantically reversible sentences with noncanonical thematic roles orders is not found in all agrammatics (Nespoulous et al., 1988), and it is present in nonagrammatic patients (Caplan, Baker, & Dehaut, 1985; Hildebrandt et al., 1987; Caplan & Hildebrandt, 1988). It is true that there are several reports in the literature that do show differences between small groups of agrammatic patients and other patient types (e.g., von Stockert, 1972; von Stockert & Bader, 1976; Friederici, 1981, 1982; Shapiro, Gordon, Hack, & Killackey, 1993; Zurif et al., 1993). However, these studies do not establish that the syntactic comprehension problems of patients with and without agrammatism are different. All but one of these studies do not test syntactic processing in comprehension. In the one study that tests this function (Zurif et al., 1993), the possibility that the group effects are simply a sampling artifact must be considered. The effects seen in a given group of agrammatic aphasics might also arise in other subsets of the patients formed at random in a particular study and have nothing to do with the agrammatism of the patients. Or it could be that the results do arise in only the group of agrammatic patients, but not in all of its members or, perhaps, not in a single individual patient. The design of the Zurif et al. (1993) study precludes the analysis of individual cases, so these questions cannot be answered. None of these results have been replicated by a second research team and may prove as insecure as other studies in this field (e.g., Bradley et al., 1980). The studies fall far short of demonstrating that the syntactic comprehension problems of patients with and without agrammatism are different.

Suppose, however, that additional studies, perhaps using on-line measures of comprehension, do establish that there is a unique syntactic comprehension disorder seen in agrammatic patients. If this is not because sentence production and comprehension are functionally related, it must be due to a feature of the responsible neurological lesion. The feature that has been suggested is the location of a lesion. In this case, once again, the patient's agrammatism would be irrelevant to his or her syntactic comprehension deficit. In actual fact, the deficit-lesion corelational data currently available suggest that the presence of a lesion in Broca's area is not required for the syntactic processing deficits described in agrammatism to be present and that it may be present without such deficits. However, much more study of this question is needed. We need much better definition of lesion location and volume in stroke cases. We need to know how the etiology and duration of a neuropathological insult affect comprehension disorders and how the pathological factors of lesion location, etiology, and duration interact with neurobiological factors such as handedness, age, and sex in determining comprehension. This is a proper area for study, but it cannot be approached by selecting patients for study who are agrammatic as a short-hand way of identifying patients with certain lesion locations.

POSSIBLE CONCLUSIONS

I have briefly reviewed a number of problems with the literature on syntactic comprehension disorders in agrammatism. However, I am not making the claim that the literature on syntactic comprehension disorders in agrammatism is without value. On the contrary, my view is that the literature on comprehension deficits in agrammatism has suggested the existence of extremely interesting disorders. The intellectual effort that has gone into formulating these accounts of deficits is considerable. It is a nontrivial task to relate a set of observations to an aspect of Chomsky's theory of syntax, as has been done by Grodzinsky (this volume), Hikock and Avrutin (this volume), and other researchers. However, as I have stressed throughout this paper, however impressive this analysis and however strong Chomsky's theory, the work of aphasiologists must also include the provision of convincing empirical evidence that the analyses are correct. For the reasons explicated above, this evidence has yet to materialize.

Two other issues deserve comment. The first is whether these analyses are likely to be specifically related to agrammatism. I do not believe that this work has shown anything specific about agrammatic patients. This is not surprising if sentence production and sentence comprehension are separate processes. However, even if a sentence comprehension deficit in an agrammatic patient is not related to the patients' expressive agrammatism, studying the deficit still can provide important data about sentence comprehension. The literature that is said to be about agrammatism has begun to document the range and types of impairments in sentence comprehension that are seen after brain injury. In my view, saying that this literature is "about 'agrammatism'" acts as a serious impediment to investigating these impairments. It encourages researchers to make unwarranted assumptions about what functions are and are not effected in their patients, based on the results of other researchers' studies that do not necessarily apply to their cases. We need to stop thinking that we are studying sentence comprehension in a group of patients in which such assumptions are valid; on the contrary, we need to be conducting research into the validity of these assumptions. One way to do this would be to study individual cases in detail, whether or not they are agrammatic, and, when we have a large enough set of well-studied cases, evaluate them to determine whether there is anything special about the deficits seen in those who have expressive agrammatism. If there is, we will have to associate that set of comprehension deficits to the deficits in sentence production in these patients, to their lesions, or to both.

The second point is that I do not believe that this work has shown anything specific about patients with lesions in Broca's area. Much more information is needed in order to be able to assert with confidence that Broca's area does something in sentence comprehension that is not also accomplished by at least other parts of the perisylvian cortex and perhaps even other parts of the brain.

SUGGESTIONS FOR FUTURE RESEARCH

I would like to conclude with a set of suggestions that I believe would serve to advance our understanding of the nature of syntactic processing deficits in sentence comprehension.

1. The field should develop a series of detailed case studies of syntactic processing deficits in sentence comprehension. It should not focus research solely on the comprehension disorders seen in agrammatic patients.

2. At this point in the development of the field, no assumptions should be made about how patients would perform on tasks on which they have not been tested. All patients should be tested to establish the integrity of processes that are necessary to accomplish experimental tasks on which they are tested and that are needed to establish the specificity of a deficit in representational and processing terms.

3. Experiments should be designed that meet accepted criteria in cognitive psychology, including matching of subjects in different groups on potentially relevant parameters, the calculation of item statistics, etc.

4. Detailed neurobiological data should be provided about all patients. If possible, both behavioral and neurobiological data should be entered into a database that is accessible to all qualified researchers in the field.

5. If the present interest in the comprehension problems of agrammatic patients is pursued, the relationship between sentence production and sentence comprehension should be spelled out in detail.

6. If the present interest in the comprehension problems of agrammatic patients is pursued, the field should establish a gold standard for the diagnosis of agrammatism. I would suggest that this standard use a sentence completion task. Patients who are entered into studies as agrammatic should fall within specific levels of performance on these tasks, and their performances should be reported.

I will end by reiterating my view that the work of the past years has brought the development of theory regarding syntactic processing in sentence comprehension in aphasic patients to a high level. There is much work to do for the experimental investigation of these theories to catch up with this level of sophistication.

REFERENCES

Berndt, R. S. 1987. Symptom co-occurrence and dissociation in the interpretation of agrammatism. In G. S. a. R. J. M. Coltheart (Ed.), *The cognitive neuropsychology of language*. London: Lawrence Erlbaum. Pp. 221–232.

Berndt, R. S., & Caramazza, A. 1980. A redefinition of the syndrome of Broca's aphasia: Implications for a neuropsychological model of language. *Applied Psycholinguistics,* **1,** 225–278.

Bradley, D. C., Garrett, M. F., & Zurif, E. B. (1980). Syntactic deficits in Broca's aphasia. In D. Caplan (Ed.), *Biological studies of mental processes*. Cambridge, MA: MIT Press. Pp. 269–286.

Caplan, D. 1987. Agrammatism and the co-indexation of traces: Comments on Grodzinsky's reply. *Brain and Language,* **30,** 191–193.

Caplan, D., & Hildebrandt, N. 1986. Language deficits and the theory of syntax: A reply to Grodzinsky. *Brain and Language,* **27,** 168–177.

Caplan, D., & Hildebrandt, N. 1988. *Disorders of syntactic comprehension.* Cambridge, MA: MIT Press.

Caplan, D., & Hildebrandt, N. 1989. Disorders affecting comprehension of syntactic form: Preliminary results and their implications for theories of syntax and parsing. *Canadian Journal of Linguistics,* 33, 477–505.

Caplan, D., Baker, C., & Dehaut, F. 1985. Syntactic determinants of sentence comprehension in aphasia. *Cognition,* 21, 117–175.

Caramazza, A., & Zurif, E. 1976. Dissociation of algorithmic and heuristic processes in language comprehension: Evidence from aphasia. *Brain and Language,* 3, 572–582.

Coltheart, M., Masterson, J., Byng, S., Prior, M., & Riddoch, J. 1983. Surface dyslexia. *Quarterly Journal of Experimental Psychology,* 35, 469–495.

Friederici, A. D. 1981. Production and comprehension of prepositions in aphasia. *Neuropsychologia,* 19, 191–199.

Friederici, A. D. 1982. Syntactic and semantic processes in aphasic deficits: The availability of prepositions. *Brain and Language,* 15, 249–258.

Gordon, B., & Caramazza, A. 1982. Lexical decision for open- and closed-class words: Failure to replicate differential frequency sensitivity. *Brain and Language,* 15, 143–160.

Gordon, B., & Caramazza, A. 1983. Closed- and open-class lexical access in agrammatic and fluent aphasics. *Brain and Language,* 19, 335–345.

Grodzinsky, Y. 1986. Language deficits and the theory of syntax. *Brain and Language,* 27, 135–159.

Grodzinsky, Y. 1988. Syntactic representations in agrammatic aphasia: The case of prepositions. *Language and Speech,* 31(2), 115–134.

Grodzinsky, Y. 1990. *Theoretical Perspectives on Language Deficits.* Cambridge, MA: MIT Press.

Grodzinsky, Y., Wexler, K., Chien, Y. C., Marakovits, S., & Solomon, J. 1993. The breakdown of binding relations. *Brain and Language,* 45, 396–422.

Hart, J., Berndt, R. S., & Caramazza, A. 1985. Category-specific naming deficit following cerebral infarction. *Nature,* 316, 439–440.

Hildebrandt, N., Caplan, D., & Evans, K. 1987. The man$_i$ left$_i$ without a trace: A case study of aphasic processing of empty categories. *Cognitive Neuropsychology,* 4(3), 257–302.

Linebarger, M. C., Schwartz, M. F., & Saffran, E. M. 1983. Sensitivity to grammatical structure in so-called agrammatic aphasics. *Cognition,* 13, 361–392.

Lonzi, L., & Luzzatti, C. 1993. Relevance of adverb distribution for the analysis of sentence representation in agrammatic patients. *Brain and Language,* 45, 306–317.

Menn, L., & Obler, L. 1990. *Agrammatic aphasia: A cross-language narrative sourcebook.* Philadelphia: John Benjamins.

Miceli, G., & Caramazza, A. 1988. Dissociation of inflectional and derivational morphology. *Brain and Language,* 35, 24–65.

Miceli, G., Silveri, M. C., Romani, C., & Caramazza, A. 1989. Variation in the pattern of omissions and substitutions of grammatical morphemes in the spontaneous speech of so-called agrammatic patients. *Brain and Language,* 36, 447–492.

Milberg, W., & Blumstein, S. E. 1981. Lexical decision and aphasia: Evidence for semantic processing. *Brain and Language,* 14, 371–385.

Milberg, W., Blumstein, S. E., & Dworetzky, B. 1987. Processing of lexical ambiguities in aphasia. *Brain and Language,* 31, 138–150.

Nespoulous, J.-L., Dordain, M., Perron, C., Ska, B., Bub, D., Caplan, D., Mehler, J., & Lecours, A.-R. 1988. Agrammatism in sentence production without comprehension deficits: Reduced availability of syntactic structures and/or of grammatical morphemes? A case study. *Brain and Language,* 33, 273–295.

Prather, P., Zurif, E. B., Stern, C., & Rosen, T. J. 1992. Slowed lexical access in nonfluent aphasia. *Brain and Language,* 45, 336–348.

Rizzi, L. 1990. *Relativized minimally*. Cambridge, MA: MIT Press.

Saffran, E. M., Berndt, R. S., & Schwartz, M. F. 1989. The quantitative analysis of agrammatic production: Procedure and data. *Brain and Language, 37,* 440–479.

Shapiro, L. P., Gordon, B., Hack, N., & Killackey, J. 1993. Verb-argument structure processing in complex sentences in Broca's and Wernicke's aphasia. *Brain and Language, 45,* 423–447.

von Stockert, T. R. 1972. Recognition of syntactic structure in aphasic patients. *Cortex, 8,* 322–334.

von Stockert, T. R., & Bader, L. 1976. Some relations of grammar and lexicon in aphasia. *Cortex, 12,* 49–60.

Zurif, E. B. 1982. The use of data from aphasia in constructing a performance model of language. In M. A. Arbib, D. Caplan, & J. C. Marshall (Eds.), *Neural models of language processes*. New York: Academic Press. Pp. 203–207.

Zurif, E., Gardner, H., & Brownell, H. H. 1989. The case against the case against group studies. *Brain & Cognition,* 448–464.

Zurif, E., Swinney, D., Prather, P., Solomon, J., & Bushell, C. 1993. An on-line analysis of syntactic processing in Broca's and Wernicke's aphasia. *Brain and Language, 45,* 448–464.